Recent Results in Cancer Research

157

Springer-Verlag Berlin Heidelberg GmbH

P. M. Schlag   U. Veronesi   (Eds.)

Lymphatic Metastasis
and Sentinel Lymphonodectomy

With 62 Figures and 43 Tables

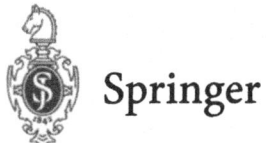

Springer

Prof. Dr. med. Dr. h. c. P. M. Schlag
Universitätsklinikum Charité
Klinik für Chirurgie und chirurgische Onkologie
Robert-Rössle-Klinik
Lindenberger Weg 80
13122 Berlin, Germany

Umberto Veronesi, MD, PhD.
Istituto Europeo di Oncologia
Via Ripamonti 435
20141 Milano, Italy

ISBN 978-3-540-66642-4
ISSN 0080-0015

Library of Congress Cataloging-in-Publication Data
Lymphatic metastasis and sentinel lymphonodectomy / P.M. Schlag (ed.). p.; cm. –
(Recent results in cancer research; 157) Includes bibliographical references and index.
ISBN 978-3-540-66642-4   ISBN 978-3-642-57151-0 (eBook)
DOI 10.1007/978-3-642-57151-0   1. Lymphatic metastasis. I. Schlag, P. (Peter),
1948- II. Series. [DNLM: 1. Lymphatic Metastasis – radionuclide imaging. 2. Lymph Node
Excision. 3. Lymph Nodes – radionuclide imaging. WH 700 L9848 2000]

© Springer-Verlag Berlin · Heidelberg 2000
Originally published by Springer-Verlag Berlin Heidelberg New York in 2000

The use of general descriptive names, registered names, trademarks, etc. in this publication
does not imply, even in the absence of a specific statement, that such names are exempt
from the relevant protective laws and regulations and therefore free for general use.

Product liability: The publisher cannot guarantee the accuracy of any information about
dosage and application contained in this book. In every individual case the user must
check such information by consulting the relevant literature.

Production: PRO EDIT GmbH, 69126 Heidelberg, Germany
Typesetting: K+V Fotosatz GmbH, 64743 Beerfelden, Germany

SPIN 10747028   21/3133göh 5 4 3 2 1 0

Preface

Metastases determine malignancy. The main attention so far has been focused upon organ metastases. The molecular mechanisms thereof, while far from being totally elucidated, are increasingly well understood. Modern diagnostic tools now enable detection and precise localization of small lesions. In contrast, our knowledge and diagnostic capabilities regarding metastatic spread to the'lymphatic system are rather limited. However, there have recently been a number of interesting advances. It is the aim of this volume to submit these developments to detailed analysis.

The therapeutic relevance of enhanced sensitivity in detection of lymph node metastases has to be considered in the light of increased morbidity versus eventual prognostic improvements by modification of therapy. An interesting concept which might improve diagnostic accuracy while reducing operative morbidity is the "sentinel node" technique. Surgical standards are lacking, however, and many fundamental questions pertaining to precise lymphatic mapping remain unanswered. Whether the sentinel node concept is of general relevance or whether it is applicable in only a few organs remains to be determined. This book offers intensive discussion of the concept from methodological and tumor biological viewpoints. World-renowned experts with long-term involvement in related basic and clinical research provide the reader with a broad survey of actual knowledge together with a critical appraisal of recent and future developments.

We sincerely hope this book succeeds in providing an outlook on future prospects and serving as a reference for all clinicians and researchers in this extremely important field.

Berlin, Milan, March 2000   PETER M. SCHLAG
UMBERTO VERONESI

Contents

III.   Principles of Lymphatic Mapping and Sentinel Node Detection

IV.   Sentinel Node Detection in Urogenital Cancer

V.   Sentinel Node Detection in Malignant Melanoma

VI.   Sentinel Node Detection in Neck and Thyroid Cancer

VII.   Sentinel Node Detection in Breast Cancer

VIII.   Sentinel Node Detection in Gastric Cancer

IX.   Sentinel Node Detection in Colorectal Cancer

List of Contributors*

Al-Yasi, A. R.[3]
Avital, S.[281]
Baratz, M.[281]
Bembenek, A.[228]
Biassoni, L.[3]
Borgstein, P. J.[130]
Brakenhoff, R. H.[90, 206]
Brazovsky, E.[281]
Britton, K. E.[3]
Cabanas, R. M.[109, 141]
Carroll, M. J.[3]
Castelijns, J. A.[206]
Chan, A. D.[161]
Chinol, M.[121]
Chu, K. U.[237]
Colnot, D. R.[90, 206]
de Cicco, C.[121]
Denkers, F.[90]
Duenne, A.-A.[82]
Ebert, B.[293]
Eccles, S. A.[41]
Eggermont, A. M. M.[178]
Gitstein, G.[281]
Giuliano, A. E.[201, 237]
Granowska, M.[3]
Haddad, R.[281]
Haigh, P. I.[201]
Handke, T.[293]
Haushofer, H.[273]

Jan, H.[3]
Kashtan, H.[281]
Katai, H.[253]
Lechner, P.[273]
Levenback, C.[150]
Lind, P.[273]
Mamelle, G.[193]
Maruyama, K.[253]
Meijer, S.[130]
Moesta, K. T.[293]
Morton, D. L.[161]
Nieuwenhuis, E. J. C.[206]
Paganelli, G.[121]
Pantel, K.[29]
Papo, M.[281]
Passlick, B.[29]
Pijpers, H. J.[206]
Pijpers, R.[130]
Rinneberg, H.[293]
Sano, T.[253]
Sasako, M.[253]
Schlag, P. M.[228, 293]
Schneebaum, S.[281]
Sendler, A.[259]
Siewert, J. R.[259]
Skornick, Y.[281]
Sleeman, J. P.[55]
Snow, G. B.[90, 206]
Snyder, M.[273]

* The address of the principal author is given on the first page
  of each contribution.
[1] Page on which contribution begins.

Strauss, L. G.[12]
Teule, G. J. J.[130]
Troitsa, A.[281]
van den Brekel, M. W. M.
[90, 206]

van Houten, V. M. M.[90]

van Diest, P. J.[90, 206]
Veronesi, U.[221]
Werner, J. A.[82]
Westerga, J.[90]
Wittekind, Ch.[20]
Zurrida, S.[221]

I. Clinical Assessment of Lymph Node Metastases

Efficacy of Immunoscintigraphy for Detection of Lymph Node Metastases

K. E. Britton, H. Jan, A. R. Al-Yasi, L. Biassoni, M. J. Carroll, and M. Granowska

Department of Nuclear Medicine, St Bartholomew's Hospital, London EC1A 7BE, UK

Abstract

The size of a lymph node is not in principle a limitation for the detection of cancer by Nuclear Medicine techniques. A radioactive pinhead is detectable if it has enough radioactivity on it. The approach of Nuclear Medicine to the demonstration of impalpable lymph nodes or to those lymph nodes detected by radiological techniques that are under 1 cm as to whether or not they contain cancer, is to increase the activity attached to cancer cells in such a lymph node as much as possible and to use sophisticated image analysis techniques to distinguish such uptake from its environment. This may be undertaken using a non specific technique such as F-18 Deoxyglucose and Positron Emission Tomography which is highly sensitive and which has been successful. The alternative approach is to use a highly specific and sensitive agent, such as a radio-labelled peptide or a radio-labelled monoclonal antibody together with image analysis. This paper describes these approaches and in particular the use of Tc-99m SM3 monoclonal antibody in the detection of impalpable axillary nodes in patients with breast cancer before surgery, using a change detection analysis providing a probability map of the significance of uptake of this radiopharmaceutical. It is a robust approach, providing the patient and the surgeon with information as to the likely need for extensive axillary surgery well prior to operation. A negative study should be followed by a sentinel node evaluation at surgery.

Introduction

Nuclear Medicine differs from Diagnostic Radiology. Radiology requires a mass in tissues, displacing tissues, infiltrating tissues for contrast. Nuclear Medicine does not require a mass. It exploits the subtle differences between the cancer cell and the normal cell for identification [1]. Radiology requires a lymph node to be a certain size "The 1 cm myth of Radiology". For cancer

Recent Results in Cancer Research, Vol. 157
© Springer-Verlag Berlin · Heidelberg 2000

in order to enlarge a lymph node beyond 1 cm diameter, cancer must have been present previously in a normal sized node. The advantage of advanced Nuclear Medicine techniques is that they can detect cancer in a node that is less than 1 cm by imaging. The symbol of cancer is the crab, rightly, with a body and fingers infiltrating tissue away from the body. Radiology can only detect the body. Nuclear Medicine can detect the ribbons, plaques or sheets of cancer cells that extend from the body or it can identify cancer when there is no body at all. This is important for the new conformal radiotherapy planning related to the CT mass, because the physical edge of the tumour is less than its biological edge. A radioactive pinhead is detectable by Nuclear Medicine if it has enough radioactivity on it. In this sense, Nuclear Medicine is not size dependent but activity dependent [2]. Nuclear Medicine has a built in amplification factor for example, there may be 5000 receptor binding sites or antigens on a single cancer cell, or even 50000. For a particular bindee such as a peptide receptor binding agent or a monoclonal antibody or fragment this amplification factor helps identification of cancer. The affinity factor is very high for antigen antibody and receptor bindee interactions and the residence time of such strongly bound bindees may be for days.

Nuclear Medicine Techniques

Nuclear Medicine has two approaches to the detection of cancer. First the "Catch all" where a technique has high sensitivity but poor specificity. These include the three phase bone scan, Gallium-67 citrate imaging and Positron emission tomography with F18 deoxyglucose, FDG. All these techniques are sensitive but do not distinguish tumour from granuloma or inflammation. Nevertheless the very high sensitivity of FDG-PET enables it to detect "Normal" size nodes that are involved with cancer. However it is context dependent. Clearly a node that shows up positive with FDG in the context of lung cancer is likely to be due to metastases of the lung cancer. This has revolutionised the management of lung cancer by usually upstaging the cancer by identifying in the mediastinum involved nodes that are CT "normal"; being less than 1 cm diameter. The same principle applies with FDG PET in Hodgkin's Disease and Melanoma. It is somewhat less successful in the abdomen in staging colorectal cancer because of gut uptake and a higher degree of non specific causes and it is relatively poor in detecting lymph nodes in prostate cancer.

The "Catch One" technique is the development of agents to bind to cancer that are as specific as possible as well as as sensitive as possible [1]. The progression has been from agents that bind to tumour and generally not to inflammation such as Thallium-201, Tc-99m-Sestamibi and Indium-111 Octreotide analogues. Class specific agents that bind to a range of cancers include anti-CEA monoclonal antibody which binds to colorectal, bladder, lung and breast cancer or I-123 MIBG which binds to neural crest tumours or I-123 vasoactive intestinal peptide, VIP, which mainly binds to gastro-intestinal tumours. The type specific bindees include anti lymphoma antibodies which will only bind in to a particular type of lymphoma for example the I-131 B1 anti CD20 antibody which binds to most non Hodgkin's lymphoma. The anti high molecular weight melanoma antigen antibody which binds almost exclusively to melanoma and the Tc-99m PR1A3 monoclonal antibody which binds almost exclusively to colorectal cancer. The development of cancer specific and cancer sensitive agents continues to progress.

Radioimmunoscintigraphy

Our work is mainly concerned with improving radioimmunoscintigraphy, RIS, so that it becomes a sensitive and specific technique for detecting primary and recurrent cancer and particularly lymph node involvement before surgery. RIS is a multi disciplinary technique using radiolabelled monoclonal antibodies fragments or genetically engineered related constructs for detecting cancer and other disease [3]. The requirements for RIS are: an antigen as specific as possible to the Cancer; a monoclonal antibody or fragment against this antigen; the best radiolabel, which is Tc-99m; a radiolabelling method that preserves binding efficiency; and a optimal imaging system and image analysis for identification of the cancer. Tumour associated antigens against which antibodies are used for RIS include those on the epithelial surface. These may be normally expressed antigens which are remote from the blood stream. It is only the architectural disruption that occurs with the malignant process that exposes them to the blood often in greater numbers per cell than the normal tissue. Such antibodies include those against polymorphic epithelial mucin, PEM antigens such as HMFG 1, HMFG 2, SM3 against the stripped mucin core protein, and PR1A3. There are oncofeotal antigens such as alphafeto protein CEA and HCG; tumour associated antigens such as B72.3 against TAG 75 and MOV 18 against a folate binding protein; antiviral antigens such as anti-hepatitis for hepatoma; synthetic antigens, such as 170 H82; or receptor antigens such as anti-epithelial growth factor receptor.

The rules of radioimmunoscintigraphy are straightforward: Specific uptake increases with time, thus an image at 5/10 min provides a tumour free template with which later images can be compared; non specific uptake after the initial distribution decreases with time; the higher the count rate the better the detection and the smaller and earlier the tumour is identified. RIS therefore can determine the presence of recurrent cancer that is sub clinical and subradiological. It can determine the presence of cancer when serum markers are still normal and it can identify the site of cancer when serum markers are elevated. It can also determine whether a radiologically detected mass contains viable tumour, for post therapy or post surgical fibrosis will not take up the antibody and enlarged lymph nodes seen radiologically due to non specific inflammation will be antibody negative. RIS can detect the effects of therapy because dormant but living cancer cells will still show antigen expression. Impalpable nodes, such as those in the axilla can be shown to be involved or not. RIS can be combined with the use of the preoperative probe to detect cancer at surgery. RIS is a necessary prelude for radioimmunotherapy.

A typical patient protocol for a Tc-99m labelled antibody is as follows:

The test is explained to the patient and an informed signed consent is obtained. Patients who are allergic to foreign protein are excluded. Provided 1 mg or less of whole antibody or fragment is used. Although human antimouse antibodies, HAMA, may develop, these have no relation to the clinical likelihood of a reaction. However when amounts over 1 mg typically 10 or 100 times this are used for therapy, then HAMA and clinical reactions are more frequent. No skin test is done as it sensitises the patient. No thyroid blockade is needed because the Tc-99m is strongly bound to the sulphurs of Cysteine and excreted as a dipeptide. A typical injection intravenously is of 600 MBq of the Tc-labelled monoclonal antibody, usually a murine IgG1, with a gamma camera peaked for Tc-99m with a 140 kev 15% window, low energy parallel hole general purpose collimator. Images are obtained for 800 000 counts per image at 10 min, 4–6 h and 18–24 h after intravenous injection together with single photon emission tomography, SPET at 4 and 22 h.

Probability Mapping

The time dependency of biological processes is one of Nuclear Medicine's greatest strengths, thus the series of images will show no abnormal uptake on the early image, possibly some uptake at the cancer site on the middle image and increased uptake at the cancer site on the next day image. Non specific uptake after the initial distribution decreases with time, thus a site of infection or inflammation will show high vascular activity on the first image, and as the blood level of the antibody decreases with time so the uptake will be less on the middle image and may have faded altogether on the late image. It is therefore clear that the kinetic analysis of the series of images improves and indeed is essential for distinguishing specific and non specific uptake. Whereas in the past subtraction techniques were used to compare one radionuclide distribution with another, these have always suffered from the inability correctly to normalise the data for the comparison so that subtraction may be too great and thus small true positives eliminated or maybe too little and thus noise blobs may be interpreted as tumours giving rise to a high false positive rate. While these may not be a problem for large tumours, the whole emphasis is to detect smaller and smaller disease, particularly disease in lymph nodes less than 1 cm. To achieve this a change detection algorithm is used. In order to do this a particular patient protocol and computer program is required. First the patient must be repositioned for each image, as accurately as possible in relation to the previous image. In order to do this indelible skin marks are made on appropriate bony prominences and up to 6 tiny cobalt-57 sources are strapped to the sites. When the patient attends for the first image, a picture of the radioactive markers is made and measurements of the patient, so that when the patient returns for the second image, then the markers are replaced, the particular image can be set up to be as close as possible to the previous one. Further marker images are obtained at each visit. These are then used in the computer program to aid superimposition of the patient images. Each marker image is analysed so that the peak marker activity is located to a single pixel. Pairs of images then undergo a translation rotation algorithm so that the marker images are superimposed. The actual patient images are then put through the same translation rotation program. Although marker images continue to be used, current versions of the program use identifiable biological edges to superimpose the images such as the outline of blood vessels, the heart and the liver.

Once the images are superimposed, and this is checked because it is easy to demonstrate negative shadows beside blood vessels if there is poor superimposition, then the change detection algorithm is applied. A 5×5 matrix of pixels is applied and centred on every pixel in the first image and similarly every pixel in the second image. Significant differences between the two images are represented as a colour scale where $P<0.001$ is shown in red, $P<0.01$ is shown in yellow, $P<0.05$ is shown in green and non significant values are shown in blue. This probability map then describes the significance of the differences between the early image which is the non-tumour template and the late image which may or may not contain tumour. If it does it will be shown as red, orange or green on the probability map (Figs. 1, 2). This approach has enabled lymph node involvement down to 3.5 mm in size to be detected in the axilla, when clinically no nodes were palpable [4].

Breast Cancer

The aim is to determine the presence of axillary node involvement when the axilla is clinically normal. Conversely the aim is to determine that clinically palpable nodes are not involved. Knowledge that axillary nodes are involved or not is essential for staging the cancer and for determining the extent of operation. With the current use of axillary clearance in association with breast tumours over 1 cm, perhaps some 30% of women undergoing surgery for breast cancer have unnecessary axillary clearance whereas no involved nodes are found. Prior knowledge of the axillary nodes status well before surgery will allow the surgeon to tailor the extent of surgery to the individual woman and will allow the woman to be prepared for extensive axillary surgery or not as the case may be. It is our intention to show that axillary node involvement using radioimmunoscintigraphy with Tc-99m labelled SM3 can predict the findings at surgery. When the axilla is clinically normal but negative on radioimmuno scintigraphy then this is an indication for sentinel node imaging since the negative is always hard to prove, and currently we combine the two modalities. Our initial evaluation of radioimmunoscintigra-

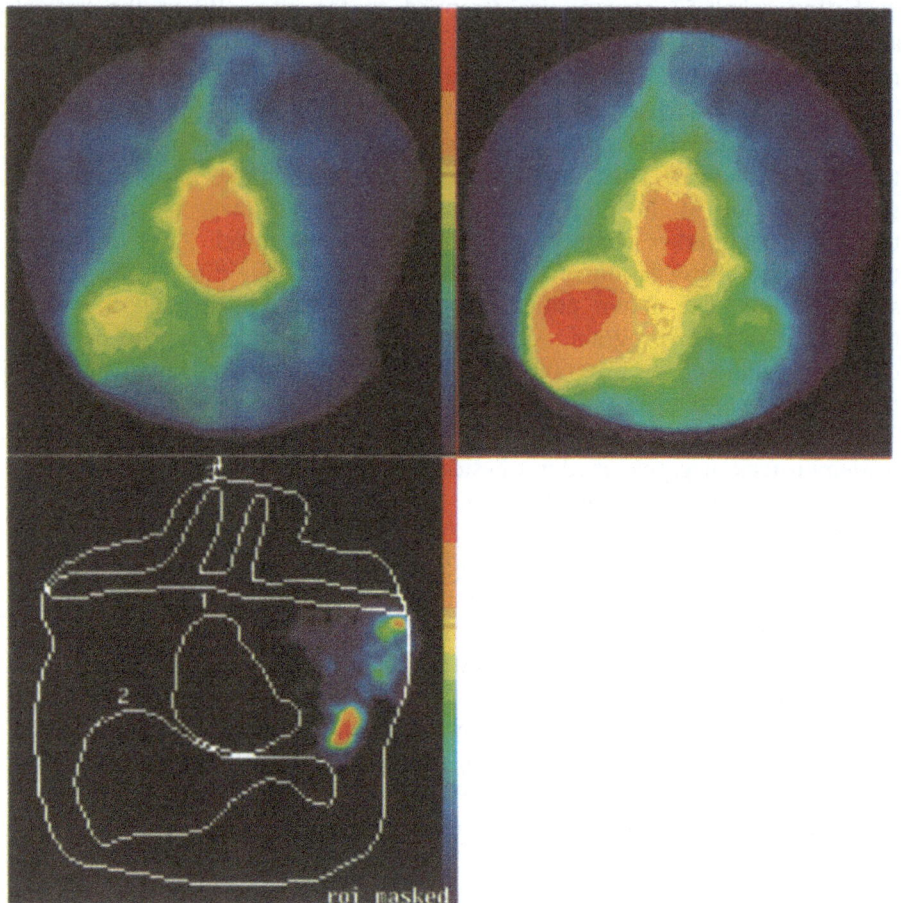

Fig. 1. Breast cancer Radioimmunoscintigraphy. *Top left:* 10-min image; *top right:* 24-h image; *bottom left:* change detection analysis applied to the two images with probability mapping: red P<0.001, orange P<0.01, green P<0.05, blue non-significant. The primary left breast cancer is clearly evident together with the involved axillary nodes. Nodal involvement was confirmed at surgery and histology

phy of the axilla in 299 surgically removed lymph nodes from 29 axilla showed 9/10 true positive and 16/19 true negative [4]. One false negative was in a micrometastases in one out of 20 involved nodes. The three false positives were: a second tumour was interpreted as an involved lymph node; a tertiary level lymph node was positive but surgery only undertook first and second level dissection; and in one a movement artefact caused the misinterpretation. Our first ten patients using Tc-99m hHMFG1, humanised antibody, has shown positive identification in 10/10, none of whom had palpable axillary nodes and one of whom had a second tumour in the axilla [5]. It is hoped that a multicentre study of this approach can be initiated. An alternative approach is FDG PET imaging [6].

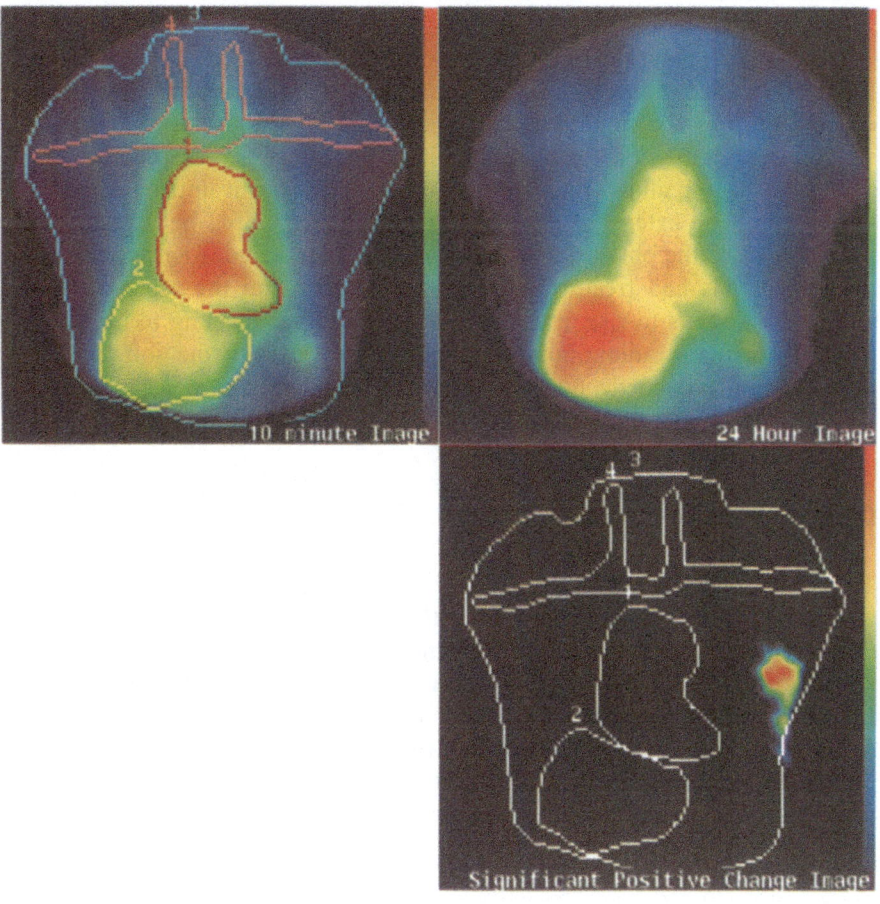

Fig. 2. Breast cancer Radioimmunoscintigraphy. *Top left:* 10-min image; *top right:* 24-h image; *bottom left:* change detection analysis comparing the two images. Key as Fig. 1. A left breast cancer is clearly identified and the axilla is shown to contain no significant uptake. Surgery and histology confirmed absence of axillary node involvement

Genito-Urinary Cancers

Ovarian Cancer

Tc-99m SM3 is used for radioimmunoscintigraphy with the same protocol but imaging the pelvis [7, 8]. The probability mapping allows distinction between malignancy and other causes of a positive ultrasound detection of a mass in the pelvis. In conjunction with CT it allows the distinction to be made between a normal size node which is involved and an enlarged node which is not involved with cancer.

Prostate Cancer

Tc-99m or In-111 anti PMSA antibody (Cytogen) is used. This reacts with the prostate membrane specific antigen which is highly selective for prostate cancer but does appear to a much lesser extent in benign hypertrophy. Early single photon emission tomography allows the tortuous vessels to be identified, late imaging allows the demonstration of significant uptake in the prostate cancer. The extension through the capsule may often be identified and involvement of the obturator or iliac nodes demonstrated. Alternatively when the patient has had treatment for prostate cancer and the prostate specific antigen PSA starts to rise, if the bone scan and other imaging techniques are negative, prostate radioimmunoscintigraphy can identify the soft tissue uptake often in paraaortic nodes which may be of normal size radiologically [9, 10].

Colorectal Cancer

Tc-99m PR1A3 for RIS is particularly useful in recurrent colorectal cancer which may present as a rising CEA with negative CT in which case focal uptake in paraaortic nodes may be demonstrated [11]. Alternatively the CT scan may be positive showing a recurrent mass in the pelvis, but be unable to identify the involvement of the iliac nodes seen by RIS. A potentially operable situation becomes inoperable due to the extra information upstaging the patient provided by RIS.

Lymphoma

Non-Hodgkin's lymphoma may be imaged using Tc-99m LL2, an anti-CD 22 antibody and the extent of lymph node involvement demonstrated using this sensitive and specific agent [12]. Alternatively FDG with PET may show context dependent involvement of nodes of less than 1 cm [13].

Lung Cancer

Mediastinal involvement is best detected using FDG with PET in primary staging, particularly when CT shows 'normal' sized glands [14]. The interpretation is context dependent since FDG uptake is not specific to cancer.

Conclusion

The new tissue characterizing Nuclear Medicine techniques have an increasingly important role to play in the staging of primary cancer and the detection of lymph node involvement when cancer recurrence occurs.

ACKNOWLEDGEMENTS. The authors acknowledge the St Bartholomew's Foundation for Research for provision of facilities, the Imperial Cancer Research Fund for the provision of the monoclonal antibodies SM3 and hHMFG1 and the Royal Hospitals NHS Trust for equipment and support.

References

1. Britton K E (1997) Towards the goal of cancer specific imaging and therapy. Nucl Med Commun 18:992–1007
2. Britton K E., Granowska M (1987) Radioimmuno scintigraphy in tumour identification, Cancer Surveys 6:247–267
3. Britton K E & Granowska M. Radioimmunoscintigraphy. In: Murray IP, Ell PJ (eds) (Edition 2) Nuclear Medicine in Clinical Diagnosis and Treatment, Vol 2, pp 871–892. Churchill Livingston, Edinburgh 1998
4. Biassoni L, Granowska M, Carroll MJ et al. (1998) Tc-99m labelled SM3 in the prospective evaluation of axillary lymph nodes and primary breast cancer with change detection statistical processing as an aid to tumour detection. Brit J Cancer 77:131–138
5. Al-Yasi AR, Jan H, Granowska M et al. (1999) Identification of lymphatic spread of breast cancer using Tc-99m labelled humanised anti human milk fat globule (MHMFG) monoclonal antibody. Nucl Med Commun 20:464 (Abstract)
7. Granowska M, Nimmon C C, Britton K E, et al. (1988) Kinetic analysis and probability mapping applied to the detection of ovarian cancer by radioimmunoscintigraphy. J Nucl Med 29:559–607
8. Granowska M, Britton K E, Mather S J, et al. (1993) Radioimmunoscintigraphy with Technetium -99m labelled monoclonal antibody, SM3, in gynaecological cancer. Eur J Nucl Med 20:483–489
9. Chengazi V U, Feneley M R, Mather S J, et al. (1997) Imaging prostate cancer with the monoclonal radioimmunoconjugate technetium-99m-7E11-C5.3 (CYT-351) J Nucl Med 38:675–681
10. Babaian, R J, Sayer J, Podoloff D A, et al. (1994) Radioimmunoscintigraphy of pelvis lymph nodes with Indium-111 labelled monoclonal antibody CYT-356. J Urol 152: 1952–1955
11. Granowska M, Britton K E, Mather S J, et al. (1993) Radioimmunoscintigraphy with Tc-99m labelled monoclonal antibody, 1A3, in colorectal cancer. Eur J Nucl Med 20: 690–698
12. Goldenberg D M, Sharkey R NM, Levine G L, et al. (1993) Initial clinical imaging results with a new monoclonal antibody agent for B cell lymphoma. Eur J Nucl Med 20:875 (Abstract)
13. Hoh CK, Glaspy J, Rosen P, et al. (1997) Whole body FDG-PET imaging for staging of Hodgkin's disease and lymphoma. J Nucl Med 38:343–348
14. Sasaki M, Ichiya Y, Kawabasa Y, et al. (1996) The usefulness of FDG positron emission tomography for the detection of mediastinal lymph node metastases in patients with non small cell lung cancer. Eur J Nucl Med 23:741–747

Sensitivity and Specificity of Positron Emission Tomography (PET) for the Diagnosis of Lymph Node Metastases

L. G. Strauss

Medical PET Group–Biological Imaging (E0105), German Cancer Research Center, Im Neuenheimer Feld 280, 69120 Heidelberg, Germany

Abstract

The introduction of Positron Emission Tomography (PET) and the use of the glucose analog F-18-Deoxyglucose (FDG) can help to improve the sensitivity of the diagnosis of lymph node metastases. Sensitivity exceeding 90% can be achieved when advanced imaging protocols and image reconstruction methods are used for PET. Superior staging information is obtained with PET as compared to morphological imaging methods for the most frequent tumor types. The accuracy of N-staging can be significantly improved by adding PET to the pretherapeutic diagnostic procedures. Limitations exist with regard to false positive results. Acute or chronic inflammation as well as unspecific reactions following radiotherapy may mimic tumor tissue.

Introduction

Positron Emission Tomography (PET) was introduced for oncological studies to detect primary tumors or tumor recurrence more than 10 years ago [1]. The use of radiolabelled pharmaceuticals provides qualitative and quantitative information about functional parameters, which can be used to predict therapy response [2–4]. The most frequently used radiopharmaceutical is F-18-deoxyglucose (FDG), which is transported and phosphorylated like glucose, but then trapped in the cells. PET images using FDG are likely to reflect tumor viability [5]. The current results with PET and FDG in oncological patients demonstrate a sensitivity exceeding 85% for most of the studies [6]. However, the specificity may be variable due to unspecific uptake of FDG in inflammatory lesions [6].

Recent Results in Cancer Research, Vol. 157
© Springer-Verlag Berlin · Heidelberg 2000

Current Results

The diagnosis of lymphatic spread is one of the most difficult tasks in tumor staging. Morphologic imaging with ultrasound (US), computed tomography (CT), and magnetic resonance tomography (MRT) has found widespread use for the detection of lymph node metastases. While morphological methods are frequently limited for the diagnosis of enlarged lymph nodes, several attempts have been made to increase accuracy. The use of contrast enhancement and spiral-CT scanners can help to delineate small lesions more accurately. However, the improvement of staging accuracy may be limited as demonstrated by Hundt et al. for the staging of colorectal carcinoma [7]. The authors evaluated contrast enhanced spiral-CT in 37 patients with proven rectum or colon carcinoma and reported correct N-classification in 64.8% of the patients [7]. Anzai et al. assessed both CT and MRI in head and neck tumors and found that MRI added little to the diagnostic accuracy of contrast enhanced CT [8]. The differentiation of borderline or slightly enlarged lymph nodes from benign hyperplasia or inflammatory lesions still remains an unsolved problem in oncology.

Head and Neck Tumors

Several studies have been performed to compare functional PET imaging with conventional imaging modalities. Adams et al. reported a study in 60 patients with head and neck tumors, examined with PET, CT, MRI, and US prior to surgery [9]. The analysis of 1284 lesions demonstrated the highest sensitivity and specificity for PET (90% and 94%), followed by CT (sensitivity 82%, specificity 85%), MRI (sensitivity 80%, specificity 79%), and US (sensitivity 72%, specificity 70%) [9]. False positive results were obtained in inflammatory lesions with uptake values within the range of metastatic masses. Therefore, the predictive value for true positive results was only 58% for PET and even lower for the morphological methods (CT 35%, MRI 27%, US 19%). Comparable results were reported by Laubenbacher et al. when PET and MRI studies were evaluated [10]. With regard to "neck sides", the sensitivity and specificity for PET was 89% and 100%, compared to MRI with 72% and 56% [10].

Breast Carcinoma

PET with FDG has limited use for the detection of lymph node metastases in breast cancer patients. Crippa et al. evaluated 567 lesions in 68 patients with breast cancer and compared the PET data to the final clinical classification according to the N-stage [11]. The study comprised 197 metastatic lesions, with 25 lesions having a diameter of less than 2 mm. The overall sensitivity

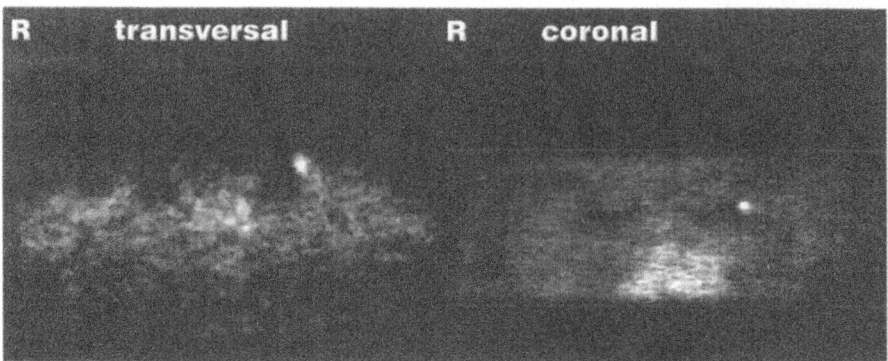

Fig. 1. Small axillary lymph node (diameter: 9.1 mm) in a patient with a breast carcinoma. The lesion has an significantly increased FDG metabolism and can be delineated due to the high image contrast

was 85% and the specificity was 91%. Small lesions classified as N_{1a} were detected in 88% of the cases, while all larger nodes were detected by PET [11]. The data demonstrate that lesion size may limit detectability.

According to our experience, PET was found especially useful for the detection of axillary lymph node metastases (Fig. 1). Avril et al. assessed PET for the detection of axillary lymph node involvement and found that the sensitivity was dependent on the primary tumor size [12]. Primary tumors smaller than 2 cm were associated with a sensitivity of 33%, while the detection rate for lymph node metastases was 94% for larger tumors [12]. Axillary PET imaging provided additional diagnostic information in 29% of the patients [12].

Lung Cancer

The diagnostic work-up of patients with lung tumors remains a difficult clinical challenge even with the use of many imaging methods. The evaluation of bronchiogenic carcinoma by current imaging techniques such as plain-film, CT, and MRI is mainly confined to morphologic information and most of the studies revealed a limited accuracy of the method. The accuracy of CT for the identification of lymph node metastases was evaluated from Matthews et al. in patients with central (n=64) and peripheral (n=66) tumors [13]. The authors reported an overall sensitivity of 86% and specificity of 78% [13]. The sensitivity was clearly dependent on the prevalence of disease and decreased to 55% when the prevalence of metastases was only 16.7% [13]. Bonomo et al. compared CT and MRI and reported that MRI may have some advantages in the detection of local spread [14]. However, the accuracy for lymph node staging was limited for both methods [14]. The authors recommend further evaluation of enlarged lymph nodes to avoid exclusion from a potentially curative resection [14].

The morphological information obtained by conventional imaging methods may be expanded by PET with FDG to assess lung tumors with a metabolically active tracer. Multitracer studies with F-18-deoxyglucose, N-13-glutamate and O-15-water demonstrated an enhanced accumulation of all tracers [15]. The analysis of 87 PET FDG studies revealed no significant difference in FDG uptake with regard to tumor histology [2,15]. Furthermore, evaluation of tumor blood flow with O-15-water showed no correlation to FDG uptake [2]. Sensitivity was high and 84 out of 87 malignant lesions showed a significantly different FDG uptake from benign lesions [2, 15]. The nodal staging was evaluated from Steinert et al. in 47 patients with non-small cell lung carcinoma [16]. The authors found a sensitivity of 89% and specificity of 99% for FDG PET, when 599 lesions were evaluated [16]. Both positive as well as negative predictive values exceeded 95%. In contrast, CT revealed a sensitivity of 57% and a specificity of 94%, resulting in a lower positive predictive value of 76% [16]. A correct N-staging was obtained with PET in 96% and with CT in 79% of the patients [16].

For routine purposes it is important to assess the gain in information when PET is added to the conventional staging methods. Vansteenkiste et al. evaluated the gain in accuracy when PET was added to the staging procedure [17]. The authors reported that CT correctly identified the nodal stage in 59% of the patients with non small cell lung cancer, while the additional use of PET increased the staging accuracy to 87% [17].

Besides FDG, other tracers have been used for the detection of malignant lesions. We investigated N-13-glutamate and found a median lesion-to-lung-ratio of 5.9 as compared to 4.7 for FDG [15]. Nettelbladt et al. used FDG and C-11-methionine in 16 patients and found a sensitivity of 93% for both tracers [18]. The authors reported that the combination of both tracers may further increase the sensitivity for detecting malignant lesions [18].

Melanoma

Whole body PET imaging is the preferential procedure for staging malignant melanomas to assess all areas of the body [19]. Macfarlane et al. performed a prospective evaluation of PET with FDG in patients with cutaneous malignant melanomas and found a sensitivity of 85% and specificity of 91% when the PET data were compared to histopathology [20]. Holder et al. compared PET and CT for the detection of melanoma metastases and reported a superior sensitivity of 94.2% for PET as compared to 55.3% for CT [21]. However, specificity was 83.3% (PET) and 84.4% (CT), because of the limitations due to other malignancies or inflammatory tissue [21]. The use of dual head Anger cameras operating in coincidence mode has found limited use for PET due to the lower costs as compared to a standard ring system. Imaging with a conventional PET system was compared to simulated images of a dual head camera [22]. The authors reported a significant difference in sensitivity with 89% true positive results for the standard PET and only 18% for the dual head camera imaging method [22]. Most lesions were missed in areas with high background activity and the tumor-to-background ratio was lower for dual head imaging. Furthermore, lesions with less than 22 mm in diameter were missed more frequently than with standard PET imaging [22].

Colorectal Carcinoma

While PET has been found useful for the detection of local recurrence [1, 23], problems may raise in the detection of lymph node metastases. Abdel-Nabi et al. evaluated PET studies in patients with primary colorectal carcinoma and reported a sensitivity of 29% for the detection of mesenteric lymph node metastases [24]. Most of the lymph nodes in patients with false negative findings were located in the vicinity of the primary tumor, therefore the high FDG uptake in the tumor area may prevent the detection of local lymphatic spread [24].

Limitations

The evaluation of PET studies requires high quality images in order to assess the activity distribution visually as well as quantitatively. While the standard filtered backprojection method provides images with severe artefacts if localized, high radioactivity concentrations are present, the iterative reconstruction procedure is superior and is finding increasing use for the reconstruction of PET images. Besides the iterative reconstruction of the emission data, the iterative calculation of absorption correction maps improve the image quality significantly. This procedure is particularly helpful for the detection of small lesions within tracer background. According to our results, we would like to emphasize that lymph nodes of less than 1.5 cm in diameter are not recognized in most cases when the standard filtered backprojection method is used.

Biological imaging with FDG implies the visualization of local glucose consumption. The FDG uptake is usually enhanced in malignant structures, but it should be kept in mind that benign lesions may also exhibit an increased tracer uptake (Fig. 2). Acute, inflammatory reactions, abscesses, etc., accumulate FDG and can be interpreted as tumors [6]. Besides acute inflammation, chronic pancreatitis, cystadenoma, retroperitoneal fibrosis and diffuse lymphocyte infiltration may result in false positive results [6]. Several attempts have been made to differentiate inflammatory and tumorous lesions with dynamic PET studies and compartmental or non-compartmental data analysis, but actually in most oncological patients it is impossible to obtain additional significant reliable information for the differential diagnosis. There is some evidence that the use of multitracer studies including C-11-aminoisobutyric acid may help to differentiate malignant lesions from inflammatory tissue [6].

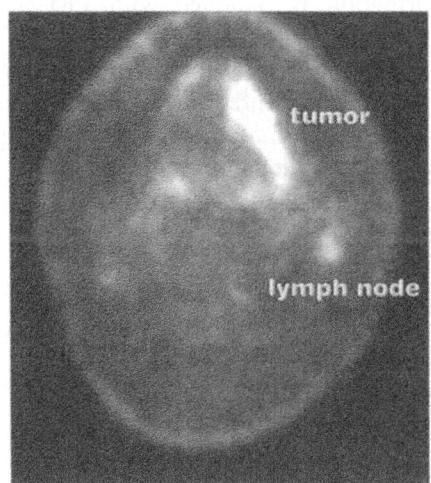

Fig. 2. Oropharynx carcinoma (label: "tumor") and suspicious FDG accumulation in a local lymph node (label: "lymph node"). The FDG uptake was only moderately increased in the lymph node (1.6 SUV). Histology revealed unspecific inflammatory changes and no signs for malignant spread

While most studies with PET and FDG are focussed on primary tumor staging or the detection of a recurrent tumor, little is known about the effects of treatment on FDG uptake. PET studies with FDG in patients with colorectal carcinomas receiving radiation therapy have shown that FDG uptake may increase up to several months following treatment [25]. The effects observed following radiation therapy may mimic inflammation and prohibit the detection of tumor areas within the treated tissue volume. There is no evidence that PET with FDG will be helpful for the assessment of possible residual tumor tissue within 6 months after completion of radiotherapy [6].

The effect of chemotherapy on the tumor metabolism has been evaluated in a few experimental studies. Minn et al. assessed the effect of doxorubicin on Lewis lung carcinoma and report enhanced FDG uptake following treatment [26]. We were able to show an initial enhancement of FDG uptake using hexadecylphosphocholine in human breast cancer cells [27]. Besides the tumor itself, normal structures, e.g., bone marrow, can show an increased FDG uptake following treatment [6]. It is still not known what effects the chemotherapy will have on lymph node metastases. Dimitrakopoulou-Strauss et al. evaluated the FDG metabolism in recurrent lymphomas and noted in patients with complete response or stable disease a moderately increased FDG tracer accumulation exceeding 1.5 SUV even after treatment [28].

Conclusion

PET with FDG is generally accepted as a second-line method for the diagnosis of lymph node metastases. The sensitivity exceeds 90% when advanced imaging protocols and reconstruction methods are used. Superior staging information is obtained with PET as compared to morphological imaging methods.

Detailed clinical information is mandatory to limit the problems concerning the differentiation of tumor and inflammation. PET studies following radiotherapy may be misleading and provide false positive results due to unspecific reactions in the tumor area.

References

1. Strauss LG, Clorius JH, Schlag P, et al. (1989) Recurrence of colorectal tumors: PET evaluation. Radiology 170:329–332
2. Strauss LG, Conti PS (1991) The applications of PET in clinical oncology. J Nucl Med 32:623–648
3. Dimitrakopoulou-Strauss A, Strauss LG, Schlag P, et al. (1998) Fluorine-18-fluorouracil to predict therapy response in liver metastases from colorectal carcinoma. J Nucl Med 39:1197–1202
4. Dimitrakopoulou-Strauss A (1996) Editorial: New approaches for the non invasive quantification of chemotherapeutic drugs in tumors and the evaluation of multidrug resistance. The Cancer Journal 9:118–120
5. Higashi K, Clavo AC, Wahl RL (1993) Does FDG uptake measure proliferative activity of human cancer cells? In vitro comparison with DNA flow cytometry and tritiated thymidine uptake. J Nucl Med 34:414–419
6. Strauss LG (1996) Fluorine-18 deoxyglucose and false-positive results: a major problem in the diagnosis of oncological patients. Eur J Nucl Med 23:1409–1415
7. Hundt W, Braunschweig R, Reiser M (1999) Evaluation of spiral CT of colon and rectom carcinoma. Eur Radiol 9:78–84
8. Anzai Y, Brunberg JA, Lufkin RB (1997) Imaging of nodal metastases in the head and neck. J Magn Reson Imaging 7:774–783
9. Adams S, Baum RP, Stuckensen T, et al. (1998) Prospective comparison of ^{18}F-FDG PET with conventional imaging modalities (CT, MRI, US) in lymph node staging of head and neck cancer. Eur J Nucl Med 25:1255–1260
10. Laubenbacher C, Saumweber D, Wagner-Manslau C, et al. (1995) Comparison of fluorine-18-fluorodeoxyglucose PET, MRI and endoscopy for staging head and neck squamous-cell carcinomas. J Nucl Med 36:1747–1757
11. Crippa F, Agresti R, Seregni E, et al. (1998) Prospective evaluation of fluorine-18-FDG PET in presurgical staging of the axilla in breast cancer. J Nucl Med 39:4–8
12. Avril N, Dose J, Janicke F, Ziegler S, et al. (1996) Assessment of axillary lymph node involvement in breast cancer patients with positron emission tomography using radiolabeled 2-(fluorine-18)-fluoro-2-deoxy-D-glucose. J Natl Cancer Inst 4:1204–1209
13. Matthews JI, Richey HM, Helsel RA, et al. (1987) Thoracic computed tomography in the preoperative evaluation of primary bronchogenic carcinoma. Arch Intern Med 147:449–453
14. Bonomo L, Ciccotosto C, Guidotti A, et al. (1996) Lung cancer staging: the role of computed tomography and magnetic resonance imaging. Eur J Radiol 23:35–45
15. Strauss LG, Clorius JH, Manke H, et al. (1987) PET in oat cell carcinoma. Radiology 165(P):212
16. Steinert HC, Hauser M, Allemann F, et al. (1997) Non-small cell lung cancer: nodal staging with FDG PET versus CT with correlative lymph node mapping and sampling. Radiology 202:441–446
17. Vansteenkiste JF, Stroobants SG, De Leyn PR, et al. (1998) Lymph node staging in non-small-cell lung cancer with FDG-PET scan: a prospective study on 690 lymph node stations from 68 patients. J Clin Oncol 16:2142–2149

18. Nettelbladt OS, Sundin AE, Valind SO, et al. (1998) Combined fluorine-18-FDG and carbon-11-methionine PET for diagnosis of tumors in lung and mediastinum. J Nucl Med 39:640–647

19. Steinert HC, Huch Buoni RA, Buck A, et al. (1995) Malignant melanoma: staging with whole-body positron emission tomography and 2-[F-18]-fluoro-2-deoxy-D-glucose. Radiology 195:705–709

20. Macfarlane DJ, Sondak V, Johnson T, et al. (1998) Prospective evaluation of 1[F-18]-2-deoxy-D-glucose positron emission tomography in staging of regional lymph nodes in patients with cutaneous malignant melanoma. J Clin Oncol 16:1770–1776

21. Holder WD Jr, Whilte RL Jr, Zuger JH, et al. (1998) Effectiveness of positron emission tomography for the detection of melanoma metastases. Ann Surg 227:764–769

22. Steinert HC, Voellmy DR, Trachsel C, et al. (1998) Planar coincidence scintigraphy and PET in staging malignant melanoma. J Nucl Med 39:1892–1897

23. Ogunbiyi OA, Flanagan FL, Dehdashti F, et al. (1997) Detection of recurrent and metastatic colorectal cancer: comparison of positron emission tomography and computed tomography. Ann Surg Oncol 4:613–620

24. Abdel-Nabi H, Doerr RJ, Lamonica DM, et al. (1998) Staging of primary colorectal carcinomas with fluorine-18 fluorodeoxyglucose whole-body PET: correlation with histopathologic and CT findings. Radiology 206:755–760

25. Engenhart R, Kimmig BN, Strauss LG, et al. (1990) Therapy monitoring of presacral recurrencies after high-dose irradiation. Value of PET, CT, CEA and pain score. Strahlenther Oncol 166:95–98

26. Minn H, Kangas L, Kellokumpu-Lehtinen P, et al. (1990) Uptake of 2-fluoro-2-deoxy-D-[U-(14)C]glucose during chemotherapy in murine Lewis lung tumor. Nucl Med Biol Int J Radiat Appl Instrum 19:55–63

27. Haberkorn U, Reinhardt M, Strauss LG, et al. (1992) Metabolic design of combined therapy: use of enhanced fluorodeoxyglucose uptake caused by chemotherapy. J Nucl Med 33:1981–1987

28. Dimitrakopoulou-Strauss A, Strauss LG, Goldschmidt H, et al. (1995) Evaluation of tumour metabolism and multidrug resistance in patients with treated malignant lymphomas. Eur J Nucl Med 22:434–442

Diagnosis and Staging of Lymph Node Metastasis

Ch. Wittekind

Institut für Pathologie der Universität Leipzig, Liebigstrasse 26,
04103 Leipzig, Germany

Abstract

The process of lymph node metastasis is not completely understood. Although we know some basic molecular mechanisms of metastasis, the exact procedure from the initiation of a primary tumour to overt lymph node metastasis remains obscure. A few morphological features of different primary tumours are known to correlate with the probability of lymph node metastasis, e.g., tumour histology (carcinoma vs. sarcoma), tumour size, T category, poor grade of differentiation and invasion of lymph vessels. Few attempts have been made to use markers of molecular differentiation such as nm23 as an additional indicator of lymph node metastasis. A drawback is the lack of an exact definition of lymph node metastasis or micrometastasis and how to include new findings such as the demonstration of cytokeratin-positive cells in "tumourfree" lymph nodes. Some of these aspects will be discussed within this review and proposals for classifications presented.

Introduction

The role of lymph node metastasis – although still far from clear in its mechanisms of development – has attracted new interest in the last few years from clinicians as well as pathologists. This relates to two topics: first, the histological findings of single cytokeratin-positive cells in lymph nodes which were conventionally diagnosed "tumourfree", i.e., lacking in metastasis and second, the concept of sentinel lymph node lymphadenectomy. The following review will deal with some of the aspects currently under discussion.

Process of Lymph Node Metastasis

The process of lymph node metastasis is influenced by a broad variety of parameters. The most important factor is the behaviour of the primary tumour, which should have the ability to grow cell clones able to disseminate and invade the surrounding stroma and lymphatic or blood vessels. Another aspect is the lymphatic system anatomy of the organ in question which may differ depending on the site of the primary tumour bearing organ. For most organs there is evidence for an orderly and predictable pattern of lymph flow. Histology of the primary tumour does influence the ability of tumour cells to grow in lymph nodes, e.g., sarcomas having less frequent lymph node metastasis than carcinomas or malignant melanomas. In some carcinomas the frequency of lymph node metastasis ranges around 70% at the time of the first diagnosis.

Possible reasons for the lower frequency of lymph node metastasis in sarcomas:

- Different molecular biology of sarcomas (expression of adhesion molecules, proteases and protease-inhibitors, etc.).
- Sarcoma cells have the ability to invade blood vessels but not lymphatic vessels.
- Sarcoma cells do not have the ability to grow in lymph nodes through which they pass.

Prediction of Lymph Node Metastasis

In looking at a primary carcinoma, one should ask oneself whether or not one has adequate parameters in order to predict the possibility of lymph node metastases. There are indeed some parameters which can be used for lymph node metastasis prediction (Table 1). Partly, they can be used as clinical parameters (tumour size, T category), others can be evaluated only after histological examination. The goal should be to predict the possibility of lymph node metastasis in biopsies of a primary tumour with such accuracy that the therapy can be designed along the probability of lymph node metastasis. The frequency of regional lymph node metastasis in rectal cancer in relation to histomorphology and depth of invasion is shown in Table 2. First attempts have been made to better predict the probability of lymph node metastasis by using immunohistology of molecular markers, i.e., nm23 (Tannapfel et al. 1995). Results are shown in Table 3.

Table 1. Parameters to predict the possibility of lymph node metastasis

Parameter	Use	
Tumour size	Clinical, pathological	
T category	Clinical, pathological	
Tumour type	Pathological	Biopsy
Tumour grade	Pathological	Biopsy
Invasion of lymphatic vessels	Pathological	Biopsy
Immunohistochemistry of nm23-H1	Pathological	Biopsy

Biopsy = parameters can be used in tumour biopsies

Table 2. Frequency of regional lymph node metastasis in rectal cancer in relation to histomorphology and depth of invasion (Hermanek et al. 1994)

Depth of invasion	Low-risk histology pN1,2	High-risk histology pN1,2
pT1	3%	12%
pT2 inner muscle	9.5%	42%
pT2 outer muscle	21%	51%
pT3 minimal invasion (pT3a)	22.6%	71.2%
pT3≥T3b and pT4	30.4%	89.2%

Low-risk-histology is defined as low-grade (G1, G2) and L0 (lymphatic invasion) of the primary tumour
High-grade-histology is defined as high-grade (G3, G4) or L1 (lymphatic invasion) of the primary tumour

Table 3. nm23-H1-Immunoreactivity, histomorphology and frequency of lymph node metastasis (Tannapfel et al. 1995)

–				n	pN1,2
pT1	Low-risk histology	nm23-IR	Strong	21	1
			Weak	22	13
pT2	High-risk histology	nm23-IR	Strong	16	2
			Weak	41	14

IR = Immunoreactivity

Diagnosis of Lymph Node Metastasis

There has been some debate about the definition of lymph node metastasis. By now, there is agreement that tumour cells in afferent or efferent lymphatic vessels or even in the sinus of the lymph nodes detected in conventional stains (e.g., HE, PAS, or others) are not considered lymph node metastasis. It should be emphasised that the latter events are very rare. It is recommended to make step sections in all cases, in which such single tumour cells or groups of tumour cells can be found in one slide. A high frequency overt lymph node metastasis can be found using this procedure.

A lymph node metastasis can be diagnosed when there has been arrest of tumour cells, extravasation, proliferation, and often a stromal reaction. According to the definition "micrometastasis" is diagnosed if the metastasis is ≤0.2 cm. Metastases >0.2 cm are called macrometastases. In the UICC TNM Classification of malignant tumours, micrometastasis are only considered in the classification of breast tumours and coded pN1a. In other tumours micrometastasis should be designated as pN1(mi).

Since the methods in detecting isolated tumour cells (ITC) have improved substantially in recent years, the number of cases in which tumour cells are detected by morphological or non-morphological techniques has increased. The findings of cytokeratin-positive cells (which are considered as tumour cells) in lymph nodes which were conventionally diagnosed as free of metastasis has been wrongly termed as "micrometastases" or in a way of substituting the latter expression as "microinvolvement". In fact, these cytokeratin-positive cells may be isolated (disseminated, circulating) tumour cells. The frequency of immunohistologically detected cytokeratin-positive cells (considered as tumour cells) in "tumourfree" lymph nodes varied in different organs (Table 4). It should be emphasised that all the technical procedures are not yet sufficiently standardised. It is generally agreed that the morphological methods, in particular immunohistochemistry (e.g., for cytokeratins), have a lower false positive rate than non-morphological methods such as flow cytometry or polymerase chain reaction (Yamamoto et al. 1997).

To promote uniform data collection essential for large scale investigation of the independent prognostic significance of ITC, an optional TNM compatible shorthand notation for describing and coding the respective findings is proposed (Hermanek et al. 1999). For analysis, it is necessary to register not only positive but also negative findings. In cases where there is morphological examination for ITC in regional lymph nodes the symbol "i" is used in parentheses after pN0. For non-morphologic examinations the symbol "mol" (for molecular) is used. Thus, one can distinguish between different subsets of pN0:

- pN0   No regional lymph node metastasis histologically,
              – no examination for isolated tumour cells (ITC)
- pN0(i–)   No regional lymph node metastasis histologically,
              – negative morphologic findings for ITC
- pN0(i+)   No regional lymph node metastasis histologically,
              – positive morphologic findings for ITC
- pN0(mol–)   No regional lymph node metastasis histologically,
              – negative non-morphological findings for ITC
- pN0(mol+)   No regional lymph node metastasis histologically,
              – positive non-morphologic findings for ITC

Table 4. Detection of isolated tumour cells in "tumourfree" regional lymph nodes. Relation to site of primary (only patients without distant metastasis) (Hermanek et al. 1999)

Site	Regional lymph nodes	Reference
Breast carcinoma	≈ 15%	Wells et al. 1984, Stosiek et al. 1996
Gastric carcinoma	90%	Fellbaum et al. 1997
Colorectal carcinoma	≈ 25–30%	Greenson et al. 1994, Jeffers et al. 1994
Prostate carcinoma	≈ 45%	Edelstein et al. 1996
Non-small cell lung carcinoma	≈ 15%	Passlick et al. 1996
Ductal pancreatic carcinoma	≈ 75%	Hosch et al. 1997
Oesophageal carcinoma	≈ 50%	Izbicki et al. 1997

Principles of Classification

In the general rules of the UICC TNM Classification there are some principles outlined on how to classify particular forms of lymph node metastasis:

- Direct extension of the primary tumour into lymph nodes is classified as lymph node metastasis.
  Example: A direct invasion of lung carcinoma in an intrapulmonary lymph node is classified as pN1 and is not considered additional by tumour size (T category).
- A tumour nodule greater than 3 mm in the connective tissue of a lymph node drainage area without histological evidence of residual lymph node is classified in the pN category.
  - Example: In rectal carcinoma such tumour nodules may be found in the adjacent perirectal fatty tissue. Tumour nodules ≤3 mm are classified as discontinuous extension of the primary tumour and are classified as pT3.
- When size is a criterion for pN classification, e.g., in breast carcinoma, measurement is made of the metastasis, not of the entire lymph node.
- Metastasis in any lymph node other than regional is classified as distant metastasis.
  - Example: Histologically proven lymph node metastasis of rectal carcinoma in paraaortic lymph nodes or lymph nodes of the hepatoduodenal ligament are classified as distant metastasis (pM1 LYM).
- In case of tumour involvement of more than one site or subsite, the regional lymph nodes are those of the involved sites and subsites.
  Example: Carcinoma of the oesophagus involving the upper thoracic portion and the cervical oesophagus: the regional lymph nodes are those for intrathoracic oesophagus, i.e., the mediastinal and perigastric nodes (excluding the coeliac nodes), as well as those for cervical oesophagus, i.e., the cervical nodes.
- Metastasis in lymph nodes which drain an organ directly invaded by the primary tumour are classified as regional.
  - Example: A sigmoid carcinoma with invasion of small bowel and occurrence of lymph node metastasis in mesenterial lymph nodes is classified as pN1 or pN2 according to the total number of nodes, not as distant metastasis.

Lymph Node Metastasis in TNM Stage Grouping

As a rule in the TNM classification of lymph node metastasis lymph node metastases are assigned to stage III. However, there are several exceptions which are listed in Table 5. Furthermore, in few instances non-regional lymph nodes which are classified as distant metastasis in most tumour sites form a separate M category as M1a, e.g., in tumours of the lower thoracic oesophagus, prostate, and testis, and malignant melanoma of the skin.

Table 5. Exceptions of assigning lymph node metastasis to stage III. (UICC TNM Classification of Malignant Tumours 1997)

Site	Lowest stage
Nasopharynx	IIB
Papillar/follicular thyroid carcinomas (younger than 45 years)	I
Oesophagus	IB
Stomach	IB
Lung	IIA
Pleural mesothelioma	II
Bone and soft tissues	IV
Breast	IIA
Penis	II
Prostate	IV
Testis	II
Renal pelvis and ureter	IV
Urinary bladder	IV

No N classification in gestational trophoblastic tumours

Number of Nodes

It has been clearly shown in several tumour entities that the frequency of lymph node metastasis is dependent on the number of the examined nodes. These observations have prompted the TNM Project Committee of the UICC in the 5th edition to recommend numbers of nodes which should be removed and examined histologically to provide a reliable indication of a negative lymph node status:

The pathological assessment of the regional lymph nodes (pN) entails removal of the nodes adequate to validate the absence of lymph nodes metastasis and sufficient to evaluate the highest pN category. The necessary number of nodes is shown in Table 6.

Some technical issues in histological examination of lymph nodes have to be considered:

- There are some controversies about the best method to detect all lymph nodes in a dissection specimen.
- How many histological sections per collected lymph node are necessary to detect all metastases? Is serial sectioning necessary?
- What is the role of immunohistology?
- Which antibodies should be used and if so, on how many slides?
- Are there any other special techniques?

Generally, there are at present no recommendations or standards. An overview with the methods employed to find the maximum number of lymph nodes by conventional preparation and staining techniques was described by Hermanek (1979). In accordance with these descriptions Zhang et al. (1998) have recently shown in a retrospective study that thorough histological examination on properly prepared sections is the most efficient and cost-effective way to detect the vast majority of axillary lymph node metastases.

Table 6. pN0 histological examination of a lymphadenectomy specimen will ordinarily include the following number of nodes

Site	Number of nodes
Thyroid gland	6
Oesophagus	6
Stomach	15
Small intestine	12
Colon and rectum	12
Anal canal	3
Liver	3
Gallbladder, extrahepatic bile ducts	3
Ampulla of Vater	10
Pancreas	10
Lung, pleural mesothelioma	6
Skin (carcinoma, malignant melanoma)	6
Breast	6
Vulva, vagina (upper 1/3)	6
Vagina (lower 2/3)	10
Cervix and corpus uteri	10
Ovary and fallopian tube	10

(UICC TNM Classification of Malignant Tumours 1997)

Further Development of Lymph Node Metastasis Classifications

In the TNM Supplement (1993, 2000) some proposals have been made to further develop the classification of lymph node metastasis. For some sites, new telescopic ramifications have been proposed, e.g., for tumours of the lung, breast, cervix uteri, prostate, and malignant melanoma of the skin. For example, the ramification proposal for carcinoma of the cervix uteri is shown:

- N1a   Metastasis in 1–2 regional lymph nodes below the common iliac artery.
- N1b   Metastasis in 3 or more regional lymph nodes below the common iliac artery.
- N1c   Metastasis in any lymph node along the common iliac artery.

Sentinel Node

There has been some debate concerning the concept of the sentinel node. Considering reports with varying definitions the UICC TNM Project Committee has provided a definition to be published in the TNM Supplement 2000:

The sentinel lymph node is the first lymph node to receive the lymphatic drainage from a primary tumour. If it contains metastatic tumour this indicates that other lymph nodes may contain tumour. If it does not contain metastatic tumour, other lymph nodes are not likely to contain tumour. Occasionally, there is more than one sentinel lymph node.

The following designations are applicable when sentinel lymph node assessment is attempted:

- pNX (sn) Sentinel lymph node could not be assessed
- pN0 (sn) No sentinel lymph node metastasis
- pN1 (sn) Sentinel lymph node metastasis

Concepts of sentinel node based surgery in several organs will be discussed in other chapters of this book.

Conclusion

There has been considerable activity in the discussion of lymph node metastasis. However, before a successful concept can universally be adopted, some basic questions will have to be clearly defined. Some attempts have been made by the UICC but need to be substantially widened with growing knowledge on the process of lymph node metastasis.

References

Edelstein RA, Zietman AL, De las Morenas A, Krane RJ, Babayan RK, Dallow KC, Traish A, Moreland RP (1996) Implications of prostate micrometastasis in pelvic lymph nodes: an archival tissue study. Urology 47:370–375

Fellbaum Ch, Kestlmeier R, Busch R, Böttcher K, Siewert JR, Höfler H (1997) Prognostic relevance of microcarcinosis ("microinvolvement") in lymph nodes in gastric cancer. In: Progress in Gastric Cancer Research 1997 (Siewert JR, Roder JD, eds) Monduzzi Editore, Bologna, pp 235–236

Greenson JK, Isenhart CE, Rice R, Mojzisik C, Houchens D, Martins jr EW (1994) Identification of occult micrometastasis in pericolic lymph nodes of Dukes B colorectal cancer patients using monoclonal antibodies against cytokeratin and CC49. Cancer 73:563–569

Hermanek P (1979) Lymphknotenuntersuchung. In: Hermanek P, Gall FP (Hrsg) Kompendium der klinischen Tumorpathologie. Band 1: Grundlagen der klinischen Onkologie. Witzstrock, Baden-Baden Köln New York, S 132–135

Hermanek P (1994) Onkologische und histopathologische Grundlagen einer lokalen Therapie in kurativer Intention. In: Hermanek P, Marzoli GP (Hrsg) Lokale Therapie des Rektumkarzinoms. Verfahren in kurativer Intention. Springer, Berlin Heidelberg New York Tokyo, S 7–14

Hermanek P, Hutter RVP, Sobin LH, Wittekind Ch (1999) Classification of isolated (disseminated, circulating) tumor cells and micrometastasis. Cancer 86:2668–2673

Hosch STB, Knoefeld WT, Metz S, Stoecklein N, Niendorf A, Broelsch ChE, Izbicki JR (1997) Early lymphatic tumor cell dissemination in pancreatic cancer: frequency and prognostic significance. Pancreas 15:154–159

Izbicki JR, Hosch STB, Pichlmeier U, Rehders A, Bsuch C, Niendorf A, Passlick B, Broelsch ChE, Pantel K (1997) Prognostic value of immunohistochemically identifiable tumor cells in lymph nodes with completely resected oesophageal cancer. New Engl J Med 337:1188–1194

Jeffers MD, O'Dowd GNI, Mulcahy H, Stagg M, O'Donoghue DP, Toner M (1994) The prognostic significance of immunohistochemically detected lymph node micrometastases in colorectal carcinoma. J Pathol 172:183–187

Passlick B, Izbicki JR, Kubuschok B, Thetter O, Pantel K (1996) Detection of disseminated lung cancer cells in lymph nodes: Impact on staging and prognosis. Am Thorac Surg 61:177–183

Stosiek P, Gerber B, Kasper M (1996) Zur prognostischen Bedeutung von Mikrometastasen in axillären Lymphknoten beim Mammakarzinom. Pathologe 17:433–439

Tannapfel A, Köckerling F, Katalinic A, Wittekind Ch (1995) Expression of nm23-H1 predicts lymph node involvement in colorectal carcinoma. Dis Colon Rectum 38:651–654

UICC (1993) TNM Supplement 1993. A commentary on uniform use. (Hermanek P, Henson DE, Hutter RVP, Sobin LH, eds) Springer, Berlin Heidelberg New York Tokyo

UICC (1997) TNM Classification of malignant tumours, 5th ed. Sobin LH, Wittekind Ch, (eds) John Wiley & Sons, New York

UICC (2000) TNM Supplement 2000. A commentary on uniform use, 2nd ed. Wittekind Ch, Henson DE, Hutter RVP, Sobin LH (eds) John Wiley & Sons, New York, in preparation

Wells CA, Heryet A, Brochier J, Gatter KC, Mason DY (1984) The immunocytochemical detection of axillary micrometastases in breast cancer. Br J Cancer 50:193–197

Yamamoto N, Kato Y, Yanagisawa et al. (1997) Predictive value of genetic diagnosis for cancer micrometastasis. Cancer 80:1393–1398

Zhang PJ, Reisner RM, Nangia R, Edge SB, Brooks JJ (1998) Effectiveness of multiple-level sectioning in detecting axillary nodal micrometastasis in breast cancer. Arch Pathol Lab Med 122:687–690

Detection and Relevance of Immunohistochemically Identifiable Tumor Cells in Lymph Nodes

B. Passlick[1] and K. Pantel[2]

[1] Department of Surgery, University of Munich, Klinikum Innenstadt,
Nussbaumstrasse 20, 80336 Munich, Germany
[2] Molekulare Diagnostik und Therapie, Universitäts-Frauenklinik, Hamburg,
Germany

Abstract

Lymph node metastasis is a well-known feature of poor prognosis in potentially resectable solid epithelial tumors. However, a significant number of apparently lymph node negative patients die early of metastatic disease. Therefore, it has to be assumed that in some patients an early tumor cell dissemination has occurred which is clearly underestimated by current staging procedures. Recently, it has been shown, that an early dissemination of individual carcinoma cells to regional lymph nodes can be detected by using sensitive immunocytochemical techniques with monoclonal antibodies against
epithelium-specific proteins. The incidence of immunohistochemically positive patients varies between 12% and 70% depending on the type of primary
tumor, the immunohistochemical staining procedure used, and especially on
the primary monoclonal antibody. The detection of disseminated tumor cells
in lymph nodes by immunocytochemistry is associated with a poorer prognosis in different types of epithelial tumors such as lung cancer or esophageal cancer. The immunocytochemical method might also be useful in the
detection of occult tumor cells in sentinel lymph nodes. In conclusion, the
immunohistochemical detection of disseminated tumor cells in lymph nodes
can help to obtain a more exact identification of patients with an unfavorable prognosis. Whether the identified patients will gain from an adjuvant
therapy has to be evaluated in further studies.

Introduction

The dissemination of malignant cells to distant organs via lymph nodes or
blood vessels in solid tumors can occur at an early stage of primary tumor
growth and is regularly underestimated by currently available clinical and
pathological staging procedures [1]. For example, approximately 40% of patients who undergo surgical resection of non-small-cell lung cancer (NSCLC)

without overt metastases (pT_{1-2}, N_0, M_0, R_0), relapse within 24 months after surgery [2]. This is also reflected in a poor 5-year survival rate of about 60% and suggests that an occult tumor load is the major reason for the high mortality in surgically treated lung cancer patients [3]. Indeed, several groups, including ours, have shown that the early dissemination of individual lung carcinoma cells to regional lymph nodes [4-6] and distant organs like the bone marrow [7-9] can be detected by immunocytochemical techniques using monoclonal antibodies against epithelium-specific proteins. In bone marrow the occurrence of cytokeratin-positive cells has recently demonstrated to be indicative for a later clinical relapse [7-9] and the malignant nature of these cells have further been supported by their tumor-associated genetic characteristics and their metastatic capacity after transplantation in immunodeficient mice [10].

Herein, we give an overview on the occurrence and significance of disseminated tumor cells in lymph nodes detected by immunohistochemical methods with a special focus on NSCLCs as an example of a solid tumor.

Detection of Tumor Cells in Lymph Nodes: Methodological Aspects

Minimal tumor-cell dissemination to regional lymph nodes has been previously assessed by serial sectioning of lymph nodes (HE staining and routine histopathologic examination of an extensive number of consecutive sections) [11]. Using this approach the number of positive lymph nodes can be increased in about 8%-30% of the specimens [12]. However, the method is time-consuming and thus not practicable as a routine procedure for tumor staging. Thus, sensitive immunocytochemical assays with antibodies to epithelial antigens might be more reasonable alternatives.

Monoclonal antibodies to epithelial cytokeratins have been successfully used to identify individual metastatic cells in bone marrow of patients with various epithelial tumors [13].

However, since reticulum cells express cytokeratins [14, 15], antibodies directed against these proteins are not the best choice for the identification of individual carcinoma cells in lymph nodes, because somewhat subjective morphological criteria must be imposed.

To develop an observer-independent assay solely based on the assessment of immunoreactivity we used mAb Ber-Ep 4 for the detection of micrometastatic tumor cells. Ber-Ep 4 (IgG1; Dako, Hamburg, Germany) is directed against two glycopolypeptides of 34 and 49 kD present on the surface and in the cytoplasm of all epithelial cells except the superficial layers of squamous epithelia, hepatocytes, and parietal cells [16, 17]. The antibody does not react with mesenchymal tissue, including lymphoid tissue [16] and can also be used on paraffin sections.

The high sensitivity of mAb Ber-Ep 4 for detection of NSCLC cells was supported by positive staining of 81 out of 82 (99%) primary tumors (45 adenocarcinomas and 37 squamous cell carcinomas). The majority of these samples (73/

Table 1. Expression of Ber-Ep 4 on primary non-small cell lung carcinomas (modified from [6])

Staining pattern[a]	Adenocarcinoma ($n = 45$)	Squamous cell carcinoma ($n = 37$)
None	1	0
Heterogeneous, focal	3 (6.6%)	5 (13.5%)
Homogeneous	41 (91.1%)	32 (86.5%)

[a] Cryostat sections were stained with mAb Ber-Ep using the APAAP technique. Specimens were analyzed by light microscopy

81) displayed a homogeneous staining (Table. 1). The consistent staining of 15 lymph nodes with overt metastases (stage N_1), further indicated that the corresponding antigens remain preserved during the process of metastases [6].

To demonstrate the specificity of our method, 28 lymph nodes from 24 control patients with non-epithelial tumors (neurofibroma, malignant melanoma, lymphoma, hamatochondroma, $n = 7$) or inflammable diseases (tuberculoma, abscesses, aspergillosis, empyema, $n = 17$) were also studied by immunocytochemistry with Ber-Ep 4. These lymph nodes were consistently negative for Ber Ep 4-positive cells.

In order to compare the effectiveness of the immunohistochemical analyses directly with the conventional Hematoxylin-Eosin (HE) method two additional sections consecutive to those displaying Ber-Ep 4-positive cells were studied. One section was stained by routine HE staining, the other was immunostained with Ber-Ep 4. Both sections were then compared with the original positive section by an experienced pathologist without having knowledge of the initial results. As a control, consecutive sections from Ber-Ep 4-negative lymph nodes were stained under the same conditions and incorporated into the evaluation. Repeated immunostaining resulted in a redetection of Ber-Ep 4-positive cells in a neighboring section in 93.3% (14/15) of the nodes and in 90.9% (10/11) of the patients, respectively. In contrast, repeated HE staining and histopathologic examination did not reveal any tumor cells. Lymph node sections initially negative for Ber-Ep 4 cells remained negative in the adjacent sections [6]. In our studies on early lymph node dissemination in lung and esophageal cancer from each lymph node 4–6 m cryostat sections were cut from three different levels and analyzed. One section per level was stained with the alkaline phosphatase anti-alkaline phosphatase (APAAP) technique.

Immunohistochemistry of Lymph Nodes: Detection Rates and Prognostic Significance

NSCLC

In NSCLC the immunohistochemical staining with the monoclonal antibody Ber-Ep 4 revealed disseminated epithelial cells in 35 (6.2%) of 565 lymph

Table 2. Presence of isolated tumor cells in lymph nodes of NSCLC patients (modified from [31])

	Number of patients per group	Number of patients with isolated tumor cells in lymph nodes
Total	125	27 (21.6%)
pT status		
pT_{1-2}	104	23 (22.1%)
pT_{3-4}	21	4 (19.0%)
pN status		
pN_0	70	11 (15.7%)
pN_1	25	4 (16.0%)
pN_2	30	12 (40.0%)
pN_{1+2}	55	16 (29.1%)*
Histological type		
Adenocarcinoma	55	13 (23.6%)
Squamous-cell carcinoma	52	10 (19.2%)
Miscellaneous[a]	18	4 (22.2%)

*$p = 0.019$ (pN_0 versus pN_{1-2} patients, Chi^2-test)
[a] Adenosquamous carcinoma ($n = 6$) and large cell carcinoma ($n = 12$)

nodes that were negative by routine histopathology and 27 (21.6%) of 125 patients with resectable NSCLC (Table 2). These cells occurred as either isolated, single cells or as cell cluster up to three cells present in the sinuses (60%) and the lymphoid tissue of the node (40%). A single positive finding of isolated tumor cells in one section of one lymph node of the investigated patient was a rare event. In 80% of cases minimal tumor cell spread were found in more than one of the three lymph node sections (31%) or more than one lymph node (55%).

By conventional histopathology 70 of 125 patients were staged as having pN_0 disease and 55 as pN_{1-2} disease according to the International Union Against Cancer TNM classification (Table 2). In pN_{1-2} patients, immunohistochemical staining exposed tumor cell dissemination to resected lymph nodes in 16 cases (29.1%). This was clearly higher in comparison with pN_0 patients, who had Ber-Ep 4-positive cells in their lymph nodes in 11 cases (15.7%) ($p = 0.019$, chi^2-test). Other pathological parameters were not associated with an increased rate of disseminated tumor cells in univariate analysis.

These rates are considerably lower than the frequencies obtained in a recent retrospective study [4], in which 17% of the lymph nodes and 63% of the patients analyzed were judged as positive. This discrepancy may in part reflect an increased rate of false-positive findings in the latter study due to the use of a polyclonal anti-keratin antiserum, which may also explain the failure to obtain a prognostic significance.

Our study on NSCLC patients revealed that after an observation time of 64 months patients with immunohistochemically proven disseminated tumor cells in regional lymph nodes had a significantly reduced overall survival

Table 3. Prognostic significance of disseminated tumor cells in lymph nodes in 125 NSCLC patients (modified from [31]): uni- and multivariate statistics of overall survival

Variable	Univariate p^a	Multivariate analysis (Cox model)			
		Estimated coefficient	SE	p	Relative risk (95% CI)
Lymphatic tumor cell dissemination (positive vs. negative)	0.0001	0.935	0.300	0.002	2.5 (1.4–4.6)
pT stage (pT_{1-2} vs. pT_{3-4})	0.002	0.602	0.350	0.068	1.8 (0.9–3.6)
pN stage (pN_0 vs. pN_{1-2})	0.0001	0.824	0.234	0.011	2.3 (1.2–4.3)
Age (years) (≤ 60 vs. >60)	0.075	0.518	0.294	0.078	1.7 (0.9–3.0)

[a] Log-rank test

(p = 0.0001 by log rank test, Table 3, univariate analysis). Correspondingly, patients with disseminated tumor cells experienced a higher rate of disease relapse than patients without such cells (p<0.0001). Because of the elevated frequency of Ber-Ep 4-positive cells in higher pN stages (Table 2), a stratification for pN stage was done. In pN_0 disease, patients with disseminated tumor cells had a significant overall survival disadvantage over those without disseminated tumor cells (p = 0.010). In pN_{1-2} disease, the overall survival rate was also definitely reduced in the presence of these cells and the impact of minimal tumor cell spread on overall survival was comparably strong (p = 0.027).

A Cox regression model was applied to analyze the influence of lymphatic tumor cell dissemination, pT stage, pN stage and age on overall survival (Table 3). Because there was no evidence for a dependence of survival rates on grading, tumor histology, or sex, these covariates were excluded from the linear predictor (data not shown). In contrast to univariate analysis, pT stage failed to prove prognostic significance for recurrence or survival in multivariate analysis. However, the multivariate analysis showed a 2.5 times increased risk for shorter survival (Table 3) and a 2.7 times increased risk for tumor relapse in patients with disseminated tumor cells versus patients without such cells. Pathological N stage had a prognostic value for reduced survival in the same range (relative risk 2.3).

Other Solid Tumors

Using the same protocol [immunocytochemical technique (APAAP method) with the epithelial specific monoclonal antibody Ber-Ep 4] as in NSCLC our group analyzed lymph nodes which were negative by routine histopathology from patients with apparently operable esophageal carcinoma for dissemi-

Table 4. Immunohistochemistry in nodal examination

Author	Year	Carcinoma	mAb	No. of patients.	Incidence of disseminated cells (%)	Prognostic significance	Ref.
Chen	1993	NSCLC	Cytokeratin	60	63.0	–	[4]
Passlick	1996	NSCLC	Ber-Ep 4	125	21.6	DFS/OS	[32]
Maruyama	1997	NSCLC	Cytokeratin	44	70.5	DFS	[5]
Dobashi	1997	NSCLC	Anti-p53	31	45.0	OS	[33]
Byrne	1992	Breast	CA15–3, MCA	39	12.8	DFS	[34]
Cutait	1991	Colon	CEA, Cytokeratin	46	23.8	–	[35]
Jeffers	1993	Colon	Cytokeratin	77	25.0	–	[36]
Greenson	1993	Colon	TAG 72, Cytokeratin	55	28.0	OS	[37]
Adell	1996	Colon	Cytokeratin	100	39	–	[38]
Sievert	1996	Gastric	Ber-Ep 4	100	21.8	OS	[39]
Izbicki	1997	Esophagus	Ber-Ep 4	68	62	DFS	[18]
Glickman	1999	Esophagus	Cytokeratin	49	31	–	[19]

nated tumor cells [18]. Individual Ber-Ep 4-positive cells were detected in 67 (17%) out of 399 lymph nodes and in 42 out of 69 (62%) esophageal cancer patients, respectively. There was no correlation between the presence of micrometastatic cells in lymph nodes and the histology or localization of the primary tumor as well as the age and sex of the patient. However, nodal micrometastases was more frequent in advanced primary tumors (T1–2 vs. T3–4) and less differentiated carcinomas (G1–2 vs. G3). Following a median observation time of 21 months (range 2–51), patients with lymph node micrometastases showed a significantly shorter disease-free survival than patients without nodal micrometastases (p = 0.001; log rank test). In a Cox regression model multivariate analysis demonstrated that the occurrence of these cells is an independent, significant determinant of early relapse. In contrast, Glickman et al., failed to confirm a prognostic relevance of occult lymphatic dissemination in esophageal cancer [19]. However, they used a different detection assay, i.e., an anti-cytokeratin antibody that can bind to normal lymph node cells and therefore cause false-positive findings.

Similar to NSCLC and esophageal cancer, lymph nodes of many other solid tumors have been screened by immunohistochemistry for disseminated tumor cells or micrometastases. An overview on recently published articles is given in Table 4.

The incidence of immunohistochemically positive patients varies between 12 and 70% depending on the type of primary tumor, the immunohistochemical staining procedure used and especially on the primary monoclonal antibody. As has been mentioned earlier, the use of cytokeratin antibodies in lymph nodes often results in some unspecific staining, due to the expression of cytokeratins by, for example, reticulum cells. This might increase the number of immunohistochemically positive lymph nodes and might reduce the specificity of the assay.

Occult Tumor Cells in Sentinel Lymph Nodes

An important advance in the evaluation of regional lymph nodes has been the development of a more limited dissection, the sentinel lymph node dissection, that is based on the identification, with dyes or radioactivity, of the specific lymph node that drains the tumor and the removal of this lymph node for analysis. This approach was pioneered by Morton and colleagues [20–22] and has been extensively evaluated in patients with melanoma and breast cancer [20–24]. Although the advantages of a more limited lymph node dissection are clear (in particular the potential for decreasing the rate of postoperative complications), there is less material available for staging evaluation. The use of sensitive methods to detect micrometastases may allow the identification of metastases in more limited amounts of material, such as lymph nodes, and thus may influence the subsequent therapeutic approach (e.g., more extensive lymph node dissection and the administration of adjuvant therapy). The use of immunohistochemistry can change the status of a negative node to a positive node in 5%–20% of the sample tested, and thus inclusion of an immunohistochemical evaluation may reduce the false-negative rate of the sentinel node technique to almost zero [25]. Thus, detection of occult tumor cells may be an important adjunct to the use of limited lymph node dissection for staging and for therapy [26].

Conclusions

In conclusion, the immunohistochemical detection of disseminated tumor cells in lymph nodes can help to obtain a more exact identification of patients with an unfavorable prognosis. Thus this information should be incorporated into the current pTNM classification system [27]. Whether the identified patients will gain from an adjuvant therapy has to be evaluated in further studies. Since most of the disseminated tumor cells appear to be in a dormant (i.e., non-proliferating) state [28] immunotherapeutic approaches might be an alternative to S-phase-specific chemotherapeutic agents. In this context the EpCam antigen (also called 17–1A antigen) appears to be an interesting target because of its expression on a variety of different epithelia tumor cells, including NSCLC cells [29].

Acknowledgements. This work was supported by grants from the Deutsche Krebshilfe, Bonn, the Deutsche Forschungsgemeinschaft (SFB 469), Bonn, the K.L. Weigand-Stiftung, Munich and the MMW-Herausgeberstiftung, Munich, Germany.

References

1. Pantel K, Riethmüller G (1996) Micrometastasis detection and treatment with monoclonal antibodies. Curr Top Microbiol Immunol 213:1–18
2. Mountain CF (1997) Revisions in the international system for staging lung cancer. Chest 111:1710–1717
3. Passlick B, Pantel K (1996) Prognostic factors in stage I non-small cell lung cancer. Zentralbl Chir 121:851–860
4. Chen ZL, Perez S, Holmes CE, et al. (1993) Frequency and distribution of occult micrometastases in lymph nodes of patients with non-small cell lung cancer. J Natl Cancer Inst 85:493–498
5. Maruyama R, Sugio K, Mitsodomi T, Saitoh G, Ishida T, Sugimachi K (1997) Relationship between early recurrence and micrometastases in the lymph nodes of patients with stage I non-small cell lung cancer. J Thorac Cardiovas Surg 114:535–543
6. Passlick B, Izbicki JR, Kubuschok B, et al. (1994) Immunohistochemical assessment of individual tumor cells in lymph nodes of patients with non-small cell lung cancer. J Clin Oncol 12:1827–1832
7. Cote RJ, Beattie EJ, Chaiwun B, et al. (1995) Detection of occult bone marrow micrometastases in patients with operable lung carcinoma. Ann Surg 222:415–425
8. Ohgami A, Mitsodomi T, Sugio K, et al. (1997) Micrometastastic tumor cells in the bone marrow of patients with non-small cell lung cancer. Ann Thorac Surg 64:363–367
9. Pantel K, Izbicki JR, Passlick B, et al. (1996) Frequency and prognostic significance of isolated tumour cells detected in bone marrow of non-small cell lung cancer patients without overt metastases. Lancet 347:649–653
10. Pantel K, Dickmanns A, Zippelius F, et al. (1995) Establishment of carcinoma cell lines from bone marrow of patients with minimal residual cancer: A novel source of tumor cell vaccines. J Natl Cancer Inst 87:1162–1168
11. International Breast Cancer Study Group (1990) Prognostic significance of occult axillary lymph node micrometastases from breast cancers. Lancet 335:1565–1568
12. Dowlatshahi K, Fan M, Snider HC, Habib FA (1997) Lymph node micrometastases from breast carcinoma: reviewing the dilemma. Cancer 80:1188–1197
13. Pantel K, Braun S, Passlick B, Schlimok G (1996) Minimal residual epithelial cancer: Diagnostic approaches and prognostic relevance. Prog Histochem Cytochem 30:1–46
14. Domagala W, Bedner E, Chosia M, Weber K, Osborn M (1991) Keratin-positive reticulum cells in fine needle aspirates and touch imprints of hyperplastic lymph nodes. Acta Cytol 36:241–245
15. Doglioni C, Dell'Orto P, Zanetti G, Iuzzolino P, Coggi G, Viale G (1990) Cytokeratin-immunoreactive cells of human lymph nodes and spleen in normal and pathological conditions. Virchows Archiv A Pathol Anat 416:479–490
16. Momburg F, Moldenhauer G, Hämmerling GJ, Möller P (1987) Immunohistochemical study of the expression of a Mr 34 000 human epithelium-specific surface glycoprotein in normal and malignant tissues. Cancer Res 47:2883–2891
17. Latza U, Niedobitek G, Schwarting R, Nekarda H, Stein H (1990) Ber-EP4: new monoclonal antibody which distinguishes epithelia from mesothelia. J Clin Pathol 43:213–219
18. Izbicki JR, Hosch SB, Pichlmaier H, et al. (1997) Prognostic value of immunohistochemically identifiable tumor cells in lymph nodes of patients with completely resected eosophageal cancer. N Eng J Med 337:1188–1194
19. Glickman JN, Torres C, Wang HH, et al. (1999) The prognostic significance of lymph node micrometastasis in patients with esophageal carcinoma. Cancer 85:769–678
20. Morton DL, Wen DR, Wong JH, et al. (1992) Technical details of intraoperative lymphatic mapping for early stage melanoma. Arch Surg 127:392–399
21. Giuliano AE, Kirgan DM, Guenther JM, Morton DL (1994) Lymphatic mapping and sentinel lymphadenectomy for breast cancer [see comments]. Ann Surg 220:391–398

22. Giuliano AE, Dale PS, Turner RR, Morton DL, Evans SW, Krasne DL (1995) Improved axillary staging of breast cancer with sentinel lymphadenectomy [see comments]. Ann Surg 222:394–399
23. Veronesi U, Paganelli G, Galimberti V, et al. (1997) Sentinel-node biopsy to avoid axillary dissection in breast cancer with clinically negative lymph-nodes [see comments]. Lancet 349:1864–1867
24. Krag D, Weaver D, Ashikaga T, et al. (1998) The sentinel node in breast cancer–a multicenter validation study. N Engl J Med 339:941–946
25. Giuliano AE, Jones RC, Brennan M, Statman R (1997) Sentinel lymphadenectomy in breast cancer. J Clin Oncol 15:2345–2350
26. Van-der-Velde ZD, Roijers JF, Bouwens RA, et al. (1996) Molecular test for the detection of tumor cells in blood and sentinel nodes of melanoma patients. Am J Pathol 149:759–764
27. Hermanek P (1995) pTNM and residual tumor classifications: Problems of assessment and prognostic significance. World J Surg 19:184–190
28. Pantel K, Schlimok G, Braun S, et al. (1993) Differential expression of proliferation-associated molecules in individual micrometastatic carcinoma cells. J Natl Cancer Inst 85:1419–1424
29. Passlick B, Seen-Hilber R, Wöckel W, Häussinger K, Thetter O, Pantel K (1998) The 17-1A antigen is expressed on primary, metastatic and disseminated non-small cell lung carcinoma cells. Ann Oncol 9:89–89 (Abstract)
30. Riethmüller G, Holz E, Schlimok G, et al. (1998) Monoclonal antibody therapy for resected Dukes C colorectal cancer: Seven year outcome of a multicenter trial. J Clin Oncol 16:1788–1794
31. Kubuschok B, Passlick B, Izbicki JR, Thetter O, Pantel K (1999) Disseminated tumor cells in lymph nodes as a determinant for survival in surgically resected non-small cell lung cancer. J Clin Oncol 17:19–24
32. Passlick B, Izbicki JR, Kubuschok B, Thetter O, Pantel K (1996) Detection of disseminated lung cancer cells in lymph nodes: Impact on staging and prognosis. Ann Thorac Surg 61:177–183
33. Dobashi K, Sugio K, Osaki T, Oka K, Yasumoto K (1997) Micrometastatic p53-positive cells in the lymph nodes of non-small cell lung cancer: Prognostic significance. J Thorac Cardiovas Surg 114:339–346
34. Byrne J, Horgan PG, England S, Callaghan J, Given HF (1992) A preliminary report on the usefulness of monoclonal antibodies to CA 15-3 and MCA in the detection of micrometastases in axillary lymph nodes draining primary breast carcinoma. Eur J Cancer ;28:658–660
35. Cutait R, Alves VA, Lopes LC, et al. (1991) Restaging of colorectal cancer based on the identification of lymph node micrometastases through immunoperoxidase staining of CEA and cytokeratins. Dis Colon Rectum 34:917–920
36. Jeffers MD, O'Dowd GM, Mulcahy H, Stagg M, O'Donoghue DP, Toner M (1994) The prognostic significance of immunohistochemically detected lymph node micrometastases in colorectal carcinoma. J Pathol 172:183–187
37. Greenson JK, Isenhart CE, Rice R, Mojzisik C, Houchens D, Martin EW (1994) Identification of occult micrometastases in pericolic lymph nodes of Dukes' B colorectal cancer patients using monoclonal antibodies against cytokeratin and CC49. Cancer 73:563–569
38. Adell G, Boeryd B, Franlund B, Sjodahl R, Hakansson L (1996) Occurrence and prognostic importance of micrometastases in regional lymph nodes in Dukes' B colorectal carcinoma: an immunohistochemical study. Eur J Surg 162:637–642
39. Siewert JR, Kestlmeier R, Busch R, et al. (1996) Benefits of D2 lymph node dissection for patients with gastric cancer and pN0 and pN1 lymph node metastases [see comments]. Br J Surg 83:1144–1147.

II. Principles of Lymphatic Metastasis

Cell Biology of Lymphatic Metastasis
The Potential Role of c-*erb*B Oncogene Signalling

S. A. Eccles

Tumour Biology and Metastasis, Section of Cancer Therapeutics,
Institute of Cancer Research, Cotswold Rd, Sutton, Surrey SM2 5NG, UK

Abstract

Lymphatic metastases are an important indicator of the malignancy of epithelial cancers. Empirical clinical observations associating specific genetic abnormalities with tumour progression, allied with basic laboratory investigations, are providing not only improved prognostic and diagnostic opportunities, but also a detailed understanding of the molecular machinery of metastasis. One such association – between the c-*erb*B oncogene family and metastasis – has proved particularly instructive. Functional links between overexpression (and occasionally mutational activation) of c-*erb*B-1 (EGFR) and c-*erb*B-2 and specific phenotypes of metastatic cells have been elucidated. Activated c-*erb*B oncogenes potentiate tumour cell adhesion to endothelial cells and upregulate VEGF, potentially facilitating angiogenesis and vascular invasion. In addition, cells over-expressing these oncogenes frequently show aberrant cell-cell and cell-matrix interactions, mediated by changes in integrin and cadherin function. Thirdly, both EGFR and c-*erb*B-2 signalling can significantly upregulate specific matrix metalloproteinases, key enzymes involved in angiogenesis and invasion. Finally, c-*erb*B receptors linked to the actin cytoskeleton and highly expressed on invadopodia, are thought to assist cell migration. Taken together, these observations suggest that such receptors can act as "master switches" in metastasis, whose activation co-ordinately controls events normally utilised in development, now subverted by the metastatic cell. As such, they represent ideal targets for therapeutic intervention.

Introduction

Lymphatic metastases are frequently the first indication of cancer spread and are an extremely important factor in staging and prognosis of many carcinomas. In some cases (e.g., breast cancer) it is possible to sample regional nodes during surgery to test for the presence of disseminated cells. However, detection depends upon either histological examination of a limited number of sections, which may miss small tumour deposits, or genetic techniques such as PCR or RT-PCR which (at least with some primers) may give false positive results, (Bostick et al. 1998). Recently, attention has turned to molecular profiling of primary tumours in an effort to obtain additional prognostic information. Empirical data have indicated associations between expression of certain molecules in human cancers (for example the c-erbB family of proto-oncogenes) and increased risk of metastasis. These clinical observations, combined with fundamental laboratory research, are now leading to a greater understanding of how such molecules may contribute to key processes involved in tumour dissemination.

The process of metastasis begins with the dissociation of cancer cells from the primary mass, invasion of surrounding tissues and their infiltration into blood vessels and/or lymphatic channels. Frequently (but not inevitably) metastases arise in the first tissue or lymph node encountered, and a cascade of tertiary sites may subsequently be colonised "downstream" of this initial focus or sentinel node. However, interactions between tumour cells and endothelial cells of the vascular and lymphatic channels may significantly affect both the extent and location of metastases. Key factors involved in metastasis have been identified as:

- Angiogenesis: prior to the vascularisation of a small focus of transformed cells, dissemination cannot occur; it is also critical for sustained growth of micrometastases.
- Adhesion: critical alterations in cell-cell and cell-matrix adhesion can promote dissemination and influence sites of attachment and invasion.
- Proteolysis: localised proteolysis assists tumour cell invasion, intravasation, and extravasation and is also required for capillary outgrowth in neoangiogenesis.
- Motility: contributes to tumour cell invasion when coupled to proteolytic activity.

This paper briefly outlines some of the basic mechanisms involved in tumour cell invasion and metastasis, with special reference to the possible role of c-erbB oncogenes in lymphatic dissemination.

Associations Between c-erbB Oncogene Expression and Metastasis

We have been interested in the significant associations between over-expression of the c-erbB oncogene family and poor prognosis in a variety of cancers (reviewed in Modjtahedi and Dean 1994, Gullick 1998, Eccles et al. 1995, 1998) and have been exploring the possible molecular bases for these observations. The c-erbB type 1 receptor tyrosine kinase family comprises four known members; epidermal growth factor receptor (EGFR/c-erbB-1) c-erbB-2, c-erbB-3 and c-erbB-4. A large family of ligands can bind to and activate EGFR (EGF, HB-

Table 1. Associations between c-*erb* oncogene expression and lymphatic metastasis

Tumour	Observation	Reference(s)
Breast	EGFR in primary tumour correlates with LNM and DFI	Okamura 1997
	Correlation between decreased E-cadherin, increased EGFR and LNM	Jones 1996
	ErbB-2/CK18+ disseminated cells found in bone marrow aspirates	Pantel 1993
	Erb-B2 correlates with LNM	Querzoli 1990
	Increased levels of shed ECD of erb-B2 in patients with LNM and/or BMM	Gebhardt 1998
	Levels of erb-B2 mRNA increased in tumours with LNM	Anan 1998
	Plasma erb-B2 levels higher with LNM	Mehta 1998
Lung	EGFR expression correlates with metastases in hilar and mediastinal LN	Fontanini 1995
	Erb-B2 expression correlates with LNM	Kern 1990, Shi 1992
Head & neck squamous cell carcinoma (HNSCC)	EGFR correlates with MMP-3 expression and with LNM	Kusukawa 1996
	EGFR and TGFα correlate with higher risk of LNM	Grandis 1998
Bladder	Erb-B2 expression correlates with LNM	Moriyama 1991, Wright 1991
Oesophagus	EGFR gene amplification correlated with extensive LNM	Kitagawa 1996
Nasopharynx	Erb-B2 expression correlates with LNM	Roychowdury 1996
Gastric	Erb-B2 expression correlates with LNMErb-B2 gene amplification associated with LNM	Mizutani 1993, Tsugawa 1998
Colon	Erb-B2 expression correlates with LNM	Yang 1997
Endometrium	Erb-B2 expression correlates with LNM	Sakamoto 95

LNM, lymph node metastasis; *BMM*, bone marrow metastasis; *ECD*, extracellular domain of c-*erb*B-2 p185; *DFI*, disease-free interval; *TGFα*, transforming growth factor α

EGF, TGFα, betacellulin, amphiregulin and epiregulin), the latter three can also bind to c-*erb*B-4. The heregulins bind to c-*erb*B-3 and c-*erb*B-4 and there are no known ligands for c-*erb*B-2. However, this molecule plays a key role in receptor signalling, since it is a preferred partner in heterodimer formation with all other *erb*B family members (Graus-Porta 1997) and can potentiate recycling of receptors rather than their degradation, thus enhancing signal potency (Lenferink 1998). This type of transactivation may explain the particularly poor prognosis associated with tumours which over-express both c-*erb*B-2 and EGFR.

It is postulated that co-expression of c-*erb*B receptors and one or more ligands leads to receptor activation and autocrine or paracrine growth stimulation of tumour cells, thus providing a survival advantage. In addition, both clinical and experimental evidence suggests a link, not just to tumour cell proliferation, but also to dissemination. Examples where expression has been associated specifically with lymphatic metastasis are illustrated in Table 1, although it must be noted that this is not an exclusive correlation, and haematogenous metastasis is also enhanced in many cases.

Direct evidence for a causal link between c-erbB expression and tumour progression has come from several experimental studies: cells transfected with c-erbB-2 or EGFR have been shown to be more invasive in vitro, and highly metastatic in vivo, and tumours arising in transgenic mice are also capable of metastasis. Inhibition of oncogene function (e.g., by adenovirus 5 E1a gene product, antisense constructs or monoclonal antibodies) reverses the malignant phenotype (Guy 1992, Yu 1992, Eccles 1995). Next I will consider evidence for functional links between c-erbB oncogene over-expression and specific phenotypes of metastatic cells, which may explain the above observations.

Angiogenesis

There are many excellent reviews attesting to the importance of neoangiogenesis in metastasis. This topic will not be covered here because the data relating to the role of angiogenic factors in lymphatic metastasis are few and contradictory, however, some positive associations have been observed in lung cancer (Ohta 1997) and gastric cancer (Xiangming 1998b). Nevertheless, it has been shown that activated c-erbB oncogenes potentiate tumour cell adhesion to microvessel endothelial cells (Yu 1992), and induce VEGF expression (Petit 1997) suggesting the possibility of involvement of these oncogenes in tumour-endothelial interactions and neoangiogenesis.

Alterations in Cell-Cell and Cell-Matrix Adhesion Molecules

One of the earliest changes in the evolution of an invasive cancer is the loss of normal tissue architecture, and in some cases tumour cells may undergo transient changes in shape (epithelial-mesenchymal transformation, EMT) as they acquire migratory capability. Many of these changes are associated with changes in adhesive interactions between cells and their surrounding extracellular matrix (ECM). The patterns of change are complex, and few generalisations can be drawn, although examples of common aberrations associated with the presence of lymphatic metastasis are shown in Table 2. A key feature in many carcinomas is down-regulation or altered localisation of one of the major cell-cell adhesion molecules, E-cadherin and/or the associated catenins that link it to the cytoskeleton. It is hypothesised that the resulting reduction in cellular cohesion may increase the probability of dissociation from the primary tumour mass (Jiang 1996, Pignatelli 1998). Activation of EGFR has been shown to alter the distribution of E-cadherin on the cell surface and to counteract junctional assembly via alterations in its association with catenins. These processes resulted in loss of epithelioid morphology, decreased aggregation and increased motility (Shiozaki 1995, Hazan 1998). Transfection of E-cadherin down-regulates EGFR expression, restores epithelial morphology and reverses the invasive phenotype. Similarly, inhibition of

Table 2. Associations between alterations in adhesion molecules and lymphatic metastasis

Adhesion system	Cancer	Observation	Reference
E-Cadherin catenins	Oesophagus	Lack of expression correlates with LNM	Natsugoe 1998
	Stomach	Reduced expression of E-cadherin and α-catenin associated with LNM	Xiangming 1998 a
	Colon	Reduced α-catenin expression associated with LNM	Raftopoulos 1998
	Lung	Inverse correlation between E-cad expression and LN stage	Sulzer 1998
	Breast	Significant reduction in E-cadherin in LNM+ tumours compared with matched LNM–	Hunt 1997
Desmosomal proteins	Squamous cell carcinomas	Loss of desmosomal components correlated with reduced E-cad and LNM	Shinohara 1998
Integrins	Melanoma	$\beta1$ expression in primary tumour predicts occult LNM, $\beta3$ expression related to lung metastases	Hieken 1999
	Breast	$\beta1$ and $\alpha V\beta5$ loss related to presence of LNM	Gui 1995
	Lung	Loss of $\alpha2$ and $\alpha3$ related to increased αV and MMP-2 expression, and LNM	Clarke 1997
	Colon	Alterations in expression of $\beta1$ associated with LNM	Fujita 1995
	Stomach	Expression of $\alpha2\beta1$ associated with LNM and liver metastasis	Ura 1998
CD44	Stomach	CD44 V6 isoform related to LNM	Streit 1996
	Ovary	CD44 V6 more frequently expressed in patients with LNM	Yorishima 1997
	Breast	CD44 expression correlated with LNM or distant metastases	Ozer 1997
	Melanoma	LNM displayed elevated levels of CD44 V5	Seiter 1996
	Lung	Expression of CD44 V6 associated with increased risk of LNM	Miyoshi 1997
	Cervix	CD44 V6 frequently expressed in LNM	Kainz 1996

the association between β-catenin and the c-*erb*B2 encoded oncoprotein p185 resulted in suppression of invasion and metastasis of a human gastric cancer cell line (Shibata 1996). These data indicate a functional link between c-*erb*B activation and loss of normal cell-cell interactions.

Many cell-matrix interactions are mediated by integrins, and although it seems that cancers of different histogenic origin utilise different sets of integrins to adhere to various ECM components, again alterations in expression of these molecules (either up or down-regulation) is a common feature of metastatic cancer. Following release of cells from the primary site (in which it is assumed that *decreased* cell-cell and cell-ECM adhesion is required) cells which can efficiently bind to endothelium in target tissue potentially have more probability of successfully extravasating and forming a metastasis. Indeed, cell attachment is not just a passive process, but triggers critical further events which may stimulate both tumour cell growth and neoangiogenesis (Brodt 1996). Regarding the role of specific integrins; $\alpha V\beta3$ has been frequently found to be upregulated during progression of melanoma and other neural crest-derived tumours, and it is hypothesised that this molecule adheres to vitronectin which is found in the reticular fibres of lymph nodes, and which is itself (together with fibronectin) upregulated following invasion by tumour cells (Nip et al. 1992). In contrast, breast carcinoma cells appear preferentially to adhere to fibronectin using integrin $\alpha3\beta1$ (Tawil 1996), although in patients, $\beta1$ *loss* has been associated with LNM (Gui 1995), suggesting that further work is required to reconcile experimental and clinical observations.

There is some evidence for functional links between c-erbB oncogene activation and integrins. Transfection of the c-erbB-2 gene into immortalised human mammary epithelial cells resulted in decreased expression of the $\alpha2$ integrin subunit and reduced ability to undergo morphogenic differentiation, and laminin (acting via $\alpha6\beta4$ integrins) can activate c-erbB2 p185. Also, HB-EGF increases the expression of $\beta1$ integrins in oesophageal cancer cells, increasing their adhesion to collagen 1 and endothelial cells, and EGF alters the function of $\alpha6\beta4$ integrin, potentiating tumour cell migration towards laminins.

Finally, there are some interesting observations regarding the association between different splice variants of CD44 and metastasis. Again, not all data are consistent, but at least in some cancers there is evidence that the V6 (and in some cases V5) variant is related to lymphatic metastasis (Table 2). CD44 binds to hyaluronic acid, an ECM proteoglycan, and the variant forms are associated with a migratory phenotype. Recently it has been shown that EGF stimulates cell binding to hyaluronate by regulating CD44 expression (Zhang 1996). Taken together, these observations provide compelling evidence that complex alterations in cell-cell and cell-matrix adhesive interactions can contribute to lymphatic metastasis, and that, at least in some cancers, activation of c-erbB oncogenes may play a key role.

Proteolysis

There has been a great deal of interest in the role of proteolytic enzymes in metastasis, with evidence for many different classes of enzymes facilitating tumour cell invasion. Since lymphatic endothelia lack a complete basal lamina, it has been proposed that these vessels provide less of a barrier to tumour cell invasion than blood capillaries. Nevertheless, there are reports of clinical associations between expression of matrix metalloproteinases (MMPs) and lymph node metastases in a variety of cancers (Table 3), although their precise role in lymphogenous dissemination has not been defined. Since our own work has focussed on MMPs, I will confine my discussion primarily on this class of enzymes, while recognising that many others (e.g., cathepsins, uPA) may be equally important.

MMP-2 and MMP-9 (gelatinases A and B) have been found to be upregulated in many cancers. Since one of their main substrates is collagen IV

Table 3. Associations between expression of matrix metalloproteinases and lymph node metastases

Tumor	Observations	References
Lung	Levels of active MMP-2 correlate with MT1-MMP and LNM	Tokuraku 1995
HNSCC	LNM correlates with MMP-3 and EGFR	Kusukawa 1993
	LNM+ expressed high MMP-2, low TIMP-2	Kawamata 1998
Oesophagus	MMP-2 and MMP-3 correlate with LNM	Shima 1992
Prostate	MMP-7 mRNA correlates with LNM	Hashimoto 1998
Stomach	MMP-2 correlates with LNM	Otani 1990
Cervix	Ras p21 correlated with high MMP-2 expression and lymphatic spread	Garzetti 1998
Breast	Ratio of MMP-2:TIMP-2 mRNA is increased in LN+ tumours	Onisto 1995
	MT1-MMP (not MT2-MMP) correlates with LNM, active MMP-2 and distant metastases	Ueno 1997
Colon	RT-PCR for MMP-7 detects LNM	Ichikawa 1998
Pancreas	Active MMP-2 in 100%; MMP-9 in 21%; activation ratio highest with LNM and distant metastases	Koshiba 1998

(found in the basal laminae of blood vessels) it has been proposed that these enzymes may assist in tumour cell intravasation and extravasation. However, some experiments with MMP inhibitors have failed to show effects on the passage of tumour cells through capillary walls, suggesting that their major role may be in post-extravasation events. Since MMP-9 and MMP-2 (Moses 1997) and also MMP-1 and plasminogen activators (Mignatti and Rifkin 1996) have been implicated in angiogenesis, an indirect role may be to assist in vascularisation of micrometastases in lymph nodes or organs. We have shown that long-term post-surgical therapy with an MMP inhibitor could prevent the outgrowth of lymphatic and haematogenous metastasis in a rat mammary carcinoma model (Eccles 1994), consistent with this hypothesis. In addition, direct inhibition of angiogenesis and hemangioma growth have been observed (Taraboletti 1995) and MMP-2 deficient mice show reduced angiogenesis and tumor progression (Itoh 1998). Interestingly, MMP-2 has been shown to localise on the surface of angiogenic blood vessels and invasive melanoma cells by binding to $\alpha V \beta 3$ integrin (Brooks 1996) providing evidence of functional associations of molecules involved in angiogenesis, adhesion, migration and invasion. In addition, there is evidence for a membrane-bound MMP (MT1-MMP) binding to, and activating MMP-2 in association with TIMP-2 in invasive cells, and these molecules have been found to be co-expressed in LNM+ breast and lung cancers (Tokuraku 1995, Onisto 1995, Ueno 1997). Other MMPs whose expression is frequently upregulated in association with lymphatic metastasis include MMP-3 (stromelysin 1) and MMP-7 (matrilysin). These enzymes have a broad substrate range, including collagens, proteoglycans, fibronectin, laminin, and are also involved in activation of other MMPs, including MMP-9.

We and others have shown that activation of c-*erb*B oncogenes results in increased expression of subsets of MMPs. In particular, EGF ligands induce high levels of MMP-9 in squamous cell carcinomas (O-charoenrat et al. 1998 and unpublished observations) and over-expression of c-*erb*B-2 is also associated with upregulated gelatinases (Yu 1992). A possible mechanism linking c-*erb*B oncogenes with increased proteolytic activity is via activation of the Ets family of transcription factors. Many protease gene promoters (including MMP-1, MMP-9 MMP-11 and uPA) contain such binding sites, and co-ordinate expression of c-*erb*B-2 p185 or EGFR with PEA-3, Ets-1 and Ets-2 have been observed in invasive cancers (Watabe 1998). Thus there are several lines of evidence to support the view that one of the major mechanisms linking activated c-*erb*B receptors with increased malignancy is via upregulation of proteolytic enzymes of the MMP family and possibly other classes.

Motility

Proteolytic activity is necessary but not sufficient for tumour cell invasion, since inhibitors of cell motility will also abort this process. Hence it is generally accepted that tumour cell migration in response to chemotactic factors is an important determinant of metastatic capacity. Since the c-*erb*B receptor tyrosine kinases are connected to the actin cytoskeleton, it is not surprising that their activation has been linked to changes in cell motility. EGF has been shown to stimulate lamellipod extension in mammary carcinoma cells, (Segall 1996), and keratinocyte migration in response to EGF was shown to be coincident with induction of MMP-9 and enhanced invasive capacity (McCawley 1998). Interestingly, HB-EGF (a ligand for both EGFR and c-*erb*B-4) has been shown to stimulate chemotaxis independently of proliferation (Elenius 1997) and c-*erb*B-2 is also localised to cell organelles involved in motility (De Potter 1993), where it presumably responds to heregulins and/or EGFR ligands by heterodimerisation with other c-*erb*B receptors. Indeed, antibodies directed against EGFR and/or c-*erb*B-2 have been shown to inhibit cell migration and invasion, in some cases without effects on cell proliferation (De Corte 1994, Eccles unpublished data).

Tyrosine Kinase Growth Factor Receptors: A Master Switch in Progression?

Taken together, the data briefly summarised above suggest that activation of cell membrane receptor tyrosine kinases can result in a cascade of cellular processes which collectively contribute to tumour cell invasion and metastasis. An early event (which in normal cells may be linked to the mitosis) is down-regulation of cell-cell adhesion molecules (exemplified by E-cadherin), and changes in the expression of integrins. Some integrins (e.g., $\alpha V\beta 3$ when ligated to lymph node vitronectin) have been implicated in the regulation of specific matrix metalloproteinases (Bafetti 1998) and the uPA receptor. Increased motility (signalled by heregulins and/or EGFR ligands) coupled with

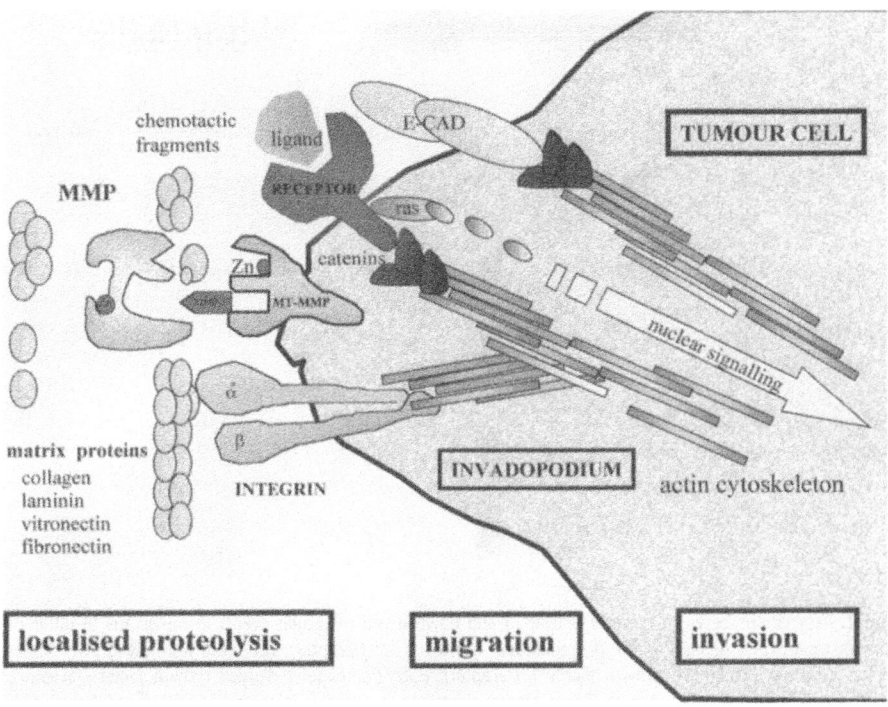

Fig. 1. Integrated functional links between receptor signalling, adhesive interactions and proteolysis in tumour cell invasion exemplified by reference to the c-*erb*B family

enhanced proteolytic activity provide the tumour cell with invasive potential, and proteolytic fragments of ECM components (e.g., laminin 5) are potent chemoattractants. Proteolysis may also release matrix-bound growth factors (including angiogenic cytokines) resulting in a positive feedback loop of both autocrine and paracrine receptor activation, providing further amplification of the adhesion-proteolysis-invasion pathways and in addition, inducing neoangiogenesis (reviewed in Brodt 1996). Figure 1 illustrates (as an example) some of the molecular networks which may be induced simply by activation of members of the c-*erb*B family, suggesting that they may act as "master switches" inducing multiple aspects of the metastatic phenotype.

It must be stressed, however, that the c-*erb*B family is just one of many whose over-expression (notably in adenocarcinomas and squamous cell carcinomas) has been linked with tumour progression. In other tumours, different ligand-receptor systems may predominate. Figure 2 illustrates examples of some associations that have been observed, although this is by no means proscriptive, and (for simplicity) does not include other important adhesion molecules such as CD44 and other protease families such as the cathepsins. However, this simple exercise illustrates that in most cases, a combination of decreased cell-cell adhesion, altered cell-matrix interactions, and increased

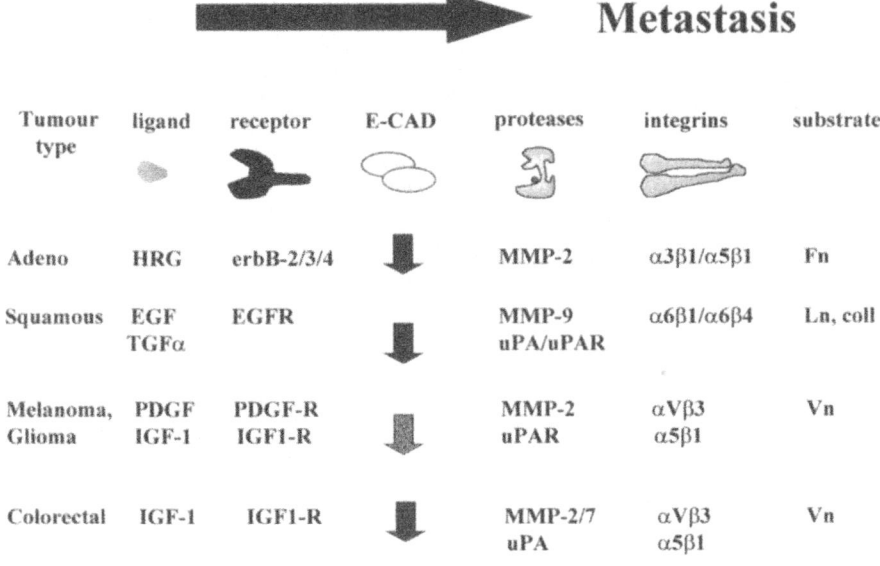

Fig. 2. Associations between receptor activation and downstream molecular events in metastasis of different tumour types. *HRG*, heregulin; *EGF (R)*, epidermal growth factor (receptor); *TGFα*, transforming growth factor alpha; *IGF-1-(R)*, insulin-like growth factor 1 (receptor); *PGDF-(R)*, platelet derived growth factor (receptor); *MMP*, matrix metalloproteinase; *uPA (R)*, urokinase plasminogen activator (receptor); *E-CAD*, E (epithelial) cadherin; *Fn*, fibronectin; *Vn*, vitronectin; *Coll*, collagen; *Ln*, laminin

proteolytic activity are required for acquisition of a metastatic phenotype, although "team players" may be substituted in different cancers.

Many of the molecules described have been the target of therapeutic intervention, and at least in experimental studies, it has been shown that inhibition of MMP activity, restoration of E-cadherin function, or inhibition of integrin-mediated binding of tumour cells to host tissues can reduce invasion and metastasis. However, the pivotal role of the receptor tyrosine kinases, (upstream of these other processes?) and their accessible position on the cell membrane, suggests that they provide ideal targets for therapy. Indeed, several antibodies directed against EGFR have been shown to be able to inhibit tumour cell proliferation, and also MMP expression, invasion, organ colonisation and angiogenesis (Eccles 1995, Petit 1997, O-charoenrat 1998). Although these receptors have not specifically been explored as targets in lymphogenous metastasis, I believe that the data are sufficiently compelling to contemplate such a strategy. Our own work has shown that monoclonal antibodies specific for c-erbB-2 p185 can be localised in axillary nodes of breast carcinoma (Allan 1993), and the antibody employed (ICR12) while not directly cytostatic, is an ideal vehicle for 2-stage targeted therapy such as ADEPT (Eccles 1994b). In addition, monoclonal antibody ICR62 has been shown to localise in lymph node metastases of squamous cell carcinomas (Modjtahedi 1996) and is now in an extended phase 1b trial. We are optimistic that these antibodies will provide the basis for future therapies targeting disseminated disease, and that they may have a significant role to play in cancers where lymphatic metastasis causes significant clinical problems (e.g., cancers of the head and neck) and/or the risk of further spread.

References

Allan SM et al (1993) Radioimmunolocalisation in breast cancer using the gene product of c-erbB2 as the target antigen. Br J Cancer 67:706–712

Anan K et al (1998) Assessment of c-erbB2 and vascular endothelial growth factor mRNA expression in fine-needle aspirates from early breast carcinomas: pre-operative determination of metastatic potential. Eur J Surg Oncol 24:28–33

Bafetti LM, Young TN, Itoh Y, Stack MS (1998) Intact vitronectin induces matrix metalloproteinase-2 expression and enhanced cellular invasion by melanoma cells. J Biol Chem 273:143–149

Bostick P et al (1998) Limitations of specific reverse-transcriptase polymerase chain reaction markers in the detection of metastases in the lymph nodes and blood of cancer patients. J Clin Oncol 16: 2632–2640

Brodt P. (1996) Adhesion receptors and proteolytic mechanisms in cancer invasion and metastasis. In: Cell Adhesion and Invasion in Cancer Metastasis. P. Brodt (ed) RG Landes Company, pp 167–242

Brooks B et al (1996) Localization of matrix metalloproteinase MMP-2 to the surface of invasive cells by interaction with integrin $aV\beta3$. Cell 85:683–693

Clarke MR et al (1997) Extracellular matrix expression in metastasizing and nonmetastasizing adenocarcinomas of the lung. Hum Pathol 28:54–59

De Corte V et al (1994) A 50 kDa protein present in conditioned medium of COLO-16 cells stimulates cell spreading and motility, and activates tyrosine phosphorylation of neu/HER-2 in human SK-BR-3 mammary cancer cells. J Cell Science 107:405–416

De Potter C, Quatacker J (1993) The p185[erbB2] is localized on cell organelles involved in cell motility. Clin Exp Metastasis 11:453–461

Eccles et al (1994) Control of lymphatic and haematogenous metastasis of a rat mammary carcinoma by the matrix metalloproteinase inhibitor, batimastat (BB-94) Cancer Res 56: 2815–2822

Eccles et al (1994b) Regression of established breast carcinoma xenografts with antibody-directed enzyme prodrug therapy directed against c-erbB-2 p185. Cancer Res 54:5171–177

Eccles SA et al. (1995) Significance of the c-erbB family of receptor tyrosine kinases in metastatic cancer and their potential as targets for immunotherapy. Invasion Metastasis 14:337–348.

Eccles SA (1998) c-erbB-2 as a target for immunotherapy. Exp Opinion Invest Drugs 7: 1879–1896

Elenius K, Paul S, Allison G, Sun J, Klagsbrun M (1997) Activation of HER4 by heparin-binding EGF-like growth factor stimulates chemotaxis but not proliferation. EMBO J 16: 1268–1278

Fontanini G et al (1995) Epidermal growth factor receptor (EGFr) expression in non-small cell lung carcinomas correlates with metastatic involvement of hilar and mediastinal lymph nodes in the squamous subtype. Eur J Cancer 31A:178–183

Fujita S, Watanabe M, Kubota T, Teramoto T, Kitajima M (1995) Alteration of expression in integrin b1 subunit correlates with invasion and metastasis in colorectal cancer. Cancer Lett 91:145–149

Garzetti GG et al (1998) Ras p21 immunostaining in early stage squamous cervical carcinoma: relationship with lymph node involvement and 72 kDa-metalloproteinase index. Anticancer Res 18:609–613

Gebhardt F, Zanker KS, Brandt B (1998) Differential expression of alternatively spliced c-erbB-2 mRNA in primary tumours, lymph node metastases and bone marrow. micrometastases from breast cancer patients. Biochem Biophys Res Commun 247:319–323

Grandis JR et al (1998) Levels of TGF-a and EGFR protein in head and neck squamous cell carcinoma and patient survival. J Natl Cancer Inst 90:824–832

Graus-Porta D, Beerly R, Daly JM, Hynes NE (1997) ErbB2, the preferred heterodimerization partner of all ErbB receptors, is a mediator of lateral signalling. EMBO J 16:1647–1655

Gui GP et al (1995) Integrin expression in primary breast cancer and its relation to axillary node status. Surgery 117:102–108

Gullick WJ (1998) Type 1 growth factor receptors: current status and future work. Biochem Soc Symp 63:193–198

Guy C et al (1992) Expression of the *neu* proto-oncogene in the mammary epithelium of transgenic mice induces metastatic disease. Proc Natl Acad Sci USA 89:10587–10582

Hashimoto K, Kihira Y, Matuo Y, Usui T (1998) Expression of matrix metalloproteinase 7 and tissue inhibitor of metalloproteinase 1 in human prostate. J Urol 160:1872–1876

Hazan RB, Norton L (1998) The epidermal growth factor receptor modulates the interaction of E-cadherin with the actin cytoskeleton. J Biol Chem 273:9078–9084

Hieken TJ et al (1999) Molecular prognostic markers in intermediate thickness cutaneous malignant melanoma. Cancer 85: 375–382

Hunt NC, Douglas-Jones AG, Jasani B, Morgan JM, Pignatelli M (1997) Loss of E-cadherin expression associated with lymph node metastases in small breast carcinomas. Virchows Arch 430:285–289

Ichikawa Y et al (1998) Detection of regional lymph node metastases in colon cancer by using RT-PCR for matrix metalloproteinase 7, matrilysin. Clin Exp Metastasis 16:3–8

Itoh T et al (1998) Reduced angiogenesis and tumor progression in gelatinase A-deficient mice. Cancer Res 58:1048–1051

Jiang W (1996) E-cadherin and its associated protein catenins, cancer invasion and metastasis. Br J Surg 83: 437–446

Jones JL, Royall JE and Walker RA (1996) E-cadherin relates to EGFR expression and lymph node metastasis in primary breast carcinoma. Br J Cancer 74:1237–1241

Kainz C et al (1996) Immunohistochemical detection of adhesion molecule CD44 splice variants in lymph node metastases of cervical cancer. Int J Cancer 69:170–173

Kawamata H et al (1998) Active MMP-2 in cancer cell nests of oral cancer patients: correlation with lymph node metastasis. Int J Oncol 13:699–704

Kern JA et al. (1990) p185[neu] expression in human lung adenocarcinoma predicts shortened survival. Cancer Res 50:5184–5191

Kitagawa Y et al (1996) Further evidence for prognostic significance of epidermal growth factor receptor gene amplification in patients with oesophageal squamous cell carcinoma. Clin Cancer Research 2:909–914

Koshiba T et al (1998) Involvement of matrix metalloproteinase 2 in invasion and metastasis of pancreatic carcinoma. Cancer 82: 642–650

Kusukawa J et al (1996) The significance of epidermal growth factor receptor and matrix metalloproteinase-3 in squamous cell carcinoma of the oral cavity. Eur J Cancer B Oral Oncol 32B:217–221

Kusukawa J, Sasaguri Y, Shima I, Kameyama T, Morimatsu M. (1993) Expression of matrix metalloproteinase-2 related to lymph node metastasi of oral squamous cell carcinoma. Am J Clin Pathol 99:18–23

Lenferink A et al (1998) Differential endocytic routing of homo- and hetero-dimeric ErbB tyrosine kinases confers signalling superiority to receptor heterodimers. EMBO J 17: 3385–3397

McCawley LJ, O'Brien P, Hudson LG (1998) Epidermal growth factor (EGF) and scatter factor (SF/HGF)-mediated keratinocyte migration is coincident with induction of matrix metalloproteinase (MMP)-9. J Cell Physiol 176:255–265

Mehta RR et al (1998) Plasma c-erbB-2 levels in breast cancer patients: prognostic significance in predicting response to chemotherapy. J Clin Oncol 16:2409–2416

Mignatti P, Rifkin D (1996) Plasminogen activators and matrix metalloproteinases in angiogenesis. Enzyme Protein 49:117–137

Mizutani T, Onda M, Tokunage A, Yamanaka N, Sugisaki Y (1993) Relationship of c-erbB-2 protein expression and gene amplification to invasion and metastasis in human gastric cancer. Cancer 72:2083–2088

Miyoshi T, Kondo K, Hino N, Uyama T, Monden Y (1997) The expression of the CD44 variant exon 6 is associated with lymph node metastasis in non-small cell lung cancer. Clin Cancer Res 3:1289–1297

Modjtahedi H, Dean CJ (1994) The receptor for EGF and its ligands: expression, prognostic value and target for therapy in cancer. Int J Oncol 4:277–296

Modjtahedi H et al (1996) Phase 1 trial and tumour localisation of the anti-EGFR antibody ICR62 in head and neck or lung cancer. Br J Cancer 73:228–235

Moriyama M et al. (1991) Expression of c-erbB-2 gene product in urinary bladder cancer. J Urol 145:423–427.

Moses M (1997) The regulation of neovascularisation by matrix metalloproteinases and their inhibitors. Stem Cells 15:180–189

Natsugoe S et al (1998) Micrometastasis and tumor microenvolvement of lymph nodes from oesophageal carcinoma: frequency associated tumor characteristics and impact on prognosis. Cancer 83:858–866

Nip J et al (1992) Human melanoma cells derived from lymphatic metastases use integrin αVβ3 to adhere to lymph node vitronectin. J Clin Invest 90:1406–1413

O-charoenrat P et al (1998) Differential upregulation of MMP-9 in squamous cell carcinomas of head and neck by EGFR. Br J Cancer 78:15

Ohta Y et al (1997) Vascular endothelial growth factor and lymph node metastasis in primary lung cancer. Br J Cancer 76: 1041–5

Okamura K et al (1997) Immunohistochemical localization of cathepsin D, proliferating cell nuclear antigen and epidermal growth factor receptor in human breast carcinoma analysed by computer image analyser: correlation with histological grade and metastatic behaviour. Histopathol 31:540–548

Onisto M et al (1995) Gelatinase A/TIMP-2 imbalance in lymph-node-positive breast carcinomas as measured by RT-PCR. Int J Cancer 63:621–626

Otani Y et al (1990) Collagenolytic activity against type IV collagen in human gastric cancer: correlation with lymphovascular invasion and lymph node metastasis. Progress in Lymphology XII. Proceedings of the XIIth International Congress of Lymphology, pp 371–372

Ozer E, Canda T, Kurtodlu B (1997) The role of angiogenesis, laminin and CD44 expression in metastatic behaviour of early stage low grade invasive breast carcinomas. Cancer Lett 121:119–123

Pantel K, Schlimok G, Braun S et al (1993) Differential expression of proliferation-associated molecules in individual micrometastatic carcinoma cells. J. Natl. Cancer Inst. 85: 1419–1423.

Petit AM et al (1997) Neutralising antibodies against epidermal growth factor and erbB-2 receptor tyrosine kinases down-regulate vascular endothelial growth factor production by tumour cells in vitro and in vivo. Am J Pathol 151:1523–1531

Pignatelli M (1998) Integrins, cadherins, and catenins: molecular cross-talk in cancer cells. J Pathol 186:1–2

Querzoli P et al (1990) Immunohistochemical expression of c-erbB-2 in human breast cancer by monoclonal antibody: correlation with lymph node and ER status. Tumori 76: 461–464

Raftopoulos I, Davaris P, Karatzas G, Karayannacos P, Kouaklis G (1998) level of alpha catenin expression in colorectal cancer correlates with invasiveness, metastatic potential and survival. J Surg Oncol 68:92–99

Roychowdury D, Tsong A, Weinberg V, Weidner N (1996) New prognostic factors in nasopharyngeal carcinoma. Cancer 77:1419–1426

Sakamoto H et al (1995) ErbB-2, a c-erbB-2-coded protein, is expressed in metastatic cells of adenocarcinoma of endometrium, cervix and ovaries. Int J Gynecol Cancer 5:411–415

Segall JE et al (1996) EGF stimulates lamellipod extension in metastatic mammary adenocarcinoma cells by an actin-dependent mechanism. Clin Exp Metastasis 14:61–72

Seiter S et al. (1996) Expression of CD44 variant isoforms in malignant melanoma. Clin Cancer Res 2:447–456

Shi D, He G, Cao S et al (1992) Overexpression of the c-erbB-2/neu-encoded p185 protein in primary lung cancer. Molec Carcinogenesis 5:213–218

Shibata T et al (1996) Dominant negative inhibition of the association between β-catenin and c-erbB-2 by N-terminally deleted b-catenin suppresses the invasion and metastasis of cancer cells. Oncogene 13:883–889

Shinohara M et al (1998) Immunohistochemical study of desmosomes in oral squamous cell carcinoma: correlation with cytokeratin and E-cadherin staining and with tumour behaviour. J Pathol 184:369–381

Shima I et al (1992) Production of matrix metalloproteinase-2 and metalloproteinase-3 related to malignant behaviour of esophageal carcinoma. (1992) Cancer 70:2747–2753

Shiozaki H et al (1995) Effect of epidermal growth factor on cadherin-mediated adhesion in a human oesophageal cancer cell line. Br J Cancer 71:250–258

Streit M, Schmidt R, Hilgenfeld R, Thiel E, Kreuser E (1996) Adhesion receptors in malignant transformation and dissemination of gastrointestinal tumours. J Mol Med 74:253–268

Sulzer MA, Leers MP, van Noord JA, Bollen EC, Theunissen PH (1998) Reduced E-cadherin expression is associated with increased lymph node metastasis and unfavorable prognosis in non-small cell lung cancer. Am J Respir Crit Care Med 157:1319–1323

Taraboletti G et al (1995) Inhibition of angiogenesis and murine hemangioma growth by batimastat, a synthetic inhibitor of matrix metalloproteinases. J Natl Cancer Inst 87: 293–297

Tawil NJ et al (1996) Integrin α3β1 can promote adhesion and spreading of metastatic breast carcinoma cells on the lymph node stroma. Int J Cancer 66: 703–10

Tokuraku M et al (1995) Activation of the precursor of gelatinase A/72 kDa type IV collagenase/MMP-2 in lung carcinomas correlates with the expression of membrane-type matrix metalloproteinase (MT-MMP) and with lymph node metastasis. Int J Cancer 64: 355–359

Tsugawa K et al (1998) Amplification of the c-met, c-erbB-2 and epidermal growth factor receptor gene in human gastric cancers: correlation to clinical features. Oncol 55:475–481

Ueno H et al (1997) Expression and tissue localisation of membrane-types 1,2, and 3 matrix metalloproteinases in human invasive breast carcinomas. Cancer Res 57:2055–60

Ura H, Denno R, Hirata K, Yamaguchi K, Yasoshima T (1998) Separate functions of α2β1 integrins in the metastatic process of human gastric carcinoma. Surg Today 28:1001–1006

Watabe T et al (1998) The Ets-1 and Ets-2 transcription factors activate the promoters for invasion-associated urokinase and collagenase genes in response to epidermal growth factor. Int J Cancer 77:128–137

Wright C et al (1991) Expression of mutant p53, c-erbB-2 and the epidermal growth factor receptor in transitional cell carcinoma of the human urinary bladder. Br J Cancer 63: 967–970.

Xiangming C et al (1998a) The expression of cadherin-catenin complex in association with the clinicopathological features of early gastric cancer. Surg Today 28:587–94

Xiangming C et al (1998b) Angiogenesis as an unfavorable factor related to lymph node metastasis in early gastric cancer. Ann Surg Oncol 5:585–9

Yang JL et al (1997) In vivo over-expression of c-erbB-2 oncoprotein in xenografts of mice implanted with human colon cancer cell lines. Anticancer Res 17:3463–3468

Yorishima T, Nagai N, Ohama K (1997) Expression of CD44 alternative splicing variants in primary and lymph node metastatic lesions of gynaecological cancer. Hiroshima J Med Sci 46:21–29

Yu D, Hamada J, Zhang H, Nicolson G, Hung M-C. (1992) Mechanisms of c-erbB-2/neu oncogene-induced metastasis and repression of metastatic properties by adenovirus 5 E1 A gene products. Oncogene 7:2263–2270

Zhang M, Singh R, Wang M, Wells G, Siegal G (1996) Epidermal growth factor modulates cell attachment to hyaluronic acid by the cell surface glycoprotein CD44. Clin Exp Metastasis 14:268–276

The Lymph Node as a Bridgehead
in the Metastatic Dissemination of Tumors

J. P. Sleeman

Forschungszentrum Karlsruhe, Institut für Toxikologie und Genetik,
Postfach 3640, 76021 Karlsruhe, Germany

Abstract

The metastatic spread of tumors is not a random process. Distinct patterns of metastasis can be discerned which vary from tumor type to tumor type. A common pattern, particularly for carcinomas, is that regional lymph nodes are often the first organs to develop metastases. This pattern of metastasis is central to the utility of the sentinel lymphonodectomy surgical technique. However, not all tumors and tumor types metastasize first to the regional lymph nodes. The mechanisms which determine whether regional lymph nodes or other sites first develop metastases remain poorly understood. In this article I review the anatomical, cellular and molecular factors which play a role in metastatic dissemination and determine patterns of metastasis. I then explore the importance of tumor heterogeneity and the selection of metastatically competent tumor cells during systemic dissemination, and suggest that some secondary sites are more readily colonised by metastasizing cells than others. Metastases at these sites act as bridgeheads, constituting a reservoir of tumor cells which, because they have already successfully metastasized, possess many of the properties required for metastasis to further sites. These tumor cells are therefore more likely than cells in the primary tumor to acquire all of the properties required for metastasis to less favourable secondary sites. To illustrate the bridgehead concept, I argue that features of the design and function of the lymphatic system make it highly amenable to the entry of metastasizing tumor cells and the formation of lymph node metastases, and suggest that lymph node metastases form a bridgehead for further metastatic spread.

Introduction

The metastatic spread of tumor cells is ultimately responsible for the majority of cancer deaths. Clinically, the most critical point in tumor progression is therefore the acquisition of metastatic potential. The mechanisms which

Recent Results in Cancer Research, Vol. 157
© Springer-Verlag Berlin · Heidelberg 2000

regulate metastasis formation are only partly understood. Understanding these mechanisms will open new avenues for diagnosis and therapy.

The majority of human carcinomas give rise to regional lymphatic metastases, and for many tumors, metastatic spread to the regional lymph nodes is often the first sign that metastasis has occurred (Willis, 1975; Carr, 1983; Brodt, 1991). This pattern is the foundation of tumor staging schemes and assessment of prognosis for many tumor types (Beahrs and Myers, 1983). Established lymph node metastases are a source of tumor cells capable of metastasizing to further sites. An important question which arises is what is the relative contribution to distant metastasis formation of tumor cells disseminated directly from the primary tumor compared to tumor cells disseminated from regional lymphatic metastases? The answer to this question is of more than academic interest: if a given tumor type generally initially metastasizes via the regional lymphatics before giving rise to distant metastases, then therapies targeted at preventing the entry and spread of tumor cells in the lymphatic system are likely to be effective at early stages of tumor development in inhibiting metastasis. Furthermore, surgical techniques such as sentinel lymphonodectomy will be successful in accurately predicting patient prognosis.

The concept of the sentinel lymph node is the basis of sentinel lymphonodectomy (Cabanas, 1977). The sentinel node (or nodes) is the first lymph node in a lymphatic basin which receives lymph flow from a primary tumor, and should therefore be the first to receive metastatic cells from the primary tumor. Analysis of the sentinel node for the presence of metastases is proving itself highly valuable for predicting metastatic involvement of the lymphatic basin in which the tumor is situated, and in tumor staging as the pathological status of regional nodes has very significant implications for prognosis and adjuvant therapy (Gulec et al., 1998). Thus, if a tumor initially metastasizes only via the lymphatic system, sentinel node status will be a good indication of whether more distant metastases are likely. However, there are many examples of tumors which do not, or do not strictly follow a primary tumor – regional lymph node – systemic dissemination pattern. It has been reported, for example, that melanomas of the trunk metastasize to distant sites without detectable involvement of regional lymph nodes in about 10% of cases (Kulakowski et al., 1984). To understand the significance and scope of sentinel node analyses, it is therefore critical to understand the usual routes of metastasis taken by a particular tumor and what factors determine its pattern of metastasis.

A Conceptual Framework to Explain Patterns of Metastasis

Tumor cells metastasize via three main routes: by direct extension, through the blood stream and through the lymphatic system. Primary metastasis by direct extension into body cavities is a feature of only a few tumor types such as lung mediastinal tumors, malignant ovarian tumors and primary tumors of the central nervous system, and will not be addressed in great detail here. With regard to disseminating tumors cells which enter the circulatory system, the experiments of Fisher and Fisher (1966, 1970) and others demonstrate that tumor cells in the lymphatic system can recirculate and enter the blood system via lymphaticovenous anastomoses or the thoracic duct, and that blood-borne tumor cells can also recirculate into the lymphatics. At face value, these observations would suggest that metastatic deposition might be random. However, this is not the case, and patterns of metastatic deposition can be discerned.

Patterns of Metastasis

Clinical observations in the last century led to the concept that tumors first metastasize via anatomically related regional lymph nodes. Subsequent metastatic deposits were observed to follow known lymphatic connections and enter the blood stream via the thoracic duct. Similarly, the anatomical location of a venous circulatory connection in relation to the primary tumor accounted for patterns of metastasis after direct entry of tumor cells into the blood stream. Mechanical entrapment of tumor cells in regional lymph nodes and in the capillary beds of the first organ which tumors cells encounter in the blood circulation such as the lung and liver was viewed as the mechanism leading to metastatic deposition (Goldman, 1906). These concepts were summarized in the anatomical/mechanical theory of metastasis formation (Ewing, 1928). Many experimental observations are consistent with this theory. For example, the ability of tumor cells to form metastases is promoted by their ability to form emboli, which would favor mechanical entrapment (e.g., Updyke and Nicolson, 1986).

Numerous observations concerning metastasis formation are incompatible with the anatomical/mechanical theory. In experimental models, it has been shown that tumor cells can pass through lymph nodes without forming metastases (e.g., Fisher and Fisher, 1966). Additionally, tumor cells can pass through the first capillary bed they encounter and form metastases in subsequent beds (e.g., Zeidman and Buss, 1952; Tarin et al., 1984). Furthermore, multiple clinical and experimental studies demonstrate that several tumor types show preferential metastatic colonization of certain organs (reviewed in Nicolson, 1982; Nicolson, 1988). For example, clear cell carcinoma of the kidney shows a high proclivity for forming metastases in the thyroid gland, which is inexplicable according to the anatomical/mechanical theory. Based on patterns of metastasis obtained at autopsy, Paget (1889) proposed that tumor cells are seeds which grow more readily in certain types of soil (organs). The seed and soil hypothesis and the anatomical/mechanical theory should be viewed as complementary rather than contradictory. As lucidly pointed out by Sugarbaker (1981), the anatomical/mechanical theory is highly relevant to regional metastatic spread, while the seed and soil hypothesis is more pertinent to the formation of distant metastases (see Fig. 1). This reflects the data sources on which the two theories were developed.

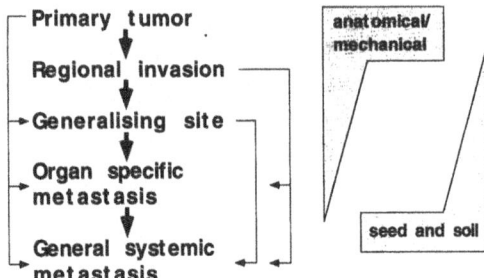

Fig. 1. Schematic outline of metastatic progression. A generalized pattern of metastatic spread is indicated by *thick arrows*. However, different tumor types may take one or several of the alternative routes identified by *thin arrows*, either in a percentage of cases or as the major metastasis pathway. The relative contribution of "anatomical/mechanical" and "seed and soil" considerations at each phase of the progression series is indicated

An important general principle is that tumor cells need to acquire altered cellular properties in order to metastasize. The nature and number of such properties will determine the range of secondary sites to which the tumor cells can metastasize. Subsequent acquisition of additional cellular properties by tumor cells which have already metastasized may permit these cells to metastasize again to further sites. For example, based on autopsy data it has been shown that statistically, a primary tumor will most commonly first metastasize to an organ or organs whose venous effluent directly enters the systemic circulation (reviewed in Sugarbaker, 1981). This organ, most often the lung or liver, constitutes a "generalizing site" for further metastatic spread. Such sequential organ involvement gives rise to the important concept of metastatic progression, in which tumor cells acquire additional properties which enable them subsequently to form metastatic colonies in new "soils" (Fig. 1). A good starting place to understand patterns of metastatic dissemination is thus to define the properties which tumor cells need to acquire in order to be able to metastasize to different sites, and to analyze how these properties combine with other factors such as anatomical location to determine metastatic dissemination patterns.

Properties Required for Tumor Cells to Leave the Primary Tumor and Enter the Circulatory System

It is thought that three major tumor cell properties, namely their adhesiveness, their ability to produce and/or activate proteases, and their motility may have to change in order to allow tumor cells to leave the primary tumor. Such changes also facilitate tumor cell entry into the circulatory system. This topic has been extensively reviewed and will only be discussed briefly here.

In order to enter the circulatory system, tumor cells have to be able to detach from the primary tumor mass and bind to different structures, which requires a change in adhesive properties. A number of cell surface molecules have been reported to be gained or lost during metastatic progression. One of the most important of these is the cell adhesion molecule E-cadherin, whose function is to bind epithelial cells together. Down regulation or functional inactivation of this cell surface molecule in carcinomas correlates with tumor progression, loss of differentiation, invasion, metastatic potential, and poor prognosis (Birchmeier and Behrens, 1994). Furthermore, tumor cells may need to adhere to new surfaces such as ECM components or endothelium, requiring new adhesive properties. Thus, changes in subunit composition of the integrin family of cell surface adhesion molecules during tumor progression play an important role in the metastatic cascade, as these changes alter the range of ligands bound by the integrin heterodimers (e.g., Chan et al., 1991; Imhof et al., 1996).

The extensive barriers formed for example by stromal cells, basement membranes and the extra-cellular matrix are likely to inhibit the entry of tumor cells in the circulatory system. Therefore a common finding is that metastatic tumor cells directly or indirectly activate proteases to penetrate these barriers. Proteases implicated in tumor cell invasion include matrix metalloproteinases (MMPs), serine proteases such as uPA, and members of the cathepsin family (Duffy, 1992). For example, the matrix metalloproteinase MMP-9 has recently been demonstrated to be important for tumor cell intravasation into the circulatory system (Kim et al., 1998). Complex tumor-host interactions regulate the activity of proteases in tumors. For example, MMPs play a very important role in tumor cell invasion, but most of these are expressed by the host tissues (reviewed in Powell and Matrisian, 1996), suggesting that tumors may secrete factors which induce MMP expression. Moreover, proteases secreted by tumors such as uPA can activate latent MMPs, and thus tumors can further indirectly influence the activity of proteases required for their invasion. In the case of MMPs, endogenously expressed tissue inhibitors of metalloproteinases (TIMPs) add an extra layer of regulation of protease activity (Gomez et al., 1997).

Tumor cells may need to become actively motile in order to invade the tissue surrounding the primary tumor and enter vessels of the circulatory system. Thus tumor cells may need to acquire the ability to respond to or produce motility factors in order to be able to metastasize. Several factors have been described which stimulate the motility of tumor cells, including growth factors and cytokines. These may be secreted by the host tissue (e.g., epitaxin; Shimonaka and Yamaguchi, 1994) or by the tumor cells themselves (e.g., autocrine motility factor; Liotta et al., 1986).

The ability of tumor cells to enter into the circulatory system is not sufficient for metastasis formation. This has been demonstrated in a few studies for the lymphatic system (e.g., Ludwig and Titus, 1967; Grundmann and Vollmer, 1985), but a more extensive literature exists for blood-borne tumor cells. The detection of tumor cells in the blood has been reported over many years. Recent sensitive PCR-based assays demonstrate that tumor cells can be detected in the blood stream early on during tumor progression (e.g., Israeli et al., 1994; Mori et al., 1996; Ennis et al., 1997; Melchior et al., 1997; Weitz et al., 1988). This may reflect the fact that angiogenesis is a very early event in tumor progression, bringing tumor cells into intimate contact with thin-walled blood vessels. In contrast, metastasis is usually a late event in tumor progression. Although the sensitive detection of circulating tumor cells by RT-PCR may turn out to prove otherwise, the prevailing view is that tumor cells in the blood do not have prognostic significance (Salsbury, 1975; Fidler et al., 1978). Thus, entry of tumor cells into the blood stream does not necessarily equate with metastasis formation.

Many other observations also demonstrate that the presence of tumor cells in the blood are not inevitable indicators of metastasis formation. For example, using the well differentiated, non-metastasizing MT-W9 rat mammary carcinoma model (Kim and Furth, 1960), it has been calculated that a 1 g tumor sheds more than 10^6 tumor cells into the blood system every day (Butler and Gullino, 1975). Additionally, the analysis of metastases in patients with inoperable cancer who had peritovenous shunts to relieve the symptoms of ascites also demonstrates the same principle (Tarin et al., 1984). Despite the fact that the patients received direct infusion of tumor cells into the blood stream, not all developed metastases despite long survival times, although quiescent tumor cells were detectable in tissues of some patients. In those patients in which metastases did form, they were small and asymptomatic.

Properties Required for Circulating Tumor Cells to Form Metastases

Once within the lymphatic system, tumor cells may form metastases within the lymphatic vessels themselves (in transit metastases), within the subcapsular lumen of the lymph node, or within the parenchyma of the lymph node after invading into it. Metastasis formation by blood-borne tumor cells involves extravasation from the blood circulatory system, and the properties a tumor cell requires to do this again include adhesive functions, upregulation and/or activation of proteases, and motility. To extravasate, blood-borne tumor cells need to adhere to the luminal endothelium and breach the endothelial intercellular junctions, perhaps by inducing endothelial cell apoptosis (Kebers et al., 1998). They must then adhere to and dissolve the underlying basement membrane and migrate into and survive within the surrounding tissue.

For tumor cells extravasating from the blood system, several cell surface adhesion molecules, including integrins, selectins and members of the immunoglobulin superfamily have been shown to be involved in mediating tumor cell interactions with the vascular endothelium (Honn and Tang, 1992). Significant understanding about the molecular mechanisms underlying "seed and soil" observations has come from recent work showing that endothelial cells in different organs express different sets of adhesion molecules (McCarthy et al., 1991; Rajotte et al., 1999), and that the organ specificity of metastasis is at least in part regulated by the ability or inability of circulating tumor cells to adhere to the endothelial adhesion molecules via cognate

Table 1. Tumor cell detection in bone marrow biopsies from gastric cancer patients at surgery and during follow-up. Data taken from Heiss et al., 1995

No. of patients	Tumor cells in bone marrow at surgery	Relapse	Tumor cells in bone marrow at follow-up
34	+	18	+
16	+	0	– (+)
15	–	11	+
13	–	1	–

receptors on their surface (Pauli et al., 1990). However, other mechanisms must also be important, as results from intravital video microscopy experiments suggest that tumor cells of varying metastatic potential may not differ in their ability to extravasate, but rather in their ability to grow progressively as metastases (Chambers et al., 1995). Thus the ability of tumor cells to respond to local growth promoting factors or to grow in an autocrine fashion are also important properties required by the tumor cells if they are to successfully form metastases. For example, Folkman and collegues have elegantly demonstrated that tumor growth beyond a couple of millimeters in diameter is critically dependent on the establishment of an adequate blood supply (Hanahan and Folkman, 1996), and the ability to induce angiogenesis and establish a suitable stroma is therefore also critical if extravasated tumor cells are to go on to form metastases.

Even if tumor cells are deposited in organs distant from the primary tumor, they do not inevitably give rise to metastasis, as is demonstrated by the studies of Heiss and coworkers who examined bone marrow biopsies from gastric carcinoma patients (Heiss et al., 1995). Gastric tumors rarely metastasize to the bone, yet at curative surgery, tumor cells could be detected in the bone marrow of 60% of the patients (see Table 1). The presence of tumor cells in these first bone marrow biopsies did not significantly correlate with disease-free survival or prognosis. In subsequent bone marrow biopsies taken at follow-up, it was found that a third of the patients with tumor cells in the bone marrow at surgery no longer had positive biopsies. Interestingly, relapses were only seen in those patients who at follow-up remained bone marrow positive, and of those patients who were bone marrow negative at surgery virtually all who relapsed became bone marrow positive during follow-up. Together with the fact that of the 78 patients, only one developed overt bone metastasis, these data suggest that at least for gastric cancer, positive bone marrow biopsies reflect tumor burden rather than indicating inevitable bone marrow metastasis formation.

Thus, from the preceding discussion it is clear that metastatically competent tumor cells have acquired properties which permit them to enter and exit the circulatory system and grow as secondary deposits. Together with other factors such as mechanical and anatomical considerations, these properties contribute towards determining the patterns of metastasis which arise from a given tumor type. Clearly not all tumor cells develop these properties, as even the ability to enter the circulatory system or form micrometastases is not sufficient for progressive metastatic growth.

Tumor Cell Properties and Intrinsic Metastatic Potential

For many types of human cancer, the probability of metastasis occurring increases with primary tumor size (Sugarbaker, 1979). However, a significant number of tumors metastasize with a higher or lower frequency than would be expected from the primary tumor size. Thus tumors can be considered to have intrinsically high or low metastatic potential, respectively. Intrinsic metastatic potential must reflect the intrinsic properties of the tumor concerned which can contribute to metastasis formation. Tumors with high metastatic potential include certain leukemias and lymphomas and small cell carcinoma of the lung. Basal cell carcinomas and chondosarcomas have low metastatic potential, generally growing to large sizes without giving rise to metastases. High metastatic potential may be reflected in part by factors such as the characteristics of the cells from which a tumor originates (for example leukemias and lymphomas arise from cells which naturally disseminate through the circulatory system) and by the anatomical location of the primary tumor (for example small cell carcinoma of the lung is ideally situated to give rise to wide-spread systemic metastatic deposits). However, the molecular and cellular basis for intrinsic metastatic potential is poorly understood, and identification of the range of factors which determine whether tumors have low or high metastatic potential will be required to fully understand intrinsic metastatic potential.

The Heterogeneity of Tumor Cell Populations and Selection Drive Metastasis Formation

The critical factor determining metastasis formation is whether disseminated tumor cells die, survive but remain dormant, or have the properties required to grow progressively as metastases. Thus, tumor cells which have the necessary properties to metastasize are selected for during their metastatic journey. Two important questions arise. By what mechanism do tumor cells acquire properties required for metastasis formation? How are metastatically competent tumor cells selected?

Tumors Contain Heterogeneous Populations of Cells

The observation that during metastatic dissemination most tumor cells fail to form metastases and die has lead to the idea that tumor cells which successfully form metastases can be thought of as decathlon winners (Fidler, 1978). In other words, only very few tumor cells possess all the properties necessary for metastasis formation. The mechanistic basis for this selective process arises from the fact that tumors are heterogeneous (Fidler, 1978). They contain subpopulations of cells possessing differing properties and differing metastatic potential. Numerous animal experiments bear out this fact. In one of the first such experiments, Fidler demonstrated that tumor cells capable of metastasis formation pre-exist in tumor cells populations, and that metastases arise by selection from these subpopulations, not by adaptation to new environments (Fidler, 1978). Since then, many experiments using different animal tumor models have shown that by repeated selection for metastatic growth at a particular site or by cloning cells from a tumor cell population it is possible to generate tumor lineages which differ in their metastatic proclivity and/or organ preference (reviewed in Nicolson, 1982; Nicolson 1988). These data demonstrate that metastasis is not the result of random survival of disseminated tumor cells, but rather that processes leading to metastasis select a small subpopulation of tumor cells with the properties required for metastasis formation. Thus tumor heterogeneity generates on a continual basis a whole range of tumor cells with differing properties. Some of these tumor cells may possess a set of properties which are sufficient for metastasis formation. These tumor cells are selected for during metastatic dissemination.

The Molecular Basis for Tumor Heterogeneity

How does heterogeneity develop within a population of tumor cells? The evolution of a metastatically competent tumor from a normal non-transformed cell involves interactions between exogenous (environmental) and endogenous (genetic, immunological, hormonal) factors, and proceeds through multiple discernible stages. These include initiation, promotion (leading to the development of benign lesions) and progression (the evolution of benign to malignant tumors). Different chemical agents enhance or inhibit the transition to these different stages, suggesting that the individual stages involve qualitatively different mechanisms at the cellular and molecular levels (Weinstein, 1988). These aspects predict that evolution to a metastatically competent malignant tumor involves multiple cellular genes and changes in genomic structure and function. The study of these genes and genomic changes has and continues to be pivotal in understanding how heterogeneity arises in tumors.

The mutation, overexpression, inappropriate expression, or deletion of key regulatory genes such as proto-oncogenes and tumor suppressor genes are key events that determine the course of tumor initiation and progression. These key genes regulate proliferation, differentiation, cell cycle progression, and sensitivity to apoptosis-inducing signals amongst other things, and have been extensively reviewed (e.g., Weinberg, 1995). For example, constitutive expression of growth factors or mutations in growth factor receptors which leave them permanently activated can lead to autonomous growth properties

(Aaronson, 1991). Genetic changes in members of the signal transduction pathway and nuclear transcriptional regulators change patterns of gene expression (Karin, 1992), leading to changes in growth or other properties required for tumor formation. Tumor suppressor genes prevent the development of one or more types of cancer, and loss of function of both alleles is permissive for tumorigenesis (Knudson, 1993). Inappropriate expression of genes such as bcl-2 can render tumor cells refractory to apoptosis-inducing signals (Reed, 1998). Thus changes in these key regulatory genes alter cellular properties required for tumor initiation and progression. These properties may also ultimately be important for metastasis formation.

Several changes in these key genes are required to transform normal somatic cells, and this reflects the long-held view that tumor formation is a multistep process (Foulds, 1975). For example, in mice transgenic for activated oncogenes, very few cells of a tissue give rise to tumors despite the fact that the activated oncogene is expressed in every cell of the tissue concerned (Viney, 1995). Furthermore, tumor initiation in these animals is often considerably delayed after birth and multiple tumors often arise stochastically within the same animal. Thus further cellular and genetic changes in addition to the transgenic activated oncogene are required for tumorigenesis. One of the best described examples of multistep tumorigenesis in humans is colorectal carcinogenesis, in which mutational activation of the ras proto-oncogene together with the loss of several tumor suppressor genes such as APC and p53 are common events (Fearon and Vogelstein, 1990). Progression to metastatic competence requires further genetic alterations. At any stage, if a genetic change arising in one tumor cell confers upon it a selective advantage, then that cell type may overgrow the other tumor cells in the developing tumor leading to clonal dominance (Kerbel et al., 1988).

Changes in the gene expression patterns and growth properties of tumor cells as a result of oncogene activation cannot alone account for the rapid and diverse changes observed in tumor heterogeneity (Nicolson, 1991). Recent developments in understanding how genomic stability and integrity changes during tumor formation have revealed new insights into how tumor heterogeneity arises. It is important that genomic integrity is maintained to ensure the fidelity of transmission of genetic material from one cell generation to the next. Not surprisingly, a plethora of mechanisms have been uncovered which ensure that DNA is accurately replicated at the proper time, that damaged DNA is adequately repaired and that the duplicated chromosomes segregate correctly into daughter cells. Alterations in these control mechanisms lead to an increased mutation frequency. Tumor suppressor genes such as p53 play a critical role in the maintenance of genomic stability, and p53 is one of the most frequently altered genes in a wide variety of tumor cells (Hollstein et al., 1991). In normal cells, p53 is activated in response to DNA damage, which may either result in cell cycle delay that is thought to permit DNA repair before replication or mitosis, or may lead to apoptosis of the damaged cell (reviewed in Amundson et al., 1998). Loss or mutation of p53 therefore has the consequence that cells with damaged DNA may survive and proliferate, with the danger that mutations persist and/or genes are amplified. The mutations and chromosomal aberrations so generated will be cell specific, leading to diversification within a developing tumor. Recent studies also suggest that loss of appropriate cellular adhesion, a necessary feature of metastatic progression, leads to rapid reduction in p53 levels and activity (Tlsty, 1998). Moreover, certain dominant gain-of-function p53 mutations disrupt spindle checkpoint control, leading to polyploidy (Gualberto et al., 1998). Furthermore, loss of multiple tumor suppressor genes and mutation or disregulated expression of oncogenes such as ras (Denko et al., 1994) or myc (McCormack et al., 1998; Yin et al., 1999) also promotes genomic instability. Thus mutation, inactivation or inappropriate expression of key control genes may not only have a direct effect on cellular properties, for example through altered patterns of gene expression, but may also promote the further accumulation of genetic abberations, contributing to tumor progression and to the acquisition of properties necessary for metastasis. This is reflected in several studies which report that highly metastatic cells have a higher spontaneous gene mutation rate than poorly metastatic cells (reviewed in Nicolson, 1987), suggesting that tumors with different metastatic capacities may differ in their genomic stability.

Genomic instability is presumably reflected in a number of parameters often associated with tumor progression to metastatic competence. For example, loss of differentiation characteristics, high mitotic index, aneuploidy and gross chromosomal abberations are associated with high-grade malignancies. Accumulation of genetic lesions as a result of genomic instability may interfere with patterns of gene expression necessary for differentiation characteristics. High mitotic index may result in part from loss of cell cycle checkpoint controls, and in the context of genomic instability will promote the further accumulation of genetic lesions. Aneuploidy and chromosomal abberations may result from disregulated spindle checkpoint control.

On the basis of the rapid and often reversible changes seen in the cellular properties of tumor cells, Nicolson (1987, 1991) has argued that heterogeneity is only rarely introduced into a tumor cell population by the accumulation of genetic lesions, and that adaptive changes based on reversible quantitative changes in gene expression leads to diversification. In this model, periodic genetic lesions in key genes such as oncogenes and tumor suppressor genes result in selective advantage for the tumor cell with the lesion, which ultimately results in clonally dominant outgrowth of these cells within the tumor. Quantitative changes in gene expression provide the diversity required for progression to metastatic competence. The corollary of this model is that the effects of genomic instability outlined above should tend to specifically target genes critical to tumor progression and clonal dominance. This is unlikely: for every qualitative genetic change which is advantageous for tumor progression and clonal dominance, there will be many others which are either deleterious for the tumor cell or neutral in terms of giving a selective advantage to the tumor cell. Moreover, when tumor cells are placed under new selection pressures such as during cancer therapy, it has been demonstrated that resistant tumor cells which grow out contain qualitative genomic changes. For example, during testosterone ablation therapy to treat prostate cancer, tumor cells which develop hormone independence and are therefore able to survive often express mutated forms of the androgen receptor (Taplin et al., 1995). Furthermore, critical experimental data can often be interpreted in several ways. For example, Poste et al. (1982) found that B16 melanoma lung metastases rapidly became heterogeneous and contained non-metastatic cells, suggesting that the acquisition of cellular properties required for metastasis is reversible. At first sight, this would support the view that the critical properties required for metastasis arose through reversible quantitative changes in gene expression. However, an alternative explanation is that genomic instability resulted in further genetic changes in the revertant non-metastatic cells which ablated critical cellular properties required for metastasis in this part of the tumor cell population. Thus, while there is certainly evidence that quantitative reversible changes in gene expression contribute to the heterogeneity within tumors (e.g., Raz and Ben-Ze'ev, 1983; see also below), qualitative changes in genes due to the effects of genomic instability described above must also be major contributors to tumor heterogeneity.

Quantitative changes in gene expression leading to diversification within tumors can arise through the interaction of tumor cells with their microenvironment. For example, some tumor cells will be directly apposed to stromal cells or ECM components, while others will simply be in contact with other tumor cells. Similarly, the vicinity of tumor cells to inflammatory cells and the cytokines they release will also vary. All of these factors can modify gene expression (e.g., Lee et al., 1985, Li et al., 1987), and thus the precise nature of the contacts and stimuli a tumor cell experiences will determine its gene expression pattern. Furthermore, depending on their location within the tumor, different tumor cells will experience different levels of hypoxia and nutrient deprivation. These factors also regulate transcriptional regulation (e.g., Ratcliffe et al., 1998; Hesketh et al., 1998) and thus will also result in zonally diverse patterns of gene expression.

Tumor Cells Are Subject to Strong Selective Forces

Tumor cells experience strong selection pressures both within the primary tumor and during metastatic dissemination. The majority of disseminated tumor cells do not give rise to metastatic deposits because they fail to survive during transportation, fail to adhere to or penetrate vascular endothelium at distant sites, or fail to establish an appropriate microenvironment. If they survive at secondary sites they may lie dormant for many years without giving rise to progressively growing metastases. Selective mechanisms thus give rise to metastatic inefficiency: a tumor containing billions of cells seldom produces more than a few tens of metastases.

The interaction between tumor cell and host constitutes a selective pressure on tumor cells. New properties which tumor cells acquire may result in the host recognizing the tumor cells as foreign and mounting a cell-mediated or humoral immune response against them. Many experiments demonstrate that immunization of syngeneic animals with tumor cells confers resistance against subsequent challenge of the animals with the same tumor (reviewed in Rosenberg, 1993). Subsequently, many antigens expressed specifically on tumor cells and not in normal adult tissue have been identified from a variety of tumors induced with physical and chemical carcinogens and viruses. Spontaneous tumors also express tumor-associated antigens, and the significance of these in human neoplasia is well illustrated in melanoma, where immunosuppression increases the risk of developing the disease and the intensity of destructive lymphocytic infiltration in melanoma tumors correlates with survival (Weinstock et al., 1993). Tumor-associated antigens include viral products, antigens which are normally only expressed during development, antigens which are expressed at low levels in normal tissues but whose expression is hugely upregulated in tumor cells, and normally expressed proteins which become mutated during tumorigenesis (Searle and Young, 1996). Tumors can escape from immunological destruction by downregulating or shedding tumor-associated antigens or by decreasing or losing expression of HLA antigens (Pawelec et al., 1997). Furthermore, it has recently been shown that several tumor types express CD95L, which can induce apoptosis of CD95+ anti-tumor T cells. This may provide a further mechanism by which tumor cells escape from destruction by the immune system (Walker et al., 1997).

Since the discovery that the bcl-2 oncogene suppresses apoptosis (Hockenberry, 1990), the concept has emerged from experimental models that an important step in tumor progression is the development by tumor cells of the ability to escape from apoptotic signals (Symonds et al., 1994; Naik et al., 1996; Shibata et al., 1996; Takaoka et al., 1997). Epithelial cells are critically dependent on contacts to each other, the underlying mesenchyme and ECM for survival (reviewed in Bates et al., 1995). Loss of such contacts results in apoptosis. Thus, metastasizing carcinoma cells have to become resistant to the apoptosis-inducing signals which result when they detach from the primary tumor. This necessity to survive may be another reason why clumps of tumor cells which retain at least some contacts with other cells have a metastatic advantage.

Physical forces such as haemodynamic shear within the blood circulatory system determine that the vast majority of disseminating tumor cells die. This point is amply illustrated by animal experiments in which tumor cells were tracked after intravenous injection, which show that very few cells survive (e.g., Fidler, 1970; Price et al., 1986). Unlike blood cells, tumor cells are not sufficiently deformable to survive transcapillary passage, and they are generally larger, rendering them highly susceptible to mechanical stress (Nicolson, 1982; Nicolson and Poste, 1982). While these physical forces generally act randomly on circulating tumor cells (Weiss, 1983), there is evidence to suggest that more deformable tumor cells are better able to survive within the circulatory system (Sato et al., 1976; 1977). Thus, physical forces may select for tumor cells with higher deformability, which in turn may determine whether the tumor cells remain in the first capillary bed they encounter, or whether they are able to recirculate to other sites.

Tumor cells also come under selective pressures at the point of exit from the vasculature. As discussed earlier, they may need to express surface molecules able to dock onto adhesion molecules on the surface of capillary bed endothelium. If they are able to do this, they need to be able to penetrate the endothelial wall and underlying basement membrane. After this, they require properties enabling them to survive and grow within their new environment, such as the ability to form a suitable microenvironment or respond to local growth factors.

Selection, Tumor Heterogeneity and Bridgeheads

Heterogeneity in a population of tumor cells represents a pool of cells with different assortments of properties. The severity and breadth of selection forces acting on a population of tumor cells will determine how many properties an individual tumor cell needs to accumulate in order to be able to successfully metastasize, and thus how large the pool must be in order to contain statistically such a tumor cell. For many tumors, tumor burden correlates with metastasis formation. Larger tumors contain proportionally more cells than small tumors, meaning that the assortment of tumor cells with different properties is likely to be larger. Combined with the fact that more tumor cells are shed into the bloodstream by large tumors compared to small tumors, there is therefore a greater probability that a tumor cell possessing the properties required to form a metastasis at a given site is able to survive the physical insults of passage through the circulatory system and successfully reach the site where it has the properties necessary to form metastases. Moreover, if a given tumor type has a higher intrinsic rate of diversification compared to another tumor type, it may be expected to metastasize at an earlier point during tumor development. This may be one factor determining intrinsic metastatic potential.

If selection pressures are less for metastasis to occur down one particular route, then it is statistically more likely that metastasis will first be seen via that route. For example, ovarian carcinomas metastasize at high frequency by direct extension into the peritoneal cavity (reviewed in Young et al., 1993). Ovarian tumor cells metastasizing by direct extension in this way avoid selection pressures such as those experienced by tumor cells within the blood stream and at exit from the vasculature, and therefore they need fewer properties to metastasize via this route. Thus, some secondary sites may be more easily colonised than others by metastasizing cells, and metastasis formation at these sites is statistically more likely to occur.

Established metastases at sites which are relatively easily colonised represent the expanded progeny of tumor cells which have been selected for on the basis of their ability to metastasize. The development of diversification continues after metastases have formed (Poste et al., 1982), and although subpopulations of tumor cells may lose their metastatic potential during this process, other subpopulations retain them. Some cellular properties required for metastasis formation are common to many secondary sites. Thus these established metastases may be expected to contain subpopulations of tumor cells already containing some of the properties required for metastasis to other sites. Therefore, compared to tumor cells in the original primary tumor, these subpopulations will need to develop less heterogeneity in order to give rise to tumor cells possessing properties required to metastasize to another site, and are thus statistically more likely to do so. In this sense established metastases may act as bridgeheads on the way to the formation of metastases at secondary sites which are more difficult to colonize. The concept of the bridgehead is well illustrated by lymph node metastases.

Lymph Node Metastases as Bridgeheads

Tumor cells within the lymphatic system are subject to selection, as is attested to by tracking the fate of tumor cells within the lymphatic system (e.g., Grundmann and Vollmer, 1985). Within the lymph node, many tumor cells die or remain dormant (e.g., Ludwig and Titus, 1967). However, given that tumor cells can be detected in the blood stream relatively early in tumor progression and might be expected eventually to give rise to metastases, why is it that regional lymph node metastases are often the first sites of metastatic spread? Several biological and physical attributes make the lymphatic system a relatively easy entry site into the circulatory system for tumor cells, and also favor metastasis formation. Thus, in comparison to forming metastases at distant sites, tumor cells need to acquire fewer properties to form regional lymph node metastases. Lymph node metastases can therefore act as bridgeheads during metastatic progression.

Lymph Nodes Are a Relatively Easy Target for Tumor Metastasis

1. Biology and properties of the lymphatic endothelium.
   The lymphatic vasculature is thought to arise out of the venous system during embryogenesis (Sabin, 1902). Lymphatic capillaries are blind-ended vessels which drain lymphatic fluid from peripheral tissues into larger collecting ducts. The majority of these collecting ducts empty into the thoracic duct, by which route most of the lymphatic fluid is discharged into the venous system. Lymph nodes are found at intervals along the length of the collecting ducts. Lymph nodes are specialized structures within which the lymphatic and venous circulatory systems communicate and immune cells reside or develop.
   The lymphatic system plays a vital role in maintaining homeostasis, returning to the circulatory system around 10% of the volume of interstitial

fluid escaping from tissue capillary beds (the physiology of the lymphatic system is thoroughly reviewed in Aukland and Reed, 1993; Guyton and Hall, 1996). More importantly, it provides a route by which biological macromolecules, which cannot be reabsorbed into the venous capillaries due to their size, can exit peripheral tissues. This helps to ensure that the colloid osmotic pressure of the interstitial fluid remains constant. Failure of the lymphatic system to maintain a constant interstitial fluid volume or colloid osmotic pressure results in edema, a major clinical problem. The lymphatics also play a key role in the absorption of lipids from the intestinal tract. Furthermore, the lymphatic system has a crucial function in the immune system, acting as a filter for pathogens by means of its lymph nodes. The lymphatic system also provides ready access to the circulatory system for cells of the immune system such as dendritic cells, which when activated in peripheral tissue in response to an immunological challenge migrate into and through lymphatic capillaries. We have recently shown that CD44 plays a critical role in this process (Weiss et al., 1997).

The ultrastructure of the lymphatic endothelium (LE) which forms or lines lymphatic vessels is specialized to accomodate its function (e.g., Leak and Burke, 1968; reviewed in Ryan, 1989). Many of these characteristics also favor entry of tumor cells into the lumen of the lymphatic vessel in ways which do not apply to the entry of tumor cells into blood vessels. The endothelium has loose junctions which readily permit the passage of large biological macromolecules, pathogens and migrating cells. Furthermore, the lymphatic capillaries have no or at best only an incomplete basement membrane, in contrast to the basement membrane of blood vessels which tumor cells need to penetrate in order to enter and exit the circulatory system. These features make the lymphatic system an attractive target for tumor cell entry into the circulatory system, as less properties are required for tumor cells to enter lymphatic vessels compared to blood vessels.

2. Flow of lymphatic fluid into the draining lymph nodes.
   The high internal pressure within tumors means that interstitial fluid flows away from them into the draining lymphatics (Jain, 1989). Tumor cells which have developed the property of being able to detach from the primary tumor mass will therefore be channeled into local lymphatic vessels by the flow of lymphatic fluid. Thus the passive transport of tumor cells in the interstitial fluid flow into the lymphatics may be expected to promote tumor cell entry into the lymphatic system. Furthermore, the flow of lymphatic fluid is passive, at least in the peripheral lymphatic vessels, and therefore tumor cells in lymphatic capillaries are not subject to the same shear forces experienced by tumor cells in the blood system, reducing the selection pressure they experience.

3. Filter function of the lymph node increases local tumor cell concentration.
   After entering the lymphatic system, tumor cells eventually reach the regional (sentinel) lymph node(s). Here, they may be destroyed, grow to

form lymph node metastases or pass through. There has been much dispute about whether lymph nodes constitute a filter, inhibiting further metastatic spread, but these arguments may be addressing the wrong issue. Within the lymph nodes the tumor cells are channeled into a confined space, the subcapsular sinuses. This is in sharp contrast to cells in the blood system, which are distributed over a large capillary bed in the next organ they reach after entering the blood stream, most often the lung. This accumulation of tumor cells may be a critical factor in understanding the propensity of metastasizing tumor cells to initially colonize the regional lymph nodes.

It is well established that emboli of tumor cells much more efficiently form metastases than single tumor cells (reviewed in Nicolson, 1988). The usual explanation for this is that emboli are more likely to lodge and therefore able to extravasate out of capillary beds. This cannot be the only explanation. Tumor cells are generally considerably larger than erythrocytes and even erythrocytes have difficulty proceeding through capillary beds and require flexibility to do so. Single tumor cells are therefore more than likely to be able to lodge in capillary beds, and indeed, their inflexibility within such beds is often postulated to be the reason for their death due to shear forces (Nicolson, 1982; Nicolson and Poste, 1982). Moreover, intravital video microscopy suggests that the deciding factor whether tumor cells form metastases or not at distant sites is not whether they lodge and extravasate, but whether they are able to go on to grow at those sites (Chambers et al., 1995). The metastatic advantage given to emboli-forming tumor cells should therefore perhaps also be viewed as one of survival. As mentioned previously, many cells are dependent on cell-cell and cell-matrix contacts for survival. Embolus formation may provide such contacts required for tumor cell survival which would not be found within the circulatory system or a sites of extravasation. Furthermore, tumor cells are critically dependent on the development of stroma to form metastases. They need to establish a blood supply by angiogenesis, for example, to be able to grow beyond a couple of millimeters in diameter. The embolus may therefore also provide a critical mass of cells required for the establishment of such stroma. The metastatic advantage given to tumor cells which are able to deposit fibrin (Tsubura et al., 1983; Weiss and Ward, 1983) should perhaps also be interpreted in this way: an attractive hypothesis presented by Dvorak (1986) is that tumors are wounds which do not heal, and during wound healing fibrin clot formation is a first step in stimulating the production of a stroma containing fibroblasts, blood vessels, immune cells and ECM components such as hyaluronic acid and collagen.

The critical mass of tumor cells in the subcapsular sinuses of lymph nodes draining primary tumors is thus likely to give a stimulus to metastasis formation which would not be experienced by tumor cells in the blood stream. Furthermore, metastasis formation can occur directly within the subcapsular space, which obviates the need for metastasizing cells to acquire properties necessary for extravasation, further increasing the probability that a metastasis may form.

4. Tumor-induced lymphangiogenesis.

The entry of metastasizing tumor cells into the lymphatic system is likely to be dependent in part on the density and positioning of lymphatic vessels relative to the primary tumor. Although histological studies on tumor lymphatics are often difficult to interpret due to a lack of markers which reliably differentiate between lymphatic and other endothelium in histological sections, they generally suggest that lymphatic vessels within tumors are sparse or non-existent (Fallowfield and Cook, 1990; Deutsch et al., 1992; de Waal et al., 1997). However, these and other studies suggest that lymphatic vessels are present in the stroma surrounding tumors, and are often observed in significant numbers (Harveit, 1990; Lubach et al., 1992; Yoshizawa et al., 1994; Jussila et al., 1998). The invasive external margin of tumors is the site where invasion of lymphatic vessels is likely to occur, and thus a high density of lymphatic vessels in the periphery of a tumor may be expected to promote lymphatic metastasis.

The new growth of lymphatic capillaries is termed lymphangiogenesis. An fms-like tyrosine kinase receptor called VEGFR-3 (Flt4) is specifically expressed on LE in the adult (Kaipainen et al., 1995; Kukk et al., 1996). VEGF-C and VEGF-D, the known ligands for VEGFR-3 (Joukov et al., 1996, Lee et al., 1996; Fitz et al., 1997; Achen et al., 1998), are homologous to the VEGF/PDGF family. After binding to VEGF-C and VEGF-D, VEGFR-3 is capable of transducing signals which trigger proliferation in vivo and in vitro (Fitz et al., 1997; Jeltsch et al., 1997; Oh et al., 1997; Achen et al., 1998), suggestive of a role for VEGFR-3 and its ligands in lymphangiogenesis.

Using rat carcinoma models, we have begun to investigate the hypothesis that by producing VEGF-C or VEGF-D, tumors could cause lymphangiogenic growth towards or in the vicinity of the tumor and thereby potentiate lymphatic metastasis by increasing lymphatic vessel density (Sleeman, J.P., Steffen, A., Mandriota, S., Krishnan, J. and Pepper, M., manuscript in preparation). We have cloned and sequenced full-length rat VEGF-C and rat VEGF-D cDNAs and used these as probes to screen a panel of 34 rat tumor cell lines with defined metastatic potential for VEGF-C and VEGF-D expression. VEGF-C is expressed at various levels in more than 50% of the cell lines, while VEGF-D is expressed strongly in only one of cell lines analyzed. Furthermore, VEGF-C and VEGF-D expression was observed in tumors derived from cells which were negative for VEGF-C and VEGF-D in tissue culture. Our current data suggest that at least part of the VEGF-D expression observed in these tumors is derived from stromal fibroblasts. Our results show that the lymphangiogenic factors VEGF-C and VEGF-D are expressed in tumors, either by tumor and/or stromal cells, and support the notion that by increasing lymphatic vessel density, tumor-induced lymphangiogenesis may be another mechanism whereby metastasis via the lymphatic system could be potentiated.

The Lymph Node as a Bridgehead During Metastatic Progression

Given that the formation of metastases is largely a selective process, lymph node metastases can be thought of as bridgeheads in the formation of distant metastases. The relative ease with which tumor cells can enter the lymphatic system and form metastases within regional lymph nodes means that the selective pressure put to bear on the metastasizing tumor cells is less than that experienced by tumor cells within the blood. Put another way, the tumor cells need to acquire less properties to successfully form metastases in the regional lymph nodes than they do to form metastases at distant sites. Once established as metastatic deposits in the regional lymph nodes, subpopulations of tumor cells already have part of the properties required to colonize distant sites. Tumor cells metastasizing from these regional lymph node metastases therefore have to acquire fewer properties to colonize distant sites than tumor cells shed directly into the blood stream from the primary tumor. This concept is supported by evidence from animal studies. For example, using subcutaneously implanted Ehrlich carcinoma, Koch excised regional lymph node metastases and serially implanted these subcutaneously into further animals. After several such cycles, the frequency of lymph node metastases increased, and after additional cycles the selected tumor cells were able to metastasize to distant sites such as the lung (Koch, 1939).

Let us assume that tumor cells need to acquire two properties x and y in order to be able to form distant metastases. If tumor cells only require property x for lymph node metastasis formation, then the probability of lymph node metastasis formation is px (see Fig. 2). The tumor cells in the lymph node metastasis then have acquired part of the properties they require for

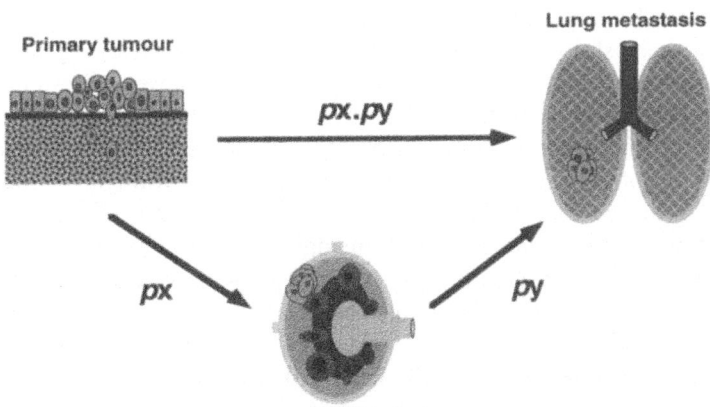

Fig. 2. Schematic diagram depicting the lymph node as a bridgehead in development of distant metastases. In the simplest case, the probability of forming a lung metastasis via a lymph node bridgehead is px + py, while the probability of forming a lung metastasis directly from a primary tumor is px.py (see text for details)

distant metastasis, and so the probability of distant metastasis formation seeded from the lymph node metastasis is py. Thus, in this (oversimplified) model, the probability of distant metastasis formation via a lymph node is px + py, whereas the probability of distant metastases forming directly from the primary tumor is px.py because both properties have to be acquired simultaneously (Fig. 2).

A useful analogy for the lymph node as a bridgehead in the formation of distant metastases is that of a lottery in which each week several numbers are randomly picked from a large pool of numbers and the punter has to correctly predict what the selected numbers will be. Suppose that 6 numbers are picked each week, and to win the jackpot (form a distant metastasis) all 6 numbers (cellular properties) need to be correctly predicted. If three correct numbers are obtained one week and these numbers can be held until the next week (metastasis via regional lymph nodes), there is a much higher probability of getting the last three numbers required for the jackpot in the next and subsequent weeks compared to getting all 6 numbers at once (metastasis directly from the primary tumor). In this analogy, primary tumors with low metastatic potential would require more correct lottery numbers to win the jackpot than tumors with high metastatic potential. For tumor types in which primary tumor size correlates with metastasis formation, tumor size represents the number of lottery tickets bought – the more guesses at what the numbers will be (number of tumor cells able to enter the lymphatic or blood systems), the higher the probability of getting the jackpot (forming metastases at regional and distant sites).

The principle of the bridgehead can be applied to the metastatic process as a whole. The concept of the "generalizing site" during metastatic progression, for example, can also be considered in these terms. Selection determines that only those tumor cells which have acquired the required properties through the processes leading to tumor heterogeneity can metastasize. Metastatic sites or routes which require tumor cells to acquire less properties to successfully metastasize are therefore more likely to be colonised, and may then function as bridgeheads. Once metastases are established by tumor cells at these more favourable sites, they already possess some properties required for metastasis to other sites where the selective pressures are more stringent. The development of heterogeneity within these metastases generates tumor cells with additional properties, some of which may suffice to permit tumor cells from the "bridgehead" to metastasize to more stringent sites. Of course, at the same time heterogeneity is continually developing in the primary tumor (and upstream bridgehead sites). There is thus also a likelihood that tumor cells may arise out of the primary tumor and/or upstream bridgehead sites which have the properties required to form metastases directly at distant sites. However, the probability of this happening is considerably smaller, as all the necessary properties need to arise at the same time. Factors which reduce the selective forces on disseminated tumor cells, such as intrinsic properties of the cells giving rise to the primary tumor, the location of the primary tumor and the kinetics of the generation of tumor heterogeneity will determine the extent to which tumors metastasize via bridgehead sites, and the range of and order in which distant sites are metastasized. Together with the partially random nature of selection and genetic changes involved in tumor heterogeneity, this concept goes a considerable way towards understanding the complex variety of metastatic patterns which nevertheless have an underlying theme, but which vary from tumor type to tumor type.

Concluding Comments: Sentinel Lymphonodectomy

If tumor cells very readily acquire the properties required to form hematogenic metastases, or only require a few properties to do so, hematogenic metastasis will be early, and the selective advantage for metastasis formation in regional lymph nodes will not be apparent. In such cases of high hematogenous metastatic potential, the prognostic significance of regional lymph node metastases will therefore be small. This has direct bearing on the relevance of sentinel lymphonodectomy as a prognostic and therapeutic tool. In tumor types with high intrinsic hematogenous potential, the use of sentinel lymphonodectomy will probably be limited to making surgical decisions about the extent of resection needed to remove tumor cells from the lymphatic basin draining the primary tumor. However, in tumors with lower hematogenous metastatic potential, the sentinel node technique has the promise of being a useful prognostic indicator, and furthermore can be expected to identify patients who can be cured of their cancer by simple excision of the primary tumor.

Lessons about the biology of the metastatic spread of different tumor types will also be learnt from on-going sentinel lymphonodectomy clinical trials. For example, currently published data suggests that if lymph node metastases are going to form, they form first in the sentinel node(s) and do not skip lymph nodes (Gulec et al., 1998). In sentinel node negative patients, the long term survival rate after surgical removal of the primary tumor will give an indication of the extent to which a given tumor type follows the primary tumor-lymph node-distant metastasis dissemination pathway. Furthermore, sites of relapse in these patients will also point out the alternative metastatic routes taken by these tumors. Thus the exciting development of the surgical technique of sentinel lymphonodectomy not only holds out the hope of improved quality of life and patient care for cancer victims, but will also teach us important lessons about the process of metastasis.

Acknowledgements. I am very grateful to Helmut Ponta and Susanne Weg-Remers for critically reading the manuscript. This article is dedicated to the memory of Martin Hoffmann.

References

Aaronson, S. (1991). Growth factors and cancer. Science 254: 1146–1153

Achen, M., Jeltsch, M., Kukk, E., Makinen, T., Vitali, A., Wilks, A., Alitalo, K. and Stacker, S. (1998). Vascular endothelial growth factor D (VEGF-D) is a ligand for the tyrosine kinases VEGF receptor 2 (Flk1) and VEGF receptor 3. Proc. Natl. Acad. Sci USA 95: 548–553

Amundson, S., Myers, T. and Fornace, A. (1998). Roles for p53 in growth arrest and apoptosis: putting on the brakes after genotoxic stress. Oncogene 17: 3287–3299

Aukland, K. and Reed, R. (1993). Interstitial-Lymphatic mechanisms in the control of extracellular fluid volume. Physiological Reviews 73: 1–75

Bates, R., Lincz, L. and Burns, G. (1995). Involvement of integrins in cell survival. Cancer Metastasis Rev. 14: 191–203

Beahrs, O. and Myers, M. (1983). Purposes and priciples of staging. Manual for staging of cancer p3–5. J. B. Lippincott Co., Philadelphia

Birchmeier, W. and Behrens, J. (1984). Cadherin expression in carcinomas: role in the formation of cell junctions and the prevention of invasiveness. Biochim Biophys Acta. 1198: 11–26

Brodt, P. (1991). Adhesion mechanisms in lymphatic metastasis. Cancer Metastasis Rev. 10: 23–32

Butler, T. and Gullino, P. (1975). Quantitation of cell shedding into efferent blood of mammary carcinoma. Cancer Research 35: 512–516

Cabanas, R. (1977). An approach for the treatment of penile carcinoma. Cancer 39: 456–466

Carr, I. (1983). Lymphatic metastasis. Cancer Metastasis Rev. 2: 307–317

Chambers, A., Macdonald, I., Schmidt, E., Koop, S., Morris, V., Khoka, R. and Groom, A. (1995). Steps in tumor metastasis: new concepts from intravital videomicroscopy. Cancer and Metastasis Reviews 14: 279–301

Chan, B., Matsuura, N., Takada, Y., Zetter, B. and Hemler, M. (1991). In vitro and in vivo consequences of VLA-2 expression on rhabdomyosarcoma cells. Science 251: 1600–1602

Denko, N., Giaccia, A., Stringer, J. and Stambrook, P. (1994). The human Ha-ras oncogene induces genomic instability in murine fibroblasts within one cell cycle. Proc. Natl. Acad. Sci. USA 91: 5124–5128

Deutsch, A., Lubach, D., Nissen, S. and Neukam, D. (1992). Ultrastructural studies on the invasion of melanomas in initial lymphatics of human skin. J. Invest Dermatol. 98: 64–67

de Waal, R., van Altena, M., Erhard, H., Weidle, U., Nooijen, P. and Ruiter D. (1997). Lack of lymphangiogenesis in human primary cutaneous melanoma. Am. J. Pathol. 150: 1951–1957

Duffy, M. (1992). The role of proteolytic enzymes in cancer invasion and metastasis. Cin. Exp. Metastasis 10: 1455–155

Dvorak, H. (1986). Tumors: wounds that do not heal. Similarities between tumor stroma generation and wound healing. N Engl J Med. 315:1650–1659

Ennis, R., Katz, A., de Vries, G., Heitjan, D., O'Toole, K., Rubin, M., Buttyan R., Benson, M. and Schiff, P. (1997). Detection of circulating prostate carcinoma cells via an enhanced reverse transcriptase-polymerase chain reaction assay in patients with early stage prostate carcinoma. Independence from other pretreatment characteristics. Cancer 79: 2402–2408

Ewing, J. (1928). Metastasis. In: Neoplastic disease, a treatise on tumors. 3rd edition, Saunders, Philadelphia

Fallowfield, M. and Cook, M. (1990). Lymphatics in primary cutaneous melanoma. Am J. Surg. Pathol. 14: 370–374

Fearon, E. and Vogelstein, B. (1990). A genetic model for colorectal tumorigenesis. Cell 61: 759–767

Fidler, I. (1970). Metastasis: quantitative analysis of distribution and fate of tumor emboli labeled with ^{125}I-5-iodo-2'-deoxyuridine. J. Natl. Cancer Inst. 45: 773–782

Fidler, I. (1978). Tumor heterogeneity and the biology of cancer invasion and metastasis. Cancer research 38: 2651–2660

Fisher, B and Fisher, E. (1966). The interrelationship of hematogenous and lymphatic tumor cell dissemination. Surg. Gynecol. Obstet. 122: 791–798

Fisher, B and Fisher, E. (1970). Significance of the interrelationship of the lymph and blood vascular systems in tumor cell dissemination. Prog. Clin. Cancer 4: 84–96

Fitz, L., Morris, J., Towler, P., Long, A., Burgess, P., Greco, R., Wang, J., Gassaway, R., Nickbarg, E., Kovacic, S., Ciarletta, A., Giannotti, J., Finnerty, H., Zollner, R., Beier, D., Leak, L., Turner, K. and Wood, C. (1997). Characterisation of murine Flt4 ligand/VEGF-C. Oncogene 15: 613–618

Foulds, L. (1975). Neoplastic development. Academic Press, New York

Goldman, E. (1906). Relation of cancer cells to blood vessels and ducts. Lancet 1: 23

Gomez, D., Alonso, D., Yoshiji, H. and Thorgeirsson, U. (1997). Tissue inhibitors of metalloproteinases: structure, regulation and biological functions. Eur. J. Cell Biol. 74: 111–122

Grundmann, E. and Vollmer, E. (1985). Early local reaction and lymph node permeation of rat carcinoma HH9-cl 14 cells. An immunohistological approach. Pathol Res Pract 179: 304–309

Gualberto, A., Aldape, K., Kozakiewicz, K. and Tlsty, T. (1998). An oncogenic form of p53 confers a dominant gain-of-function phenotype that disrupts spindle checkpoint control. Proc. Natl. Acad. Sci. USA 95: 5166–5171

Gulec, S., Moffat, F., Carroll, R., Serafini, A., Skakianakis, G., Alle, L., Boggs, J., Escobedo, D., Pruett, C., Gupta, A., Livingstone, A. and Krag, D. (1998). Sentinel lymph node localization in early breast cancer. J. Nuclear Med. 39: 1388–1393

Guyton, A. and Hall, A. (1996). Textbook of Medical Physiology (9th ed.). W. B. Saunders Company, Philadelphia, USA

Hanahan, D. and Folkman, J. (1996). Patterns and emerging mechanisms of the angiogenic switch during tumorigenesis. Cell. 86: 353–364

Harveit, F. (1990). Attenuated cells of the breast stroma: the missing lymphatic system of the breast. Histopathology 16: 533–543

Heiss, M., Allgayer, H., Gruetzner, K., Funke, I., Babic, R., Jauch, K.-W. and Schildberg, F. (1995). Individual development and uPA-receptor expression of disseminated tumor cells in bone marrow: a reference to early systemic disease in solid cancer. Nature Med. 1: 1035–1039

Hesketh, J., Vasconcelos, M. and Bermano, G. (1998). Regulatory signals in messenger RNA: determinants of nutrient-gene interaction and metabolic compartmentation. Br. J. Nutr. 80: 307–321

Hill, R., Chambers, A., Ling, V. and Harris, J. (1984). Dynamic heterogeneity: rapid generation of metastatic varinats of mouse B16 melanoma cells. Science 224: 998–1001

Hockenberry, D., Nunez, G., Milliman, C., Screiber, R. and Korsmeyer, S. (1990). Bcl-2 is an inner mitochondrial membrane protein that blocks programmed cell death. Nature 348: 334–336

Hollstein, M., Sidransky, D., Vogelstein, B. and Harris, C. (1991). p53 mutations in human cancers. Science 253: 49–53

Honn, K. and Tang, D. (1992). Adhesion molecules and tumor cell interaction with endothelium and subendothelial matrix. Cancer and Metastasis Reviews 11: 353–375

Imhof, B., Piali, L., Gisler, R. and Dunon, D. (1996). Involvement of a6 and av integrins in metastasis. Current Topics in Microbiology and Immunology 213/I: 195–203

Israeli, R., Miller, W., Su, S., Powell, C., Fair, W., Samadi, D., Huryk, R., DeBlasio, A., Edwards, E., Wise, G. et al. (1994). Sensitive nested reverse transcription polymerase chain reaction detection of circulating prostatic tumor cells: comparison of prostate-specific membrane antigen and prostate-specific antigen-based assays. Cancer Research 54: 6306–6310

Jain, R. (1989). Delivery of novel therapeutic agents in tumors: physiological barriers and strategies. J. Natl. Cancer Inst. 81: 52–58

Jeltsch, M., Kaipainen, A., Joukov, V., Meng, X., Lakso, M., Rauvala, H., Swartz, M., Fuku-mura, D., Kain, R. and Alitalo, K. (1997). Hyperplasia of lymphatic vessels in VEGF-C transgenic mice. Science 276: 1423–1425

Joukov, V., Pajusola, K., Kaipainen, A., Chilov, D., Lahtinen, I., Kukk, E., Saksela, O., Kalkki-nen, N. and Alitalo, K. (1996). A novel vascular endothelial growth factor, VEGF-C, is a ligand for the Flt4 (VEGFR-3) and KDR (VEGFR-2) receptor tyrosine kinases. EMBO J. 15: 290–298

Jussila, L., Valtola, R., Partanen, T., Salven, P., Heikkilä, P., Matikainen, M.-T., Renkonen, R., Kaipainen, A., Detmar, M., Tschachler, E., Alitalo, R. and Alitalo, K. (1998). Lymphatic endothelium and Kaposi's sarcoma spindle cells detected by antibodies against the vas-cular endothelial growth growth factor receptor-3. Cancer Res. 58: 1599–1604

Kaipainen, A., Korhonen, J., Mustonen, T., van Hinsberg, V., Fang, G.-H., Dumont, D., Breit-man, M. and Alitalo, K. (1995). Expression of the fms-like tyrosine kinase 4 gene be-comes restricted to lymphatic endothelium during development. Proc. Natl. Acad. Sci. USA 92: 3566–3570

Karin, M. (1992). Signal transduction from cell surface to nucleus in development and dis-ease. FASEB J. 6: 2581–2590

Kebers, F., Lewalle, J.-M., Desreux, J., Munaut, C., Devy, L., Foidart, J.-M., Noel, A. (1998). Induction of endothelial cell apoptosis by solid tumor cells. Exp. Cell Res 240: 197–205

Kerbel, R., Waghorne, C. and Korczak, B. (1988). Clonal dominance of primary tumours by metastatic cells: genetic analysis and biological implications. Cancer Surv. 7: 597–629

Kim, U. and Furth, J. (1960). Relation of mammotropes to mammary tumors. IV. Develop-ment of highly hormone-dependent mammary tumors. Proc. Soc. Exptl. Biol. Med. 105: 490–492

Kim, J., Yu, W., Kovalski, K. and Ossowski, L. (1998). Requirement for specific proteases in cancer cell intravasation as revealed by a novel semiquantitative PCR-based assay. Cell 94: 353–362

Knudson, A. (1993). Antioncogenes and cancer. Proc. Natl. Acad. Sci. USA 90: 10914–10921

Koch, F. E. (1939). Zur Frage der Metastasenbildung bei Impftumoren. Z. Krebsforsch. 48: 495–507

Kulakowski, A., Madej, G. and Pienkowski, T. (1984). Distribution of lymph node metasta-ses in the malignant melanoma of the trunk. Oncology 41: 242–244

Kukk, E., Lymboussaki, A., Taira, S., Kaipainen, A., Jeltsch, M., Joukov, V. and Alitalo, K. (1996). VEGF-C receptor binding and pattern of expression with VEGFR-3 suggests a role in lymphatic vascular development. Development 122: 3829–3837

Leak, L. and Burke, J. (1968). Ultrastructual studies on the lymphatic anchoring filaments. J. Cell Biol. 36: 129–149

Lee, E., Lee, W.-H., Kaetzel, C., Parry, G. and Bissel, M. (1985). Interaction of mouse mam-mary epithelial cells with collagen substrates: regulation of casein gene expression and secretion. Proc. Natl. Acad. Sci USA 82: 1419–1423

Lee, J., Gray, A., Yuan, J., Luoh, S.-M., Avraham, H. and Wood, W. (1996). Vascular endothe-lial growth factor-related protein: a ligand and specific activator of the tyrosine kinase receptor Flt4. Proc. Natl. Acad. Sci. USA 93: 1988–1992

Li, M., Aggeler, J., Farson, D., Hatier, C., Hussell, J. and Bissell, M. (1987). Influence of re-constituted basement membrane and its components on casein gene expression and se-cretion in mouse mammary epithelial cells. . Proc. Natl. Acad. Sci. USA 84: 136–140

Liotta, L., Mandler, R., Murano, G., Katz, D., Gordon, R., Chiang, P. and Schiffman, E. (1986). Tumor-cell autocrine motility factor. Proc. Natl. Acad. Sci. USA 83: 3302–3306

Lubach, D., Berens von Rautenfeld, D. and Kaiser, H. (1992). The possible role of the initial lymph vessels of the skin during metastasis of malignant tumors. In vivo, 6: 443–450

Ludwig, J. and Titus J. (1967). Experimental tumor cell emboli in lymph nodes. Arch. Pathol. 84: 304–311

McCarthy, S., Kuzu, I., Gatter, K. and Bicknell, R. (1991). Heterogeneity of the endothelial cell and its role in organ preference of tumour metastasis. Trends Pharmacol. Sci. 12: 462–467

McCormack, S., Weaver, Z., Deming, S., Natarajan, G., Torri, J., Johnson, M., Liyanage, M., Ried, T. and Dickson, R. (1998). Myc/p53 interactions in transgenic mouse mammary development, tumorigenesis and chromosomal instability. Oncogene 16: 2755–2766

Melchior, S., Corey, E., Ellis, W., Ross, A., Layton, T., Oswin, M., Lange, P. and Vessella, R. (1997). Early tumor cell dissemination in patients with clinically localized carcinoma of the prostate. Clin. Cancer Res. 3: 249–256

Mori, M., Mimori, K., Ueo, H., Karimine, N., Barnard, G., Sugimachi, K. and Akiyoshi, T. (1996). Molecular detection of circulating solid carcinoma cells in the peripheral blood: the concept of early systemic disease. Int. J. Cancer 68: 739–743

Naik, P., Karrim, J. and Hanahan, D. (1996). The rise and fall of apoptosis during multistage tumorigenesis: down-modulation contributes to tumor progression from angiogenic progenitors. Genes Dev. 10: 2105–2116

Nicolson, G. (1982). Cancer Metastasis: organ colonisation and the cell-surface properties of malignant cells. Biochim. Biophy. Acta 695: 113–176

Nicolson, G. (1987). Tumor cell instability, diversification, and progression to the metastatic phenotype: from oncogene to oncofetal expression. Cancer Res. 47: 1473–1487

Nicolson, G. (1988). Organ specificity of tumor metatasis: role of preferential adhesion, invasion and growth of malignant cells at specific sites. Cancer and Metastasis Reviews 7: 143–188

Nicolson, G. (1991). Gene expression, cellular diversification and tumor progression to the metastatic phenotype. Bioessays 13: 337–342

Nicolson, G. and Poste, G. (1982). Tumor cell diversity and host response in cancer metastasis. Curr. Prob. Cancer 7: 1–83

Oh SJ, Jeltsch MM, Birkenhager R, McCarthy JE, Weich HA, Christ B, Alitalo K, Wilting J (1997). VEGF and VEGF-C: specific induction of angiogenesis and lymphangiogenesis in the differentiated avian chorioallantoic membrane. Dev. Biol. 188: 96–109

Padget, S. (1889). Distribution of secondary growths in cancer of the breast. Lancet 1: 571–573

Pauli, B., Augustin-Voss. H., El-Sabban, M., Johnson, R. and Hammer, D. (1990). Organ-preference of metastasis: the role of endothelial cell adhesion molecules. Cancer and Metastasis Reviews 9: 175–189

Pawelec, G., Zeuthen, J. and Kiessling, R. (1997). Escape from host-antitumor immunity. Crit. Rev. Oncog. 8: 111–141

Poste, G., Tzeng, J., Doll, J., Greig, R., Rieman, D. and Zeidman, I. (1982). Evolution of tumor cell heterogeneity during progressive growth of individual lung metastases. Proc. Natl. Acad. Sci. USA 79: 6574–6578

Powell, W. and Matrisian, L. (1996). Complex roles of matrix metalloproteinases in tumor progression. Curr. Top. Microbiol. Immunol. 213/1: 1–21

Price, J., Aukerman, S. and Fidler, I. (1986). Evidence that the process of murine melanoma metastasis is sequential and selective and contains stochastic elements. Cancer Res. 46: 5172–5178

Rajotte, D., Arap, W., Hagedorn, M., Koivunen, E., Pasqualini, R. and Ruoslahti, E. (1999). Molecular heterogeneity of the vascular endothelium revealed by in vivo phage display. J. Clin. Invest. 102: 430–437

Ratcliffe, P., O'Rourke, J., Maxwell, P. and Pugh, C. (1998). Oxygen sensing, hypoxia-inducible factor-1 and the regulation of mammalial gene expression. J. Exp. Biol. 201: 1153–1162

Raz, A. and Ben-Ze'ev, A. (1983) Modulation of the metastatic capability in B16 melanoma by cell shape. Science 221: 1307–1310

Reed, J. (1998). Bcl-2 family proteins. Oncogene 17: 3225–3236

Rosenberg, S. (1993). Principles and applications of biologic therapy. In Cancer, Principles and Practice of Oncology, Fourth Edition, Eds DeVita, Hellman and Rosenberg, pp 293–324. J. B. Lippincott Co., Philadelphia

Ryan, T. (1987). Structure and function of lymphatics. J. Invest. Dermatol. 93: 18S-23 S

Salsbury, A. (1975). The significance of the circulating cancer cell. Cancer Treat. Rev. 2: 55–72

Sato, H., Khato, J., Sato, T. and Suzuki, M. (1977). Deformability and filtrability of tumor cells through "nucleopore" filter, with reference to viability and metastatic spread. Gann monogr. Cancer Res. 20: 3–13

Sato, H. and Suzuki, M. (1976). In Fundamental aspects of metastasis (Weiss, L., ed.), pp311–317. North Holland Publishing Co., Amsterdam

Searle, P. and Young, L. (1996). Immunotherapy II: antigens, receptors and costimulation. Cancer Metastasis Rev. 15: 329–349

Shibata, M., Maroulakou, I., Jorcyk, C., Gold, L., Ward, J. and Green, J. (1996). p53-independent apoptosis during mammary tumor progression in C3(1)/SV40 large T transgenic mice: suppression of apoptosis during transition from preneoplasia to carcinoma. Cancer Res. 56: 2998–3003

Shimonaka, M. and Yamaguchi, Y. (1994). Purification and biological characterisation of epitaxin, a fibroblast-derived motility factor for epithelial cells. J. Biol. Chem. 269: 14284–14289

Sugarbaker, E. (1979). Cancer metastasis: a product of tumor-host interactions. In Current Problems in Cancer, Vol. III, R. Hickey, Ed. Year Book Medical Publishers, Chicago

Sugarbaker, E. (1981). Patterns of metastasis in human malignancies. Cancer Biol. Rev. 2: 235–278

Symonds, H., Krall, L., Remington, L., Saenz-Robles, M., Lowe, S., Jacks, T. and Van Dyke, T. (1994). p53-dependent apoptosis suppresses tumor growth and progression in vivo. Cell 78: 703–711

Takaoka, A., Adachi, M., Okuda, H., Sato, S., Yawata, A., Hinoda, Y., Takayama, S., Reed, J. and Imai, K. (1997). Anti cell death activity promotes pulmonary metastasis of melanoma cells. Oncogene 14: 2971–2977

Taplin, M., Bubley, G., Shuster, T., Frantz, M., Spooner, A., Ogata, G., Keer, H. and Balk, S. (1995). Mutation of the androgen-receptor gene in metastatic androgen-independent prostate cancer. N. Engl. J. Med. 332: 1393–1398

Tarin, D., Price, J., Kettlewell, M., Souter, R., Vass, A. and Crossley, B. (1984). Mechanisms of human metastasis studied in patients with peritovenous shunts. Cancer Res. 44: 3584–3592

Tlsty, D. (1998). Cell-adhesion-dependent influences on genomic instability and carcinogenesis. Current Opinion in Cell Biology 10: 647–653

Tsubura, E., Yamashita, T. and Sone, S. (1983). Inhibition of the arrest of hematogenously disseminated tumor cells. Cancer Metastasis Rev. 2: 223–237

Updyke, T. and Nicolson, G. (1986). Malignant melanoma cell lines selected in vitro for increased homotypic adhesion properties have increased experimental metastasis potential. Clin. Exp. Metastasis 4: 273–284

Viney, J. (1995). Transgenic and gene knockout mice in cancer research. Cancer Metastasis Rev. 14: 77–90

Walker, P., Saas, P. and Dietrich, P. (1997). Role of fas ligand (CD95L) in immune escape: the tumor cell strikes back. J. Immunol. 158: 4521–4524

Weinberg, R. (1995). The molecular basis of oncogenes and tumor suppressor genes. Ann. N. Y. Acad. Sci. 758: 331–338

Weinstein, I. B. (1988). The origins of human cancer: molecular mechanisms of carcinogenesis and their implications for cancer prevention and treatment – tenty seventh G. H. A. Clowes memorial award lecture. Cancer Res. 48: 4135–4143

Weinstock, M., Clark, J. and Calabresi, P. (1993). Melanoma. In Medical Oncology, 2nd edition (Eds. Calabresi and Schein), p 545–563. McGraw-Hill, Inc., New York, USA

Weiss, J. M., Sleeman, J. P., Renkl, A. C., Termeer, C., Dittmar, H., Taxis, S., Howells, N., Hofmann, M., Schöpf, E., Ponta, H., Herrlich P. and Simon, J. C. (1997). An essential role for CD44 variant isoforms in epidermal Langerhans cell and blood dendritic cell function. J. Cell Biol. 137: 1137–1147

Weiss, L. (1983). Random and nonrandom processes in metastasis and metastatic efficiency. Invasion Metastasis 3: 193–208

Weiss, L. and Ward, P (1983). Cell detachment and metastasis. Cancer Metastasis Rev. 2: 111–127

Weitz, J., Kienle, P., Lacroix, J., Willeke, F., Benner, A., Lehnert, T., Herfarth, C. and von Knebel Doeberitz, M. (1998). Dissemination of tumor cells in patients undergoing surgery for colorectal cancer. Clin. Cancer Res. 4: 343–348

Willis, R. A. (1975). Metastasis via the lymphatics. In: The spread of tumours in the human body, third edition. Butterworths, London

Yin, X., Grove, L., Dataa, N., Long, M. and Prochownik, E. (1999). C-myc overexpression and p53 loss cooperate to promote genomic instability. Oncogene 18: 1177–1184

Yoshizawa, M., Shingaki, S., Nakajima, T. and Saku, T. (1994). Histopathological study of lymphatic invasion in squamous cell carcinoma (O-1 N) with high potential of lymph node metastasis. Clin. Exp. Metastasis 12: 347–356

Young, R., Perez, C. and Hoskins, W. (1993). Cancer of the ovary. In: Cancer, Principles and Practice of Oncology, Fourth Edition, Eds DeVita, Hellman and Rosenberg, pp 1226–1263. J. B. Lippincott Co., Philadelphia

Zeidman, I. and Buss, J. (1952). Transpulmonary passage of tumor cell emboli. Cancer Res. 12: 731–733

Functional Anatomy of Lymphatic Vessels Under the Aspect of Tumor Invasion

A.-A. Duenne and J. A. Werner

Department of Otolaryngology, Philipps-University, Deutschhausstrasse 3, 35037 Marburg, Germany

Abstract

In the human body there are about 800 lymph nodes, of which 300 are lo-cated in the head and neck area. The lymphatic system begins with initial finger-shaped lymphatic vessels consisting of valveless lymphatic capillaries and precollectors with valves. The precollectors become collectors and trans-port the lymph to the so-called lymph stems. These vessels lead into the right and left lymphatic duct and into the jugular trunk of the head and neck region. At the end they join into the blood circulation at the junction point of the jugular and subclavian veins. On the basis of the morphology of the initial lymphatics, these are probably the main port of entry of tumor cells. Investigations demonstrate the active invasion into the lymphatic sys-tem of melanoma cells. The preference of melanoma cells to adhere to the extracellular fibronectin of the endothelial cells may be a reason for the pri-vileged invasion of the melanoma cells in the lymphatic system, because the extracellular matrix is not protected by a continuous basal lamina like blood vessels. Based on the directed movement of melanoma cells towards the fiber felt, there might be regulative mechanisms influencing the process of tar-geted adhesion.

Structure of the Lymphatic System

In the human body there are about 800 lymph nodes, of which 300 are located in the head and neck area. The lymphatic system begins with initial finger-shaped lymphatic vessels (Fig. 1), which show a wide vascular lumen of 30–50 µm. The system of the initial lymph vessels consists of two sections. First, the valveless lymphatic capillary, and second the precollectors with valves (Fig. 2). In this context the following aspect should be recognized. There is an inadmissible difference between the term "lymphatic capillary" and "capil-laries" in the blood circulation because they differ enormously in morphology

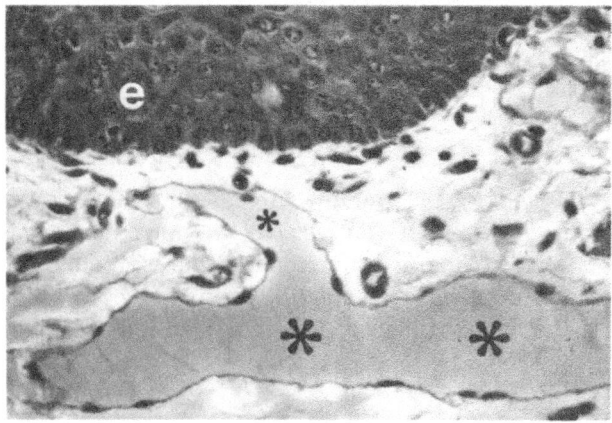

Fig. 1. Just subepithelial located initial lymphatic vessel. The lymphatic system begins with initial finger-shaped lymphatics. The system of the initial lymph vessels consists of two sections: first the valveless lymphatic capillary, and second the precollectors with valves. *, lumen; **e**, epithelium

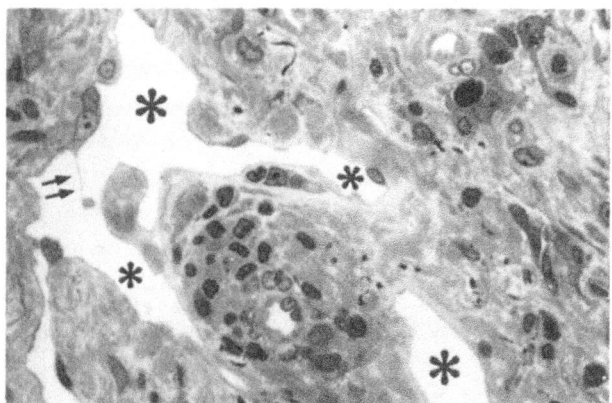

Fig. 2. Precollector with valve (*arrow*). *, lumen; →, valve

and function. The initial lymphatic vessel is able to increase the volume of its contents, compared to the resting stage, to more than fifty-fold. For this reason the term "lymph sinus" seems to be the more correct one, but it isn't well accepted. The precollectors become collectors in the adventitia of hollow viscus, in the capsule of the parenchyma, or at the boundary from dermis to the skin's subcutis. The proximal section between its initial catchment area and the first lymphatic node station is designated as the peripheral collector. The postnodal collector transports the lymph to the so-called lymph stem. These vessels lead into the right and left lymphatic duct and into the jugular trunk of the head and neck region. At the end they join into the blood circulation at the junction point of the jugular and subclavian veins [1, 2].

Morphology of the Lymphatic System

The initial lymphatic wall is made of endothelial cells and an incomplete basal lamina with interendothelial openings. The endothelium is very thin, about 0.1–0.2 µm, and only in areas of the perykaryon will larger dimensions be reached.

The ends of the endothelial cells don't have any contact by interendothelial junctions either (Fig. 3). On the other hand, it is possible that they are connected by means of interendothelial junctions and overlap each other like roofing tiles. In some cases the overlapping ends of the endothelial cells create interlocked complex interdigitations (Fig. 4). These interendothelial junc-

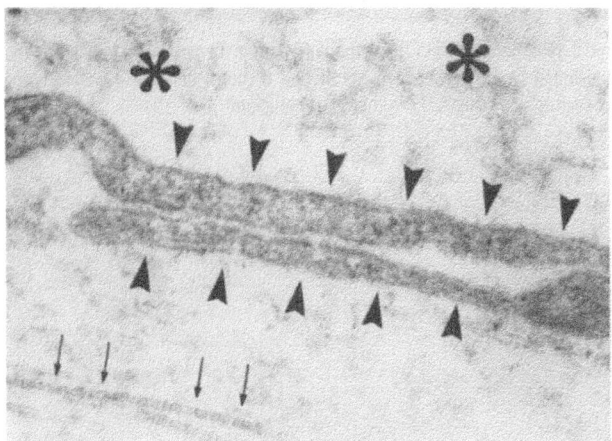

Fig. 3. Connection of the ends of the endothelial cells in the initial lymphatic wall ends of the endothelial cells (-▽-) without any contact by interendothelial junctions. *, lumen; →, collagen fibres

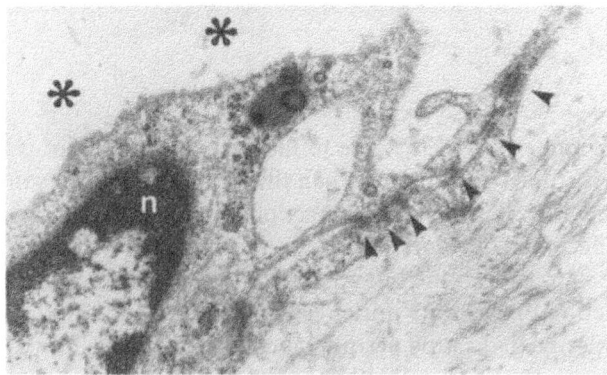

Fig. 4. Connection of the ends of the endothelial cells in the initial lymphatic wall ends of the endothelial cells (-▽-) with connection by interlocked complex interdigitations. These interendothelial junctions work like inflow and outflow valves. *, lumen; n, nucleus

tions work like inflow and outflow valves. In this context it has to be mentioned that the occlusion of side by side plasmatic membranes is usually based on macula densae and rarely on macula occludentes. Several investigations have shown that the interendothelial openings were mostly found in the area of the initial lymphatics and rarely in the section of the precollectors. The possible function of these interdigitations is to create a larger intercellular space between the lumen of the lymphatic vessel and the interstitium for an increased metabolism without a loss of continuity of the endothelial cell layer [3, 11].

In the endothelium of the initial lymphatic vessels of the aerodigestive tract, different ultrastructural features can be distinguished.

Mitochondria are predominantly located in the perinuclear cytoplasm, but occasionally also in the nucleus-distant and thin endothelial regions, as has already been described for the lymphatic vessels of the skin [5]. Furthermore, vesicles, poly and monoribosomes, centrioles, a Golgi apparatus, lysosomes as well as microfilaments running in bundles are found to occur. An actin-like function is ascribed to the cytoplasmic microfilaments that are approximately 4–6 nm thin [5, 17]. In perinuclear cytoplasm, an endoplasmatic reticulum is nearly always regularly detected. It is often more clearly developed in the upper aerodigestive tract than in the other body regions [5, 11]. The strongly developed endoplasmatic reticulum indicates an intensive protein synthesis, a high intracellular substance transport, and a sufficient membrane deposit within the endothelium cells of the lymphatic vessels of the head and neck region. The membrane deposit supplied by the endoplasmatic reticulum finds its expression in the numerous vesicles that are particularly said to have transport functions.

Weibel-Palade bodies cannot be detected in the initial lymphatic vessels [19]. These granula are also missing in the lymphatic vessels of the spleen [7], of the tonsilla palatina [12], of the appendix [10], and of the skin [5]. The lack of Weibel-Palade bodies seems to be an important differential diagnostic criterion to distinguish lymphatic vessels from blood capillaries, in whose endothelium cells these granula are detectable [7]. The differential diagnostic value, however, is called into question by the fact that Weibel-Palade bodies are described in lymphatic vessels of dogs [18] and occasionally in human tissue such as lymphatic vessels of the larynx [13] and in the dental pulp [14]. It cannot be said with certainty at the moment if the detection of endothelial specific granula in the lymphatic vessel endothelium is connected with certain sections of the lymphatic vessels or with functional or pathophysiological conditions, or if the Weibel-Palade bodies occur in such a small number that they are not detectable. So far, the exact origin and function of these granula are not exactly known. Studies indicate a storage function for histamine and the factor VIII-associated antigen [8].

In most cases, the lumen of the initial lymphatic vessels of the upper aerodigestive tract contains a flocculent material of medium electron density (Fig. 5) that has been interpreted as lymph being rich in proteins [5]. The protein content of the lymph is about three times higher than that of the in-

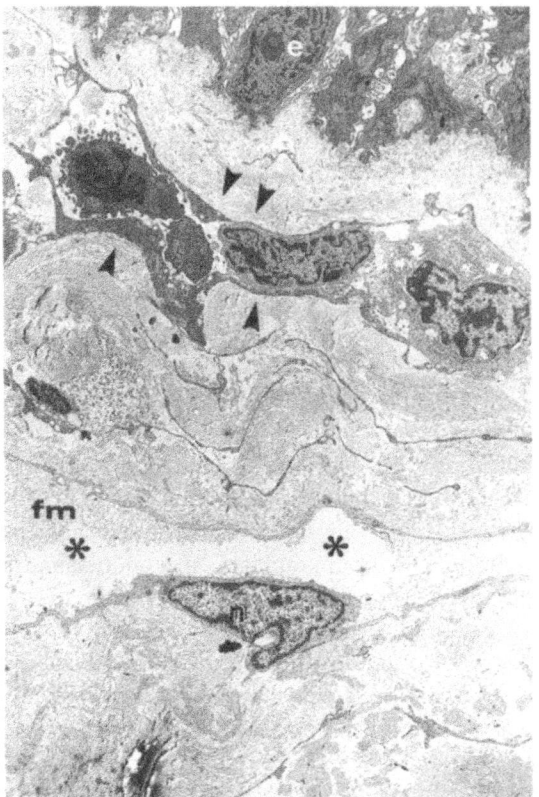

Fig. 5. Electron-microscopic view of part of an initial lymphatic vessel. *, lumen; *fm*, flocculent material; *n*, nucleus; *e*, epithelium; -▽-, blood capillary

terstitial liquid. This is due to the fact that initial lymphatic vessels are able to concentrate liquids. The protein content decreases during the inflow phase and increases during the outflow phase [4].

Furthermore, in contrast to the vessels of the blood circulation, the initial lymphatics are regularly surrounded by an elastic fiber network, the so-called subendothelial fiber felt. They are located near to the endothelial cells of initial lymphatics and it may be possible that the ends of the fibers are an element of the abluminal cell membrane. Because of the missing pericytes in the area of the lymphatic vessels, the different forces, which have an effect on the initial lymphatics, are transmitted to the wall of the lymphatic vessel by the perivascular elastic fiber network. This interaction seems to be very important in the regulation of transendothelial fluid transport and also in cellular migration of lymphocyte.

In contrast to initial lymphatics, the precollectors, the collectors as well the lymphatic stems have valves (Picture 3). The distance among the several valves is about three times to ten times the diameter of the lymphatic vessel.

At the adhering part of the valves, there are intervening layers with thin connective tissues, entering between the endothelial layers to support valves. As lymphatics are swollen a little at the location of valves, they have an appearance like beads on a rosary. There are various forms of valves in lymphatic vessels: bicuspid valves, tricuspid valves, and also quadruspid valves and valves with only one leaflet. They are necessary to prevent backflow of lymph. The direction of the flow from interstitium into the lymphatic system depends on the ratio between the hydrostatic and colloid-osmotic pressure in the different spaces. Furthermore, there are some extrinsic forces like contraction of the surrounding musculature, arterial pulsation, respiratory excursion, and tissue massage, which influence the lymphatic drainage.

The lymphatic collectors consist of three histomorphological layers. The intima contains endothelial cells, delicate collagen fibers, and several smooth muscle cells. The media is made of bundles of smooth muscles in the form of winding screwdrivers or corkscrews. The adventitia consists of longitudinal stripped bundles of connective tissue, network of elastic fibers and a few muscle cells. The lymphatic collectors and also the close-fitting lymph stems are surrounded with a continuous basal lamina [1].

Invasion of Tumor Cells into the Lymphatic System

A direct infiltration of a malignant tumor in the lymph vessel system seems to be possible in every area of the mentioned sections. This fact constitutes a potential port of entry of a direct invasion of tumor cells into the lymphatic vessel system and the following lymphatic nodes. Unfortunately, no detailed investigations exist regarding which area of the lymphatic system is the most common port of entry of tumor cells. On the basis of the morphology of the initial lymphatics this is probably the main port of entry of tumor cells.

Investigations [6, 15], showed that the tumor cells of a malignant melanoma instruct a cytodendrite in the direction to the subendothelial fiber felt. Next, the cytodendrite continues its way and reaches the space between endothelium and subendothelial fiber felt, where it forms a pseudopodia, which is directed to the endothelium. Directly after the contact between the melanoma cell and the endothelial cell, they will fuse at the place of contact and the result will be a filamental bridge. Because of the following destruction of the endothelial cell it's possible for the melanoma cell to find its direct way into the lumen of the lymphatic vessels. The endothelial junctions close to the persisting port of entry and also fragments of the destructed endothelial cells, demonstrates the active invasion into the lymphatic system of melanoma cells [15].

Typically, there are only a few melanoma cells, which invade a centrally located initial lymphatic vessel. It has already been estimated that a clear preference was given to an invasion of the initial lymphatics and not to the precollectors. The reason for this behaviour is the preference of melanoma cells to adhere to the extracellular fibronectin of the endothelial cells. This may be a reason for the privileged invasion of the melanoma cells in the lymphatic system, because the extracellular matrix is not protected by a continuous basal lamina like blood vessels. Because of the directed movement of melanoma cells towards the fiber felt the investigators came to the conclusion that there are regulative mechanisms influencing the process of targeted adhesion [9, 16].

Unfortunately, there are no corresponding investigations of the invasion of squamous cell carcinoma into the lymphatic system which is most common in the upper airway and digestive tract. Although surgical removal of the primary tumor is possible in most cases in the head and neck region based on the high frequency of lymphatic metastasis in this tumor entity, patients with squamous cell carcinoma have a very pure prognosis. It is known that 5-year-survival will be reduced by histologically proved lymph node metastasis around 50%. According to this prognostic the influence of lymph node metastasis illustrates the rank of sufficient therapy in squamous cell carcinoma in the head and neck region. This contains several forms of operating procedures, radiotherapy or their combination. Referring to this the management of clinically diagnosed (ultrasound and CT) N+ neck is less controversial than the management of clinically N0 neck. For this approach, experience with radionuclide-labeled colloid injection to identify the first draining sentinel node in malignant melanoma and breast cancer suggests a high level of accuracy to identify clinically unknown metastasis. Its sensitivity is currently still one of the most current questions in oncology. At the present time only a few publications exist engaging with sentinel node biopsy in squamous cell carcinoma of the head and neck. Based on this, investigations to evaluate more detailed information about efficacy and sensitivity of sentinel node biopsy in squamous cell carcinoma in head and neck region have started. For this approach, detailed knowledge of the anatomy and kinetics of the lymphatic system seems to be the foundation for avoiding pitfalls during sentinel node biopsy in clinical practice. According to the fact that sentinel node biopsy reflects the initial steps of lymphatic metastasis, transmission electron microscopic investigations have been started to describe the behaviour of invasion of squamous cell carcinoma into the lymphatic system.

References

1. Werner J A (1995) Untersuchungen zum Lymphgefäßsystem der oberen Luft- und Speisewege. Shaker, Aachen, pp 1–152
2. Berens von Rautenfeld D, Lüdemann W, Cornelsen H (1996) Die peripheren Lymphgefäße – eine Blackbox der anatomischen Ausbildung – der Versuch eines Kataloges von Mindestanforderungen an Medizinstudenten. In: Tiedjen K U (ed) Lymphologica, Medikon, München, pp 5–10
3. Berens von Rautenfeld D, Castenholz A (1987) Neues zur Form und Funktion der interendothelialen Öffnungen. Verh Anat Ges 81:751–752
4. Casley-Smith J R, Sims M A (1976) Protein concentration in regions with fenestrated and continuous blood capillaries and in the inital and collecting lymphatics. Microvasc Res 12:245–257
5. Daroczy J (1988) The dermal lymphatic capillaries. Springer, Berlin

6. Deutsch A, Lubach D, Nissen S (1992) Untersuchung über die Invasion von Tumorzellen des malignen Melanoms in die dermalen Lymph- und Blutgefäße. In: Berens von Rautenfeld D, Weissleder H (eds) Lymphologica, Kagerer, Bonn, pp 122–125
7. Heusermann U (1979) Morphologie der Lymphgefäße, der Nerven, der Kapsel und der Trabekel der menschlichen Milz. Habilschrift Medical Faculty, University of Kiel, Germany
8. Kagawa H, Fujimoto S (1987) Electron-microscopic and immunocytochemical analyses of Weibel-Palade bodies in the human umbilical vein durig pregnancy. Cell tissue Res 249:557–563
9. Kramer RH, Gonzalez R, Nicolson GL (1980) Metastatic tumor cells adhere preferentially to the extracellular matrix underlying vascular endothelial cells. Int J Cancer 26: 639–645
10. Labusch DM (1988) Das Lymphgefäßsystem des menschlichen Appendix. Enzymhistochemische und elektronenmikroskopische Untersuchungen zum Vorkommen und Verlauf. Medical Dissertation, University of Kiel, Germany
11. Leak LV, Burke JF (1986) Ultrastructural studies on lymphatic anchoring filaments. J Cell Biol 36:129–149
12. Loose R (1987) Das Lymphgefäßsystem der menschlichen Gaumenmandel. Enzym histochemische und elektronenmikroskopische Untersuchungen zum Vorkommen und Verlauf. Medical Dissertation, University of Kiel, Germany
13. Mann W, Beck Chl, Freudenberg N, Leupe M (1981) Der Bestrahlungseffekt auf die Lymphkapillaren des Kehlkopfes. HNO 29:381–387
14. Marchetti C, Poggi P, Calligaro A, Casasco A (1992) Lymphatic vessels in healthy and pulpitic dental pulp. In: Cluzan RV, Pecking AP, Lokiec FM (eds) Progress in lymphology – XIII. Excerpta Medica, Amsterdam, p 59
15. Platschek H, Lubach D, Deutsch A, Nissen S (1990) Transmissionsmikroskopische Untersuchungen über das Verhalten von Lymph- und Blutgefäßen in Melanomexzitaten. In: Baumeister RGH (ed) Lymphologica, Medikon, München, pp 96–97
16. Repesh LA, Fitzgerald TJ (1980) Interactions of tumor cells with intact capillaries: a modell for intravasation. Clin Expl Metastasis 2:139–150
17. Schipp R (1968) Feinbau filamentärer Strukturen im Endothel peripherer Lymphgefäße. Acta Anat 71:341–351
18. Tabuchi H, Yamamoto T (1974) Specific granules in the endothelia of the blood and lymphatic vessels in the cardiac valves of dogs. Arch Histol Jpn 27:217–224
19. Weibel ER, Palade GE (1964) New-cytoplasmatic components arterial endothilia. J Cell Biol 23:101–112

Molecular Diagnosis of Head and Neck Cancer

V. M. M. van Houten[1], M. W. M. van den Brekel[1], F. Denkers[1],
D. R. Colnot[1], J. Westerga[2], P. J. van Diest[2], G. B. Snow[1],
and R. H. Brakenhoff[1]

[1] Department of Otolaryngology–Head and Neck Surgery, Section Tumor Biology,
University Hospital Vrije Universiteit, P.O. Box 7057, 1007MB Amsterdam,
The Netherlands

[2] Department of Pathology, University Hospital Vrije Universiteit, Amsterdam,
The Netherlands

Abstract

Patients with advanced stages of head and neck cancer frequently develop locoregional recurrence as well as distant metastases. These data indicate that
traditional diagnostic methods such as histopathology and radiology are not
sensitive enough to detect the small numbers of tumor cells which are left
behind, defined as minimal residual disease (MRD). Sensitive diagnostic assays based on molecular markers appear to be powerful tools to improve the
staging of these patients. At the DNA level, tumor-specific p53 mutations
seem to have great potential for the detection of "occult" tumor cells at surgical margins and lymph nodes. At the RNA level HNSCC associated antigens like the E48 antigen, allow the detection of rare HNSCC cells in blood
and bone marrow and, it is hoped, also in lymph nodes and lymph node aspirates. However, the molecular assays which are used to detect MRD are
subject to certain (technical) problems which affect their sensitivity and
specificity. In this paper we will present examples of molecular assays such
as the plaque assay using p53 mutations and the E48 RT-PCR, and show
their use for MRD detection in cervical lymph nodes. In addition, we will
discuss the problems and pitfalls associated with these sensitive techniques.

Introduction

Head and Neck Cancer

Head and neck squamous cell carcinoma (HNSCC) are the main histologic
type of tumors of the upper aerodigestive tract. It accounts for approximately
5% of all newly diagnosed malignant tumors in Western Europe and the
United States. Annually there are approximately 500 000 new cases of HNSCC
worldwide, and in 1995 over 1800 cases in the Netherlands alone (Parkin
1988; Vokes 1993; Boring 1994; Netherlands Cancer Registry 1998). HNSCC

Recent Results in Cancer Research, Vol. 157
© Springer-Verlag Berlin · Heidelberg 2000

patients can be divided into four different clinical stages I–IV, according to the TNM classification of the International Union Against Cancer (UICC). In this classification system patients are grouped according to their tumor size and presence of lymph node or distant metastases. In general patients with stages I or II have a relatively good prognosis as they can often be cured with single modality treatment, i.e., surgery or radiotherapy. Patients with the more advanced stages III and IV are treated with combined surgery and radiotherapy. Despite advances in these treatments, these patients have a rather poor prognosis with a high incidence of locoregional recurrence and distant metastases.

Inaccurate Diagnosis of HNSCC

Local Relapse

Clinical studies provide statistical evidence that 40%–50% of the patients with resectable advanced tumors develop local recurrence, despite improvements in therapy. This failure in treatment results in part from a failure in diagnosis. This is illustrated by the fact that in approximately 15%–30% of the stage III and IV patients with histopathologically tumor-free resection margins a local recurrence develops (Leemans et al. 1994). These clinical data indicate that routine histopathology is not sensitive enough to detect the small tumor deposits that eventually develop into a recurrence (Brennan et al. 1995). These undetectable tumor cells have been defined as minimal residual disease (MRD) (Hermanek 1993; Pantel et al. 1996).

Distant Metastases

In addition to local relapse, about 15%–25% of the HNSCC patients with advanced tumor stages develop distant metastases after treatment (most commonly in the lungs, liver and skeletal system) (Hong et al. 1985; Zbaren and Lehmann 1987; Cerezo et al. 1992; Leemans et al. 1993). Like local relapses, distant relapses occur in patients who had no evidence of distant metastases at the time of locoregional therapy, again indicating that the current methods of staging have a limited sensitivity in detecting small disseminated tumor deposits. For example, spiral computed tomography (CT) of the thorax and liver or bone scintigraphy can nowadays detect distant lesions of approximately 1 cm in diameter. Currently, no curative treatment options are available for these patients.

Regional Recurrence – the N0 Neck

A particular staging problem with regard to treatment planning is the assessment of the clinically N0 neck. Routinely, the neck is staged by palpation and, if necessary, by various imaging modalities such as CT or magnetic resonance imaging (MRI). However, these staging modalities are not very accurate for the assessment of the N0 neck. Physical examination by palpation is known to be an inaccurate staging method, because both its false positive rate and false negative rate are unsatisfactorily high (Sako et al. 1964; Ali et al.; Van den Brekel et al. 1993). CT and MRI have in recent years proven to be more reliable than palpation but are still insufficient in detecting small metastases (Van den Brekel et al. 1991). Currently, the most reliable staging method for the N0 neck is Ultrasound-guided Fine Needle Aspiration Cytology (USgFNAC) (Van den Brekel et al. 1993; Van den Brekel and Snow 1994). Using this technique the lymph nodes are visualized and under ultrasound guidance aspirated by a needle. From the aspirate, cytological slides are prepared and screened by routine methods. When the cytology is negative, at our hospital we refrain from neck-dissection and a wait-and-see policy is preferred. However, Van den Brekel et al. (1999) recently showed that even with USgFNAC in some patients the staging of the neck is false negative. They retrospectively analyzed the clinical outcome of 77 HNSCC patients in whom USgFNAC had been used as initial staging method of the neck. In 14 out of 77 cases (18%) a recurrence occurred during follow-up, whereas the neck had initially been diagnosed as negative on the basis of USgFNAC.

Theoretically, false negative observations with USgFNAC result from three specific problems: (1) aspiration of the wrong node; (2) sampling error in the aspirate; (3) false negative cytological diagnosis. The first problem might be overcome by using the concept of the sentinel node (SN) (Cabanas 1977; Morton et al. 1992; Giuliano et al. 1994). The SN is the first draining lymph node in a particular lymphatic region (e.g., the cervical lymph node region) to which a tumor in that area drains. This SN will most likely be the first lymph node to receive metastatic tumor cells and if it is selectively sampled and diagnosed as free of tumor, other lymphatic metastases will most likely not exist. In a large group of breast cancer patients, Veronesi et al. (1997) showed that selective biopsy of the SN correctly predicted the status of the axillary lymph nodes in 97.5% of the cases. The second problem, sampling error, is caused by the fact that only part of the lymph node is aspirated. In theory, it can be overcome when the SN procedure for the staging of the N0 neck has shown to be a relevant, reliable and routinely applicable procedure. Excision of the SN and accurate examination will reduce the sampling error to almost zero. Finally, the sensitivity of the USgFNAC procedure might be further improved by increasing the tumor cell detection rate in the aspirate. The presence of a small number of tumor cells might be missed by routine cytology. As described, a similar problem is faced with the histopathological examination of the resection margins.

Molecular Detection of MRD2

DNA Markers

The limitations of the current diagnostic modalities triggered the development of novel technologies which are based on the molecular detection of tumor cells. These techniques are all based on the use of specific tissue or tumor markers, either at the DNA level or at the RNA/protein level (RNA/protein markers, see below). Cancer develops as a result of the accumulation of mutations and other changes in the DNA (Fearon and Vogelstein 1990; Califano et al. 1996). Some of these changes occur in specific genes which play a crucial role in the normal behavior of the cell. Other changes appear in less crucial sequences and are a reflection of the genetic instability of the tumors. Examples of DNA markers which can be exploited as tumor markers are: (1) alterations in DNA repeat sequences, known as microsatellites (Weber and May 1989; Mao et al. 1996; Steiner et al. 1997); and (2) specific mutations in oncogenes and tumor suppressor genes (Sidransky et al. 1991; Brennan et al. 1995).

Microsatellites represent a highly polymorphic class of genetic elements within the human genome, consisting of small DNA repeat sequences. PCR amplification of these repeats allows a distinction between the maternal and paternal alleles. During neoplastic transformation the cells often acquire specific alterations in these microsatellites, which can be detected in the DNA of a tumor by comparing it to the normal DNA of a patient (usually isolated from blood lymphocytes). In this way microsatellite analysis of tumor DNA can reveal loss of an allele (loss of heterozygosity, LOH) or the presence of a new allele (microsatellite instability) (Sidransky 1997). Microsatellite analysis has emerged as a relatively easy and inexpensive method for cancer detection and has been widely used for the detection of genetic alterations in various cancer types, including HNSCC (Field et al. 1995; González et al. 1995; Linn et al. 1997; Mao et al. 1996; Partridge et al. 1997; Piccinin et al. 1998). In a number of studies these changes in the tumor DNA have been exploited as marker (Boyle et al. 1994; Nawroz et al. 1996; Steiner et al. 1997). However, the sensitivity of the microsatellite technique is rather low and as a result this method seems less suitable for MRD detection.

More sensitive assays have been developed using mutations in oncogenes and tumor suppressor genes as markers. Alterations of the tumor suppressor gene p53 are the most common genetic events in human tumors, including head and neck cancer and they play an important role in the pathogenesis of HNSCC (Hollstein et al. 1991; Field 1992; Boyle et al. 1993; Greenblatt et al. 1994; Pellegata and Ranzani 1996; Raybaud-Diogene et al. 1996). Based on a genetic analysis of mucosal lesions with apparent progressive histopathological appearance, Califano et al. (1996) presented a genetic progression model for HNSCC in which p53 plays an important role. According to their model, which is supported by other investigations, p53 inactivation or mutation occurs in the transition from the early preinvasive (hyperplastic) state to the invasive state (Pavelic et al. 1994; Sauter et al. 1994; Califano et al. 1996). The role of p53 in this progression model favors its use as a molecular marker for cancer staging, as explained by Brennan and Sidransky (1996): p53 mutations are closely associated with tumor development, p53 mutations precede the stage of invasive cancer, and they are retained during clonal outgrowth. The additional observation that p53 mutations occur in a relatively large percentage (about 50%) of all HNSCC patients makes this a very suitable marker for tumor cell detection (Sakai and Tsuchida 1992; Greenblatt et al. 1994). Brennan et al. (1995) described a method (the plaque assay) in which they use p53 mutations as marker for the detection of MRD in surgical margins and lymph nodes in a pilot group of HNSCC patients. We have implemented and developed this method further for the molecular diagnosis of a large group of HNSCC patients.

Tumor Cell Detection on the Basis of p53 Point Mutations

Tumor cell detection on the basis of point mutations in the p53 gene is relatively complex. First, the presence of a mutation in the p53 gene is determined. For this purpose tumor DNA is isolated from microdissected cryosections. Subsequently, a fragment of the p53 gene is amplified by the polymerase chain reaction (PCR), using the tumor DNA as template. By PCR the initial minute amounts of DNA template are exponentially amplified as follows: initial template DNA is denatured at 95°; subsequently two short, single-stranded oligonucleotides (primers) anneal to their complementary sequences on the single-stranded template DNA. A thermostable DNA polymerase elongates the primers in both directions, using nucleotides present in the reaction mixture. By performing several successive cycles of denaturation, primer annealing and elongation in a thermal cycler, the minute amounts of initial DNA will increase exponentially. Subsequently, the amplified DNA is sequenced.

Based on the mutation found in the DNA of the primary tumor, an oligonucleotide identical to the mutated sequence is synthesized as well as an oligonucleotide corresponding to the wild type sequence on that position. These oligonucleotides can be labeled and used as probes for the detection of either mutant (tumor cell) DNA or wild type DNA, respectively.

From the samples of interest (resection margins and/or lymph nodes) DNA is extracted, the p53 gene amplified, and cloned in lambda phage vectors. After transduction to a bacterial host strain and overnight incubation, the phages infect and lyse the bacteria which results in plaques (after plating on agar). Each individual plaque consists of identical phages, derived from either a mutant or a wild type p53 strand. As a consequence, every plaque represents a single mutant or wild type DNA strand in the original mixture. These plaques are then transferred to nitrocellulose membranes and subsequently identified by differential hybridization with the tumor-specific (mutant) and wild type oligonucleotides as probes. Tumor DNA of the patient and wild type DNA are included as positive and negative controls, respectively. The percentage of mutant DNA in a tissue sample (resection margin/ lymph node) is calculated by dividing the number of hybridized mutant plaques by the number of hybridized wild type plaques. When a positive signal is observed, the assay is confirmed by stabbing the particular plaques out of the agar, replating of the phages, and rehybridization with the same mutant-specific probe. With this technique it is possible to detect a single tumor cell in 1000–10 000 normal cells, indicating that it is a rather sensitive and quantitative technique. However, there are a number of drawbacks as well. First of all, this technique can only be applied to HNSCC patients who have a p53 mutation in their primary tumor (approximately 50% of the patients). This problem might be overcome when other HNSCC tumor-specific gene alterations are discovered and could be exploited in addition to p53 mutations. Second, the plaque assay is a very laborious technique and it takes at least one week to perform all the analyses. Finally, as is the case with all sensitive assays, the plaque assay is prone to false positivity. This and other problems with sensitive techniques are further discussed below in "Problems and Pitfalls".

Patient Example

Here we describe the molecular analysis of an HNSCC patient's primary tumor and lymph nodes with the plaque assay. Patient 97–40 is a 59-year-old male with a history of a T1N0M0 SCC of the left lateral tongue, for which a resection of the primary tumor in combination with a unilateral selective neck dissection (levels I and IIa) was performed elsewhere. One year later he developed a local recurrence and surgical resection in combination with a left modified comprehensive neck dissection of the remaining levels (IIb, III–V) was carried out, followed by postoperative radiotherapy. From this patient we obtained a tumor sample, 5 histopathologically tumor-free surgical margins and a total of 7 histopathologically tumor-free lymph nodes (A–G) (sliced at intervals or, if too small, divided into half by the pathologist). Duplicate margins and one section of the lymph nodes were used for routine histopathological examination and the other parts for molecular analysis. Again, by histopathological examination the resection margins as well as the lymph nodes were diagnosed as tumor-free.

Sequencing of the primary tumor DNA revealed a p53 mutation, shown in Table 1 and corresponding Fig. 1.

Based on this mutation, oligonucleotides identical to the mutated and corresponding wild type sequences were synthesized (Table 2).

Table 1. p53 gene mutation identified in the primary tumor of patient 97–40

Patient no.	Exon	Codon	Nucleotide change	Amino acid change
97–40	8	282	CGG → TGG	Arg → Trp

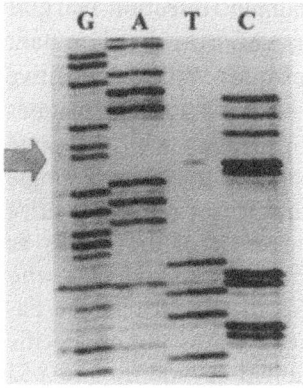

Fig. 1. Autoradiograph of sequencing analysis of DNA from the primary tumor of patient 97–40. The *lanes* represent G, A, T, and C of exon 8. To facilitate the identification of mutations, 3 patients are run in parallel, where each *2nd lane* corresponds to the DNA of patient 97–40. For the tumor in this patient a point mutation, consisting of a C → T base substitution at codon 282 (changing arginine to tryptophane) is evident (*arrow*)

Table 2. Wild type and mutant oligonucleotides selected for patient 97–40 for differential hybridization

Patient no.	Wild type oligonucleotide	Mutant oligonucleotide
97–40	5'-GGAGAGACCGGCGCACA-3'	5'-GGAGAGACTGGCGCACA-3'

Table 3. Molecular analysis of lymph nodes in patient 97–40

Patient no.	Lymph-node no.	Level	Number of mu plaques screened	Number of pos plaques with mutant-specific probing	Percentage of mutant clones (%)
97–40	A	2	900	1	0.11
	B	3	1360	0	0
	C	3	1220	1	0.08
	D	4	1000	1	0.1
	E	5	1410	1	0.07
	F	5	920	2	0.22
	G	5	500	1	0.2

Subsequently, the plaque assay was used to perform molecular analysis on the 7 lymph nodes. In all but one of the histopathologically negative lymph nodes tumor cell DNA was detected with the plaque assay, showing percentages of mutant clones ranging from 0.07% to 0.22%. Each positive plaque was confirmed by replating and rehybridizing. Details of the lymph node analysis are shown in Table 3 and Fig. 2.

The patient's 5 histopathologically negative margins were analyzed similarly and 3 margins were also positive for mutant DNA (data not shown).

Notwithstanding the apparent MRD in this patient, he is alive, 2 years after treatment, without signs of recurrence. The combined treatment of

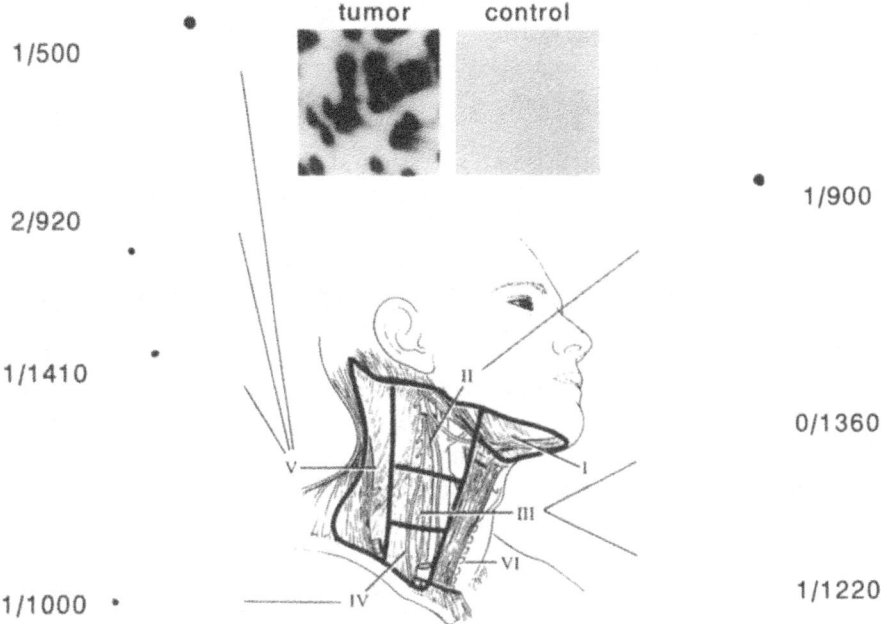

1/500

tumor   control

1/900

2/920

1/1410

0/1360

1/1000

1/1220

Fig. 2. Plaque assay on lymph nodes of patient 97–40. Insets show autoradiographs of the lymph nodes from various levels, which are differentially hybridized with the mutant-specific oligonucleotide. The assay was positive in 6/7 histopathologically negative lymph nodes of this patient, as can be seen from the *black dots*, which are hybridizing plaques. Exact data on this patient are shown in Table 3

tumor resection, comprehensive neck dissection and postoperative radiotherapy appears to have prevented locoregional recurrence effectively.

RNA/Protein Markers

In addition to alterations in DNA, changes in gene expression measured at the mRNA or protein level have also proved to be valuable tools for detection of disseminated tumor cells. Although RNA, because of its rapid degradation, is more difficult to manage as substrate for clinical diagnosis than DNA, it has equal value in distinguishing differences between cell types. Tumor cell detection at the mRNA or protein level is based on a differential expression of cellular genes as markers. Obviously, when applying these markers for the detection of residual tumor cells in particular tissues it is a prerequisite that the particular mRNA or protein is not expressed by the cells of that tissue. As an example squamous tumor cells can be detected in non-squamous/non-epithelial tissues such as blood and bone marrow. Nowadays many mRNA/protein markers have been described as being more or less restrictedly expressed by tumor cells in certain tissues. Two methods are widely being used at the moment to detect these markers: immunocytochemistry (ICC) and reverse transcriptase PCR (RT-PCR).

Immunocytochemistry

ICC detects tumor-associated gene expression at the protein level and relies on monoclonal antibodies (MAbs) against tumor-associated antigens. Most MAbs used for epithelial tumor cell detection are directed against cytokeratins (CKs) or membrane-bound glycopolypeptides. ICC has been applied in several studies to detect rare tumor cells in lymph nodes and bone marrow from patients with a variety of cancers, including cancers of the lung and esophagus (van den Brekel et al. 1992; Pelkey et al. 1996; Izbicki et al. 1997; Pantel and Ahr 1998) and HNSCC (Wollenberg et al. 1994; Gath et al. 1995). The majority of these studies show that once a tissue-specific antigen and a selective high affinity MAb recognizing this antigen have been selected, ICC is a reliable and sensitive method to detect disseminated tumor cells in bone marrow. Some limitations of ICC, when applied for tumor cell detection in bone marrow, are that the technique is quite laborious and that results are sometimes difficult to interpret because of unwanted background staining of hematopoietic cells (Nadji and Morales 1986; Borgen 1998). Therefore, attention has shifted towards the use of RNA instead of protein, using an alternative method: RT-PCR.

RT-PCR

The RT-PCR technique is at present widely used for the detection of disseminated tumor cells because of its relative rapidness and its alleged sensitivity (Pelkey et al. 1996). In short, the RT-PCR technique can be explained as follows: first, the mRNA, extracted from cells or tissue is converted to cDNA by the enzyme reverse transcriptase; the cDNA is subsequently amplified by PCR, using a sense and antisense primer; the presence of the amplified product can be identified by gel electrophoresis and ethidium bromide staining, or by Southern blotting and hybridization. The selected primers in combination with the cycle protocol and the detection method for amplimer visualization determine the sensitivity of the method. Again, these sensitive (RT)-PCR techniques suffer from a number of problems, which will be discussed in "Problems and Pitfalls".

In our group we have explored the selective expression of the E48 antigen on squamous tissues for the molecular detection of rare tumor cells in blood, bone marrow, and lymph nodes of HNSCC patients. Based on the E48 cDNA and gene sequences encoding the E48 antigen, an RT-PCR assay was developed (Brakenhoff et al. 1997). After extensive optimization with reconstruction experiments in blood we were able to reproducibly detect a single tumor cell in 7 ml of blood (approximately 2×10^7 white blood cells), indicating that it is a very sensitive technique as compared to conventional microscopy, cytology or ICC (Brakenhoff et al. 1999). However, in spite of its sensitivity, the E48 RT-PCR assay is not suitable for the detection of rare tumor cells in resection margins of HNSCC patients, because these contain normal squamous cells which also express the E48 antigen. Currently we are further optimizing the E48 RT-PCR assay to make it suitable for the detection of rare squamous tumor cells in lymph nodes of HNSCC patients. However, initial experiments have shown that in normal lymph nodes E48 antigen expression can also be detected, probably due to the presence of epithelial elements in lymph nodes expressing the antigen. This kind of "unwanted" expression is seen more often (see below), and markers which are really tumor- or tissue-specific are very rare. A very interesting family in this respect is the MAGE (melanoma antigen-encoding gene) family of antigens. These antigens are only expressed in tumors, but not in normal tissues, with the exception of testis and placenta (Coulie et al. 1993; De Plaen et al. 1994; Weynants et al. 1994; Eura et al. 1995). A drawback of these markers is that they show a more heterogeneous expression pattern, thereby influencing sensitivity of the assays for different tumors.

In general, it can be concluded that we are in fact at the beginning of nucleic acid-based detection, and due to its relatively low costs and putative high sensitivity, we expect increasingly more applications in regular health care, including tumor cell diagnosis in lymph nodes.

Problems and Pitfalls

Specificity (False Positivity)

General

Despite all the advantages of the described (RT-)PCR-based techniques for employment in MRD detection, these techniques are subject to certain (technical) problems, which could cause false positive results. This false positivity arises in general from the enormous sensitivity of the PCR reaction in amplifying not only target material, but also undesired contamination, even if the latter consists only of minute amounts of DNA or amplimers derived from prior PCR reactions. Contamination can be introduced at different time points in the procedure: either during sampling of the material by the clinician or the pathologist or during the technical processing of the material in the laboratory.

To reduce the risk of tumor cell contamination in our margin and lymph node samples to an absolute minimum, precautions are taken in the operating theatre and pathology department. The sampling of the resection margins is performed only after extensive rinsing of the operating field, and when gloves and surgical instruments have been changed. For the preparation of the lymph nodes by the pathologist, also several precautions are taken. First, the lymph nodes are dissected before a tumor sample is taken, second, the scalpel is decontaminated in 0.1 M HCl and PBS to prevent cell or DNA contamination and obviously, the working area is kept tumor cell free as much as possible.

To decrease the risk of contamination during the processing of the samples in the laboratory, the DNA is isolated directly from the snap-frozen material without cutting cryosections in order to prevent contamination with previously sectioned tumor material via the cryostat microtome. Contamination by DNA products from prior PCR reactions (amplimers), can be reduced and controlled by stringent measures, including performing PCR reactions in a separate laboratory room, maintaining clean reaction reagents and always checking for possible contamination with the use of proper negative control reactions.

DNA Markers: Taq Errors

A cause of false positivity which is specific for DNA-based assays using point mutations as marker is caused by the fact that the enzyme mostly used to replicate the DNA strands, Taq polymerase, introduces spontaneous replication errors in the amplification reaction in the range of 1 in 10 000. Because this rate is in the order of the numbers of mutant plaques we also find in HNSCC patients' resection margins and lymph nodes, screened with the plaque assay (1/1000–1/10 000), we cannot initially exclude that these mutants are caused by Taq errors. Therefore, when only a single margin is positive, the complete assay is repeated with a high fidelity polymerase, which causes less errors. As these enzymes are very expensive, not all assays are performed with this enzyme. In addition, the rate of false positivity in our assay is determined by screening large numbers of plaques which contain the p53 insert, with oligonucleotides which differ only one nucleotide from the wild type and mutant sequence at a particular position. Preliminary data suggest that these replication errors play a role in frequencies of 1/100 000. Obviously, this figure depends on the used enzyme and reaction conditions.

RNA/Protein Markers: Unwanted Expression

Apart from general contamination, "false positivity" in RT-PCR reactions can occur due to the expression of a tumor-associated marker by a small number of cells in that tissue. Besides specific expression, many cells show illegitimate, physiologically irrelevant expression of a large number of genes, which causes specificity problems in many applications (Zippelius et al. 1997). An example of this limitation of the use of RT-PCR in MRD detection has already been given when we described that the E48 RT-PCR cannot easily be used for MRD detection in lymph nodes, as they appear to contain "epithelial-like" cells which express E48 mRNA (see above). For some markers these limitations of the RT-PCR approach can be overcome if the amplification protocol of the transcribed cDNA is adapted. Liefers et al. (1998) showed how they used an adapted RT-PCR cycling program to detect micrometastases in lymph nodes of colorectal cancer patients, using carcino-embryonic

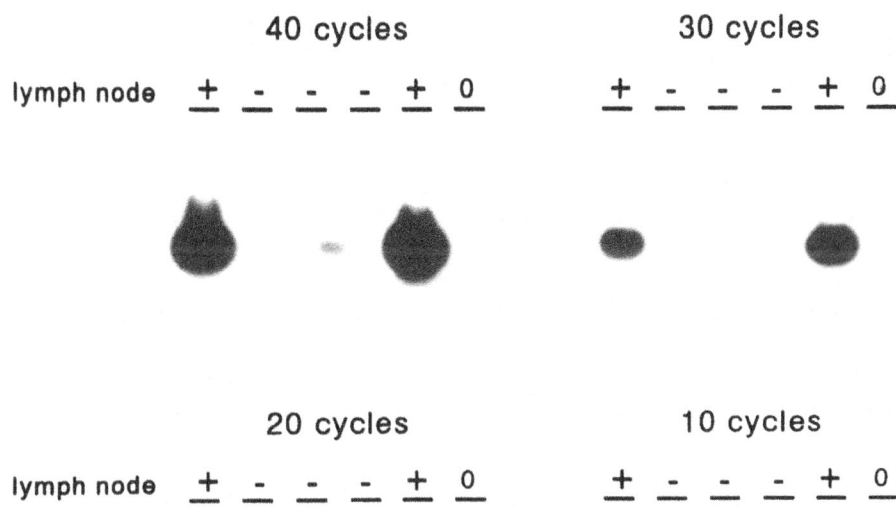

Fig. 3. Optimization of E48 RT-PCR on lymph nodes of HNSCC patients. For detailed description see text

antigen (CEA) mRNA expression as marker. By decreasing the number of cycles they could reduce the background level, and still detect clinically relevant data. A similar approach was followed by us. In an initial experiment we applied E48 RT-PCR on lymph nodes of HNSCC patients. In total we used four lymph nodes, three of which were negative according to both histopathology and molecular diagnosis, and one which was positive. We used 10, 20, 30 and 40 cycles of PCR respectively. With 40 cycles we observed unwanted positive signal in 1/3 negative nodes, probably due to the fact that cervical lymph nodes contain squamous (non-tumor) cells that express E48. When we performed 10 or 20 cycles instead, we obtained no signal at all from the positive node. Thirty cycles of PCR gave optimal results as is shown in Fig. 3. Future experiments have to show whether this adapted E48 RT-PCR protocol is suitable for reliable detection of MRD in lymph nodes of HNSCC patients.

Sensitivity

Another crucial issue that is faced in MRD detection is the problem of sensitivity. At this moment the clinical significance of sensitive detection of MRD with molecular techniques is not always clear: these techniques might either be not sensitive enough or in contrast, detect tumor loads which are not clinically relevant. The presence of low numbers of tumor cells appears to imply the eventual appearance of recurrent disease, but this is not necessarily true.

Detection limits of the E48 RT-PCR were established with reconstruction experiments, in which defined numbers of tumor cells were seeded in blood.

As mentioned before we were able to detect a single tumor cell in 7 ml of blood (approximately 2×10^7 white blood cells). The detection limit of E48 RT PCR in lymph nodes has not yet been determined. Detection limits for the plaque assay were reported to be approximately 1 tumor cell in 10^4 normal cells in surgical margins and lymph nodes (Brennan et al. 1995). Preliminary data in our lab show approximately the same figures, ranging from a single tumor cell in 10^3–10^4 normal cells. Moreover, it should be realized that the sensitivity of the plaque assay is in fact solely dependent on the numbers of plaques that are screened. If, for example, a million plaques are screened, the sensitivity might be 1/1 000 000. Obviously, the frequency of false positive signal due to Taq errors will increase accordingly.

The question concerning the clinically required sensitivity can only be answered if quantitative analyses in large studies, in combination with (long-term) follow-up have been completed. Following the clinical outcome, we can, if necessary, adapt our sensitivity limits of screening. Ideally, to gain insight into the clinically required sensitivity of MRD detection, patients should be studied for whom particular clinical interventions such as elective neck-dissection or postoperative radiotherapy is not performed and for whom a so-called wait-and-see policy is followed. This might provide insight into the clinical relevance of the presence of MRD, as detected by these sensitive techniques. For example, the detection of MRD in resection margins of patients treated only by tumor excision and no further therapy will demonstrate the clinical relevance with long-term follow-up. Similarly, in patients with a clinically N0 neck, molecular analysis of ultrasound-guided aspirates of the sentinel node might reveal small numbers of tumor cells. A wait-and-see policy is also still followed for these patients at this stage.

Conclusions and Future Perspectives

In conclusion, sensitive molecular techniques seem promising to close the gap between the current histopathological and radiological staging of HNSCC patients, and their clinical outcome. It should also be realized however, that these assays are complex and prone to misinterpretation. Moreover, most molecular techniques are still quite laborious. However, recent technological advances in PCR and sequencing will reduce the time needed to perform molecular analysis. Recently two machines have become available, the Light Cycler (Boehringer Mannheim, Almere, The Netherlands), which can process samples for (RT)PCR in less than 30 min, and the Affymetrix (Affymetrix, Santa Clara, CA 95051, USA), which can be used for rapid sequencing of p53 and other genes. These improvements in technology will be crucial to implement these assays in the clinic.

Another problem with molecular techniques is that suitable molecular markers are not always available yet. However, as more and more markers become available for head and neck cancer, and the techniques improve to identify and isolate single tumor cells from tissues, these limitations might be overcome in the future.

Finally, the major limitation of molecular staging at the moment is probably the fact that the clinical implication of sensitive molecular techniques has not yet been proven in large trials. Except for studies using immunocyto-chemical staining, the studies are usually small. Nevertheless, prospective clinical trials are underway to evaluate the predictive value of molecular staging, with respect to the clinical outcome of HNSCC patients. Once its predictive value has been established, molecular techniques might find acceptance in the clinic for improved staging and more individualized treatment of HNSCC patients.

Acknowledgements. We thank Dr. David Sidransky (Johns Hopkins University School of Medicine, Department of Otolaryngology-Head and Neck Surgery, Baltimore, USA) for his support and advice to implement the molecular assays.

References

1. Ali S, Tiwari RM and Snow GB (1985) False positive and false negative neck nodes. Head & Neck Surgery 8:78–82
2. Borgen E, Beiske K, Trachsel S, Nesland JM, Kvalheim G, Herstad TK, Schlichting E, Qvist H and Naume B (1998) Immunocytochemical detection of isolated epithelial cells in bone marrow: non-specific staining and contribution by plasma cells directly reactive to alkaline phosphatase. Journal of Pathology 185(4):427–434
3. Boring CC, Squires TS, Tong T and Montgomery S (1994) Cancer statistics, 1994. CA: a Cancer Journal for Clinicians 44(1):7–26
4. Boyle JO, Hakim J, Koch W, van der Riet P, Hruban RH, Roa RA, Correo R, Eby YJ, Ruppert JM and Sidransky D (1993) The incidence of p53 mutations increases with progression of head and neck cancer. Cancer Research 53(19):4477–4480
5. Brakenhoff RH, van Dijk M, Rood-Knippels EM and Snow GB (1997) A gain of novel tissue specificity in the human Ly-6 gene E48. Journal of Immunology 159(10):4879–4886
6. Brakenhoff RH, Stroomer JGW, ten Brink C, de Bree R, Weima SM, Snow GB and van Dongen GAMS (1999) Sensitive detection of squamous cells in bone marrow and blood of head and neck cancer patients by E48 reverse transcriptase polymerase chain reaction. Clinical Cancer Research *In press*
7. Brennan JA, Mao L, Hruban RH, Boyle JO, Eby YJ, Koch WM, Goodman SN and Sidransky D (1995) Molecular assessment of histopathological staging in squamous-cell carcinoma of the head and neck. New England Journal of Medicine 332(7):429–435
8. Brennan JA and Sidransky D (1996) Molecular staging of head and neck squamous carcinoma. Cancer & Metastasis Reviews 15(1):3–10
9. Cabanas RM (1977) An approach for the treatment of penile carcinoma. Cancer 39(2):456–466
10. Califano J, van der Riet P, Westra W, Nawroz H, Clayman G, Piantadosi S, Corio R, Lee D, Greenberg B, Koch W and Sidransky D (1996) Genetic progression model for head and neck cancer: implications for field cancerization. Cancer Research 56(11):2488–2492
11. Cerezo L, Millan I, Torre A, Aragon G and Otero J (1992) Prognostic factors for survival and tumor control in cervical lymph node metastases from head and neck cancer. A multivariate study of 492 cases. Cancer 69(5):1224–1234

12. Coulie PG, Weynants P, Lehmann F, Herman J, Brichard V, Wolfel T, van Pel A, de Plaen E, Brasseur F and Boon T (1993) Genes encoding for tumor antigens recognized by human cytolytic T lymphocytes. Journal of Immunotherapy 14(2):104–109

13. De Plaen E, Arden K, Traversari C, Gaforio JJ, Szikora JP, De Smet C, Brasseur F, van der Bruggen P, Lethe B, Lurquin C et al. (1994) Structure, chromosomal localization, and expression of 12 genes of the MAGE family. Immunogenetics 40(5):360–369

14. Eura M, Ogi K, Chikamatsu K, Lee KD, Nakano K, Masuyama K, Itoh K and Ishikawa T (1995) Expression of the MAGE gene family in human head and neck squamous cell carcinomas. International Journal of Cancer 64(5):304–308

15. Fearon ER and Vogelstein B (1990) A genetic model for colorectal tumorigenesis. Cell 61(5):759–767

16. Field JK (1992) Oncogenes and tumour-suppressor genes in squamous cell carcinoma of the head and neck. European Journal of Cancer Part B, Oral Oncology 28B(1):67–76

17. Field JK, Kiaris H, Howard P, Vaughan ED, Spandidos DA and Jones AS (1995) Microsatellite instability in squamous cell carcinoma of the head and neck. British Journal of Cancer 71(5):1065–1069

18. Gath HJ, Heissler E, Hell B, Bier J, Riethmuller G and Pantel K (1995) Immunocytologic detection of isolated tumor cells in bone marrow of patients with squamous cell carcinomas of the head and neck region. International Journal of Oral & Maxillofacial Surgery 24(5):351–355

19. González MV, Pello MF, López-Larrea C, Suárez C, Menéndez MJ and Coto E (1995) Loss of heterozygosity and mutation analysis of the p16 (9p21) and p53 (17p13) genes in squamous cell carcinoma of the head and neck. Clinical Cancer Research 1:1043–1049

20. Greenblatt MS, Bennett WP, Hollstein M and Harris CC (1994) Mutations in the p53 tumor suppressor gene: clues to cancer etiology and molecular pathogenesis. Cancer Research 54(18):4855–4878

21. Giuliano AE, Kirgan DM, Guenther JM and Morton DL (1997) Lymphatic mapping and sentinel lymphadenectomy for breast cancer. Annals of Surgery 220(3):391–401

22. Hermanek P (1993) TNM Supplement 1993. Geneva, International Union Against Cancer. Heidelberg: Springer Verlag, 1993

23. Hollstein M, Sidransky D, Vogelstein B and Harris CC (1991) p53 Mutations in human cancer. Science 253(5015):49–53

24. Hong WK, Bromer RH, Amato DA, Shapshay S, Vincent M, Vaughan C, Willett B, Katz A, Welch J, Fofonoff S et al. (1985) Patterns of relapse in locally advanced head and neck cancer patients who achieved complete remission after combined modality therapy. Cancer 56(6):1242–1245

25. Izbicki JR, Hosch SB, Pichlmeier U, Rehders A, Busch C, Niendorf A, Passlick B, Broelsch CE and Pantel K (1997) Prognostic value of immunohistochemically identifiable tumor cells in lymph nodes of patients with completely resected esophageal cancer. New England Journal of Medicine 337(17):1188–1194

26. Leemans CR, Tiwari R, Nauta JJ, van der Waal I and Snow GB (1993) Regional lymph node involvement and its significance in the development of distant metastases in head and neck carcinoma. Cancer 71(2):452–456

27. Leemans CR, Tiwari R, Nauta JJ, van der Waal I and Snow GB (1994) Recurrence at the primary site in head and neck cancer and the significance of neck lymph node metastases as a prognostic factor. Cancer 73(1):187–190

28. Liefers GJ, Cleton-Jansen AM, van de Velde CJ, Hermans J, van Krieken JH, Cornelisse CJ and Tollenaar RA (1998) Micrometastases and survival in stage II colorectal cancer. New England Journal of Medicine 339(4):223–228

29. Linn JF, Lango M, Halachmi S, Schoenberg MP and Sidransky D (1997) Microsatellite analysis and telomerase activity in archived tissue and urine samples of bladder cancer patients. International Journal of Cancer 74(6):625–629

30. Mao L, Schoenberg MP, Scicchitano M, Erozan YS, Merlo A, Schwab D and Sidransky D (1996) Molecular detection of primary bladder cancer by microsatellite analysis. Science 271(5249):659–662

31. Morton DL, Wen DR, Wong JH, Economou JS, Cagle LA, Storm FK, Foshag LJ and Cochran AJ (1992) Technical details of intraoperative lymphatic mapping for early stage melanoma. Archives of Surgery 127(4):392–399

32. Nadji M and Morales AR (1986) Immunoperoxidase Techniques: A practical approach to tumor diagnosis. American Society of Clinical Pathologists, Chicago

33. Nawroz H, Koch W, Anker P, Stroun M and Sidransky D (1996) Microsatellite alterations in serum DNA of head and neck cancer patients. Nature Medicine 2(9):1035–1037

34. Netherlands Cancer Registry (1998) Head and neck tumours in the Netherlands 1989–1995. Visser O, Coebergh JWW, Otter R, and Schouten LJ (eds.). Utrecht: Association of comprehensive cancer centres

35. Pantel K and Ahr A (1998) Immunocytochemical and molecular strategies for the detection of micrometastases in patients with solid epithelial tumours – a review. Nuclear Medicine Communications 19(6):521–527

36. Pantel K, Braun S, Passlick B and Schlimok G (1996) Minimal residual epithelial cancer: diagnostic approaches and prognostic relevance. Progress in Histochemistry & Cytochemistry 30(3):1–60

37. Parkin DM, Laara E and Muir CS (1988) Estimates of the worldwide frequency of sixteen major cancers in 1980. International Journal of Cancer 41(2):184–197

38. Partridge M, Emilion G, Pateromichelakis S, Phillips E and Langdon J (1997) Field cancerisation of the oral cavity: comparison of the spectrum of molecular alterations in cases presenting with both dysplastic and malignant lesions. Oral Oncology 33(5):332–337

39. Pavelic ZP, Li YQ, Stambrook PJ, McDonald JS, Munck-Wikland E, Pavelic K, Dacic S, Danilovic Z, Pavelic L, Mugge RE et al. (1994) Overexpression of p53 protein is common in premalignant head and neck lesions. Anticancer Research 14(5B):2259–2266

40. Pelkey TJ, Frierson HF Jr and Bruns DE (1996) Molecular and immunological detection of circulating tumor cells and micrometastases from solid tumors. Clinical Chemistry 42(9):1369–1381

41. Pellegata NS and Ranzani GN (1996) The significance of p53 mutations in human cancers. European Journal of Histochemistry 40(4):273–282

42. Piccinin S, Gasparotto D, Vukosavljevic T, Barzan L, Sulfaro S, Maestro R and Boiocchi M (1998) Microsatellite instability in squamous cell carcinomas of the head and neck related to field cancerization phenomena. British Journal of Cancer 78(9):1147–1151

43. Raybaud-Diogene H, Tetu B, Morency R, Fortin A and Monteil RA (1996) p53 overexpression in head and neck squamous cell carcinoma: review of the literature. European Journal of Cancer Part B, Oral Oncology 32B(3):143–149

44. Sakai E and Tsuchida N (1992) Most human squamous cell carcinomas in the oral cavity contain mutated p53 tumor-suppressor genes. Oncogene 7(5):927–933

45. Sako K, Pradier RN, Marchetta FC and Pickren JW (1964) Fallibility of palpation in the diagnosis of metastases to cervical nodes. Surgery Gynecology & Obstetrics 118:989–990

46. Sauter ER, Cleveland D, Trock B, Ridge JA and Klein-Szanto AJ (1994) P53 is overexpressed in fifty percent of pre-invasive lesions of head and neck epithelium. Carcinogenesis 15(10):2269–2274

47. Sidransky D, Von Eschenbach A, Tsai YC, Jones P, Summerhayes I, Marshall F, Paul M, Green P, Hamilton SR, Frost P and Vogelstein B (1991) Identification of p53 gene mutations in bladder cancers and urine samples. Science 252(5006):706–709

48. Sidransky D (1997) Nucleic acid-based methods for the detection of cancer. Science 278(5340):1054–1059

49. Somers KD, Merrick MA, Lopez ME, Incognito LS, Schechter GL and Casey G (1992) Frequent p53 mutations in head and neck cancer. Cancer Research 52(21):5997–6000

50. Steiner G, Schoenberg MP, Linn JF, Mao L and Sidransky D (1997) Detection of bladder cancer recurrence by microsatellite analysis of urine. Nature Medicine 3(6):621–624

51. Van den Brekel MWM, Stel HV, van der Valk P, van der Waal I, Meyer CJ and Snow GB (1992). Micrometastases from squamous cell carcinoma in neck dissection specimens. European Archives of Oto-Rhino-Laryngology. 249 (6):349–353.

52. Van den Brekel MW, Castelijns JA, Stel HV, Golding, RP, Meyer CJ and Snow GB (1993) Modern imaging techniques and ultrasound-guided aspiration cytology for the assessment of neck node metastases: a prospective comparative study. European Archives of Oto-Rhino-Laryngology 250(1):11–17

53. Van den Brekel MW and Snow GB (1994) Assessment of lymph node metastases in the neck. European Journal of Cancer Part B, Oral Oncology 30B(2):88–92

54. Van den Brekel MW, Castelijns JA, Reitsma LC, Leemans CR, Van der Waal I and Snow GB (1999) Outcome of observing the No neck using ultrasound guided cytology for follow up. Archives of Otolaryngology-Head & Neck Surgery 125:153–156

55. Veronesi U, Paganelli G, Galimberti V, Viale G, Zurrida S, Bedoni M, Costa A, de Cicco C, Geraghty JG, Luini A, Sacchini V and Veronesi P (1997) Sentinel-node biopsy to avoid axillary dissection in breast cancer with clinically negative lymph nodes. Lancet 349(9069):1864–1867

56. Vokes EE, Weichselbaum RR, Lippman SM and Hong WK (1993) Head and neck cancer. New England Journal of Medicine 328(3):184–194

57. Weber JL and May PE (1989) Abundant class of human dna polymorphisms which can be typed using the polymerase chain reaction. American Journal of Human Genetics 44(3):388–396

58. Weynants P, Lethe B, Brasseur F, Marchand M and Boon T (1994) Expression of MAGE genes by non-small-cell lung carcinomas. International Journal of Cancer 56(6):826–829

59. Wollenberg B, Ollesch A, Maag K, Funke I and Wilmes E (1994) Micrometastases in bone marrow of patients with cancers in the head and neck area. Laryngo-Rhino-Otologie 73(2):88–93

60. Zbären P and Lehmann W (1987) Frequency and sites of distant metastases in head and neck squamous cell carcinoma. An analysis of 101 cases at autopsy. Archives of Otolaryngology – Head & Neck Surgery 113(7):762–764

61. Zippelius A, Kufer P, Honold G, Kollermann MW, Oberneder R, Schlimok G, Riethmuller G and Pantel K (1997) Limitations of reverse-transcriptase polymerase chain reaction analyses for detection of micrometastatic epithelial cancer cells in bone marrow. Journal of Clinical Oncology 15(7):2701–2708

III. Principles of Lymphatic Mapping and Sentinel Node Detection

The Concept of the Sentinel Lymph Node

R. M. Cabanas

Attending Surgeon, Victory Memorial Hospital, Beth Israel Hospital North Division, Long Island Medical College Hospital, 1725 York Ave. 33 F. N.Y.N.Y. 10128 USA

Abstract

Lymphangiograms performed via direct cannulation of lymphatic ducts demonstrate drainage of the lymph into a specific lymph node center, the so-called SLN. Contrast materials such as lipiodol, injected directly into the tissue (e.g., tongue) can demonstrate the SLN. As the neoplastic cells can be carried through the lymphatic ducts, the SLN is the first filter in the lymphatic pathway, and the SLN is indeed the most likely regional node to harbor metastatic carcinoma. The results of these efforts challenged the surgical community worldwide to recognize the importance of the concept of SLN. This concept needs to be inexpensive and easily applied in daily practice. Recently, brilliant investigators have found that using "blue dye" and or radioactive tracers are a resourceful way in identifying SLN and have applied the benefits in their daily practice. Morton [15] using the "blue dye" and Krag [1] using radioactive tracers are pioneers in the application of these concepts in other malignant diseases. The SLN concept today is feasible to apply in the investigation, diagnosis, staging and treatment of almost all solid tumors in human pathology. Numerous elegant reports have proved the validation of the concept [2, 7–9, 11, 12, 16, 17, 20, 21, 26–28].

Introduction

Routine or prophylactic lymphoadenectomies performed, as a part of oncological surgical treatment, is potentially a source of morbidity that includes seromas or chylous fistula, scar formation, infection, numbness, nerve injury, lymphedema, restricted regional mobility, and cosmetics alterations. When the lymphatic nodes are positive for metastases, surgery fills its purpose of staging and treatment, but when it is negative for metastasis surgery is unnecessary for therapy although useful for staging. Almost everybody agrees that in human solid cancer the status of the regional lymph node is a prognostic factor for survival as well as for adjuvant therapy. In the surgical treatment of penile carcinoma we have been analyzing this therapeutic dilemma during many years [3, 4]. Therefore, twenty-two years ago, I proposed an approach for the treatment of penile carcinoma. I had studied lymphangiograms, anatomic dissections, and microscopic reports of one hundred patients in detail for eight years, including eighty cases of penile carcinomas, ten inflammatory diseases of the penis, and ten normal volunteers in whom lymphangiography was performed via the dorsal lymphatics of the penis. The basic concept derived was that the lymphatic system of the penis drains into one or a group of nodes, the "sentinel lymph node" (SLN), that appeared to be the primary site of metastases for penile carcinoma [3–5]. The SLN is the first lymph node that receives primary lymphatic fluids and neoplastic cells draining from the lesion, within the regional lymph nodes basin prior to its subsequent spread to other lymph nodes. The analysis of two hundred cases of lymphangiograms in malignant melanomas of the extremities, testicular, vulvar, anal, head and neck, breast, and cervix carcinomas also promulgate the existence of sentinel lymph node [3]. As a matter of fact, any anatomical location has a specific SLN, a potential primary site of metastasis (e.g., stomach, colon, scrotum, prostate). If the localization, excision, and pathologic evaluation of the SLN are feasible (biopsy of the SLN) we can identify patients in whom, by minimizing the approach, we can maximize the diagnosis. With minimal surgery we can maximize the local nodal control.

The purpose of this article is to review the basic studies and the anatomical findings of the past in order to demonstrate evidence of the existence of the specific lymph center, the so-called SLN [3, 4].

Anatomic Considerations

The classic teaching has always been that when a neoplastic lesion is found in the heel, the posterior portion of the sole of the foot, or in the posterior surface of the leg, and if this tumor tends to produce lymph node metastasis, then these metastases should occur in the popliteal lymph nodes.

We have studied the popliteal lymph nodes by means of lymphoadenography (LAG) performed on patients with lesions in the region, which normally drains into these nodes.

After the skin was cleaned and sterile drapes were placed, 1–2 ml of patent blue or one percent methylene blue were injected with 0.5 ml of one percent procaine in the lateral retromalleolar portion of the heel area. A 2 cm longitudinal incision was made behind the malleolus over the ankle. Upon opening the skin and subcutaneous tissues, the stained lymphatic channels with their blue color could be seen and freed. These were catheterized, and the contrast material was slowly injected.

The contrast material ascends in the deep lymphatic system between the muscle layers and opens into the popliteal lymph nodes; this represents the SLN for these lesions (Fig. 1 A, B) [3, 14].

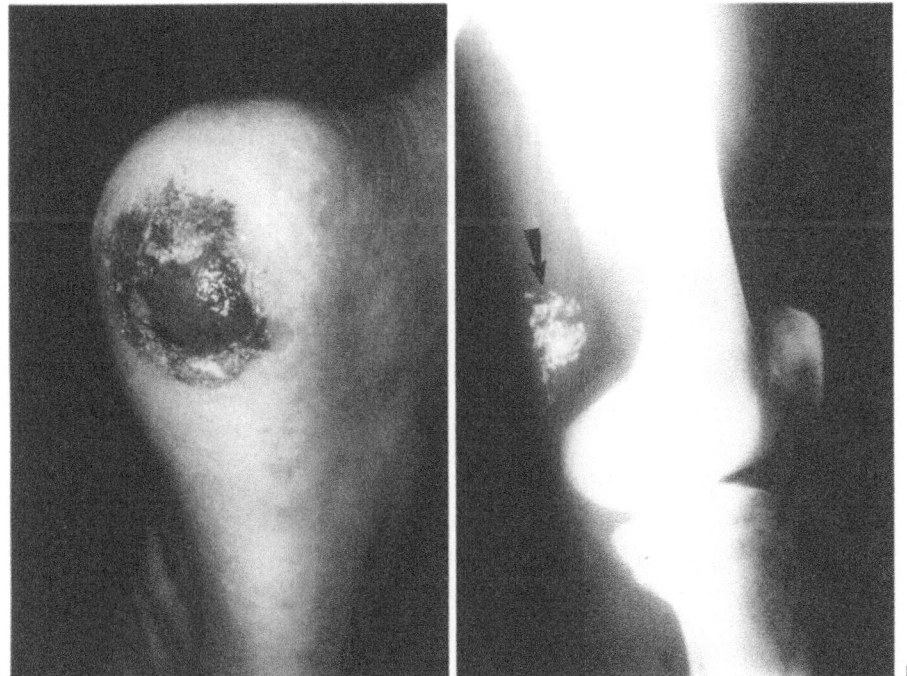

Fig. 1. a Malignant melanoma of the heel. **b** Invasion of the SLN (propliteal lymph node)

When LAG is performed to study the lymphatic pathway of the testis by direct cannulation, the lymphatic vessels drain to a specific lymph center (SLN) located closely to the aorta, vena cava as well as renal pedicle. On the left side the lymphatic channels drain into a lymph node located between vertebral body off L_1 and L_3 (Fig. 2 A–D) [3, 6, 19, 22].

There are accessory lymphatic ducts that drain into a lymph node located at the level of the bifurcation of the external iliac and hypogastric artery, close to where the urether crosses over the hypogastric artery [23]. Anatomically these SLN are located over the lateral and anterior aspect of the vena cava, aorta, and in relation with the spermatic arteries as well as the inferior border of both renal veins [3, 19, 22].

Lesions of the hands have been studied injecting Ethyodol through lymphatic ducts of the dorsal aspect of the hand, and the SLN for the lesion depicted in Fig. 3 A is located in the epitrochlear area (Fig. 3 B).

Retro auricular lymphangiograms disclosed SLN of lesions located in the scalp, head, as well as upper neck lesions. In the same manner, direct injection of ultrafluids lipiodol (iodized oil) into the tongue visualizes the SLN of the area (Fig. 4 A, B).

Cancer of the vulva similarly metastasized to the SLN located in the inguinal area (Fig. 5 A, B).

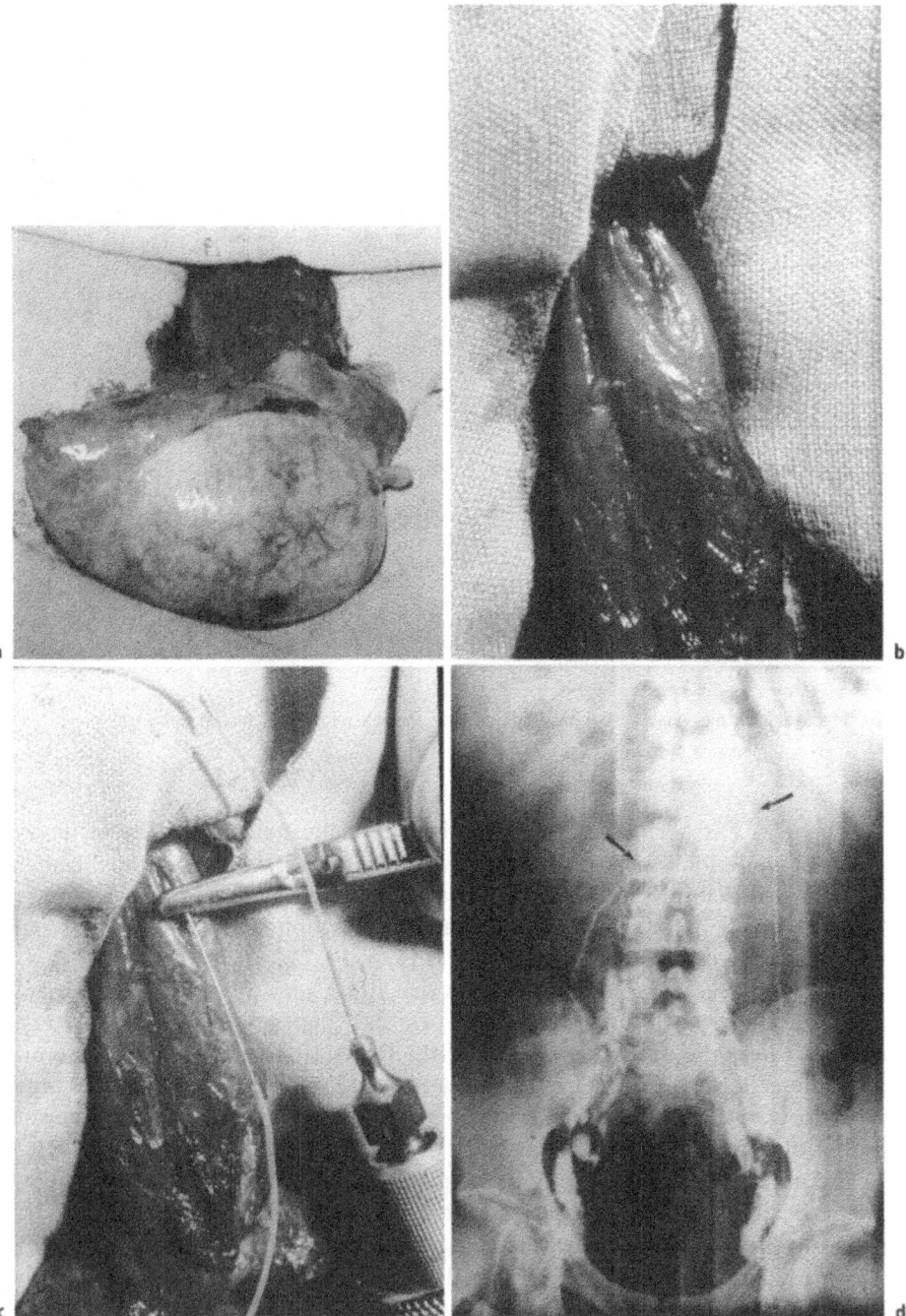

Fig. 2. a Testicular injection of Evans blue (sub-albuginea). **b** Dissection-isolation of the lymphatic duct in the spermatic cord – inguinal canal. **c** Cannulation of lymphatic duct. **d** *Arrows* indicate SLN on each side. Other opacified lymph nodes have been injected through lymphatic ducts via dorsalis pedis

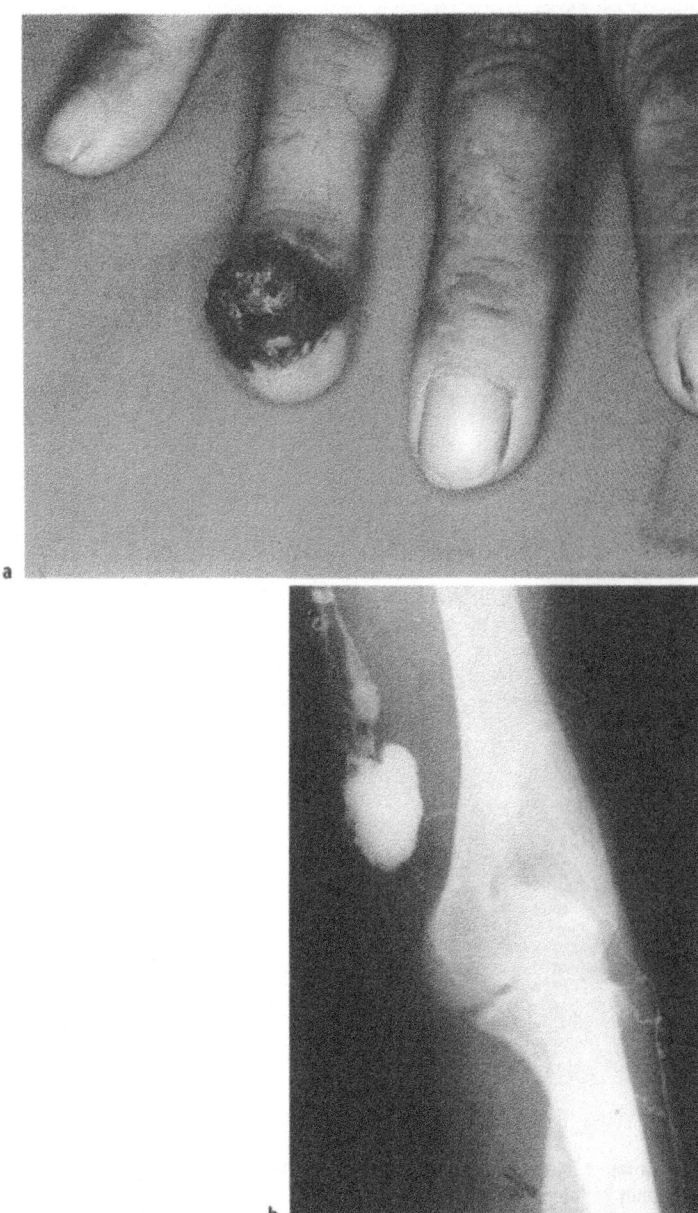

Fig. 3. a Malignant melanoma. **b** Lymphangiogram of elbow region taken after injection of radioopaque medium showing the SLN of the Epitrochlear Area

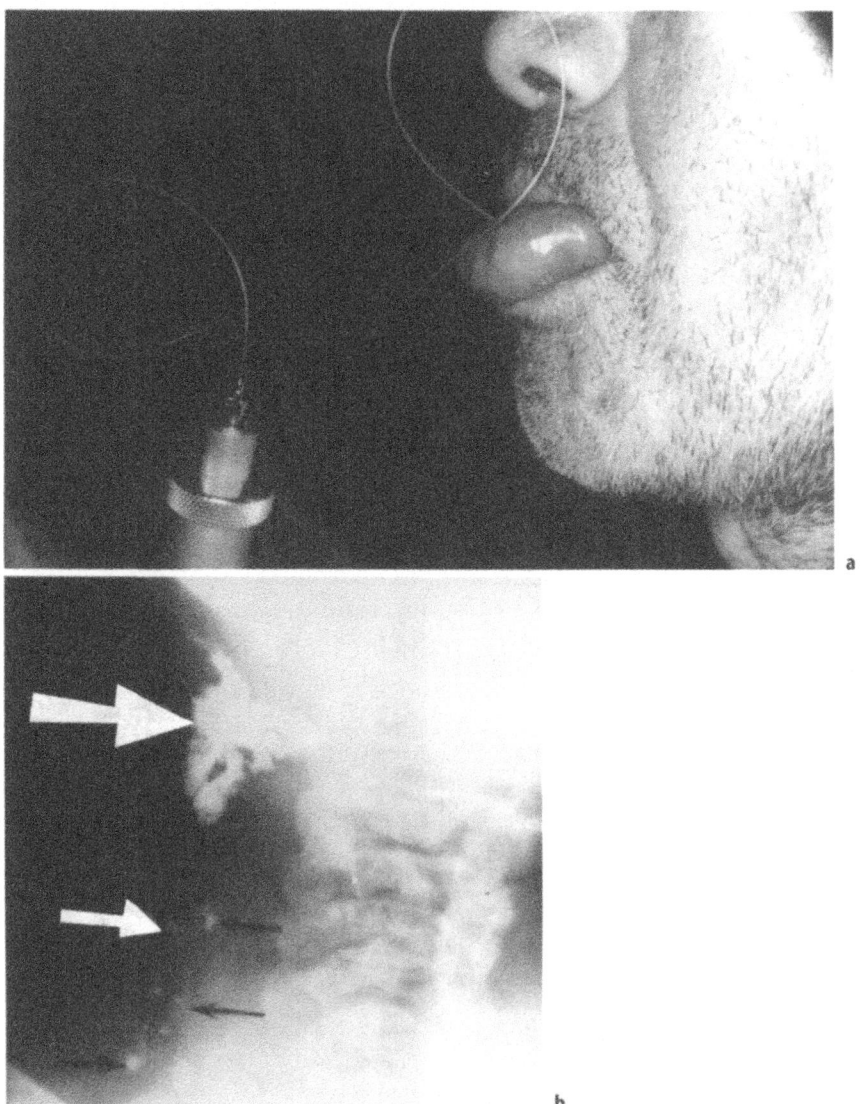

Fig. 4. a Direct injection in the tongue helps visualize the SLN. **b** *White superior arrows* visualize the SLN. Radiography of the neck

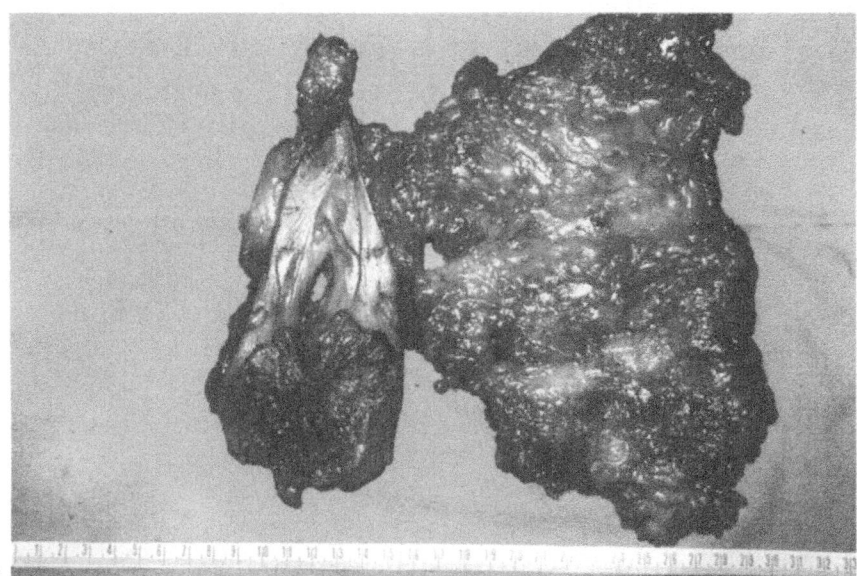

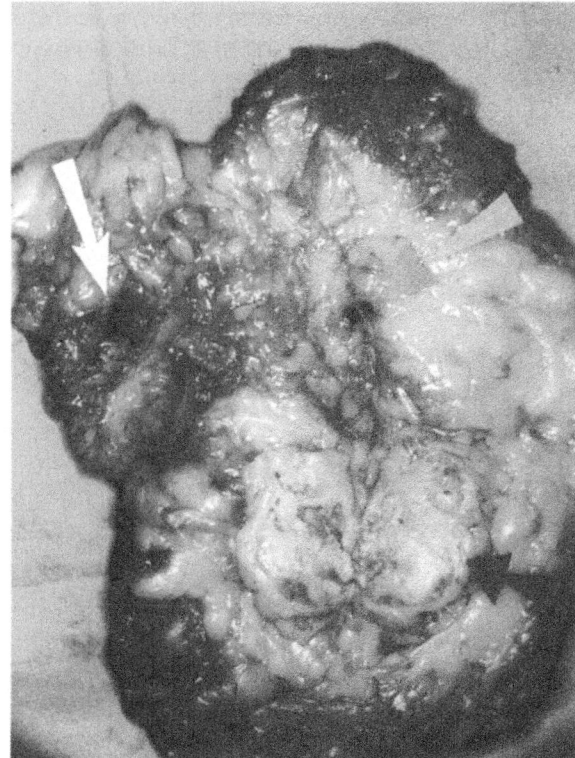

Fig. 5. a Cancer of the vulva. Surgical specimen of total vulvectomy and left groin radical lymph node dissection. **b** Same surgical specimen as 5 a. *Dark arrows* indicate SLN. *Superior arrows* indicate lymph nodes free of metastasis

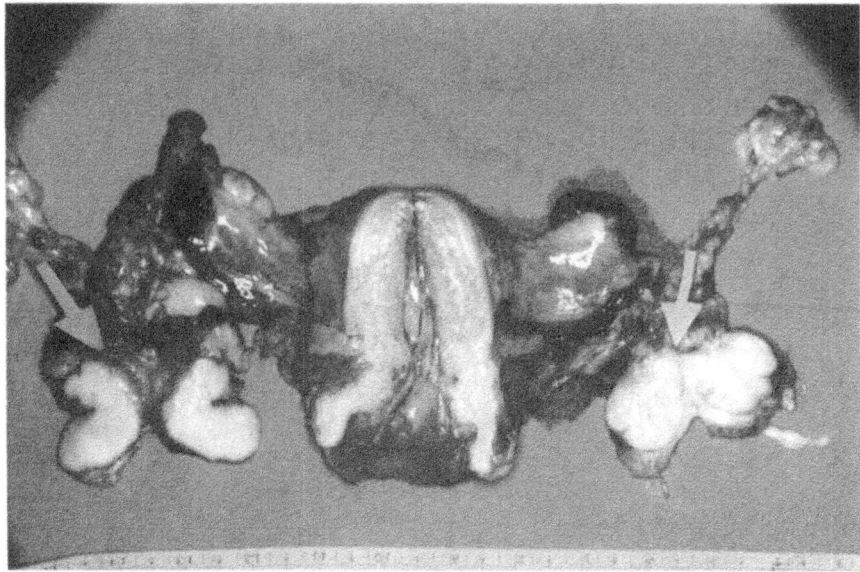

Fig. 6. Cervix carcinoma: metastasis to SLN. Both sides are attached to the obturator nerve (Leveuf, Godard) or close to the urether and cervix (Championere). *Arrows* indicate SLN invasion on each side

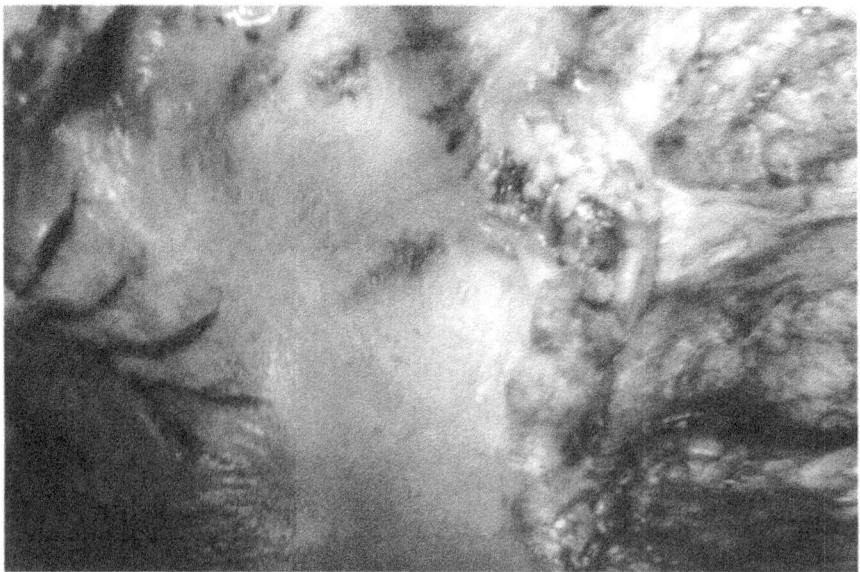

Fig. 7. Subserorsal injection of vital dye into the stomach demonstrates the "blue" SLN

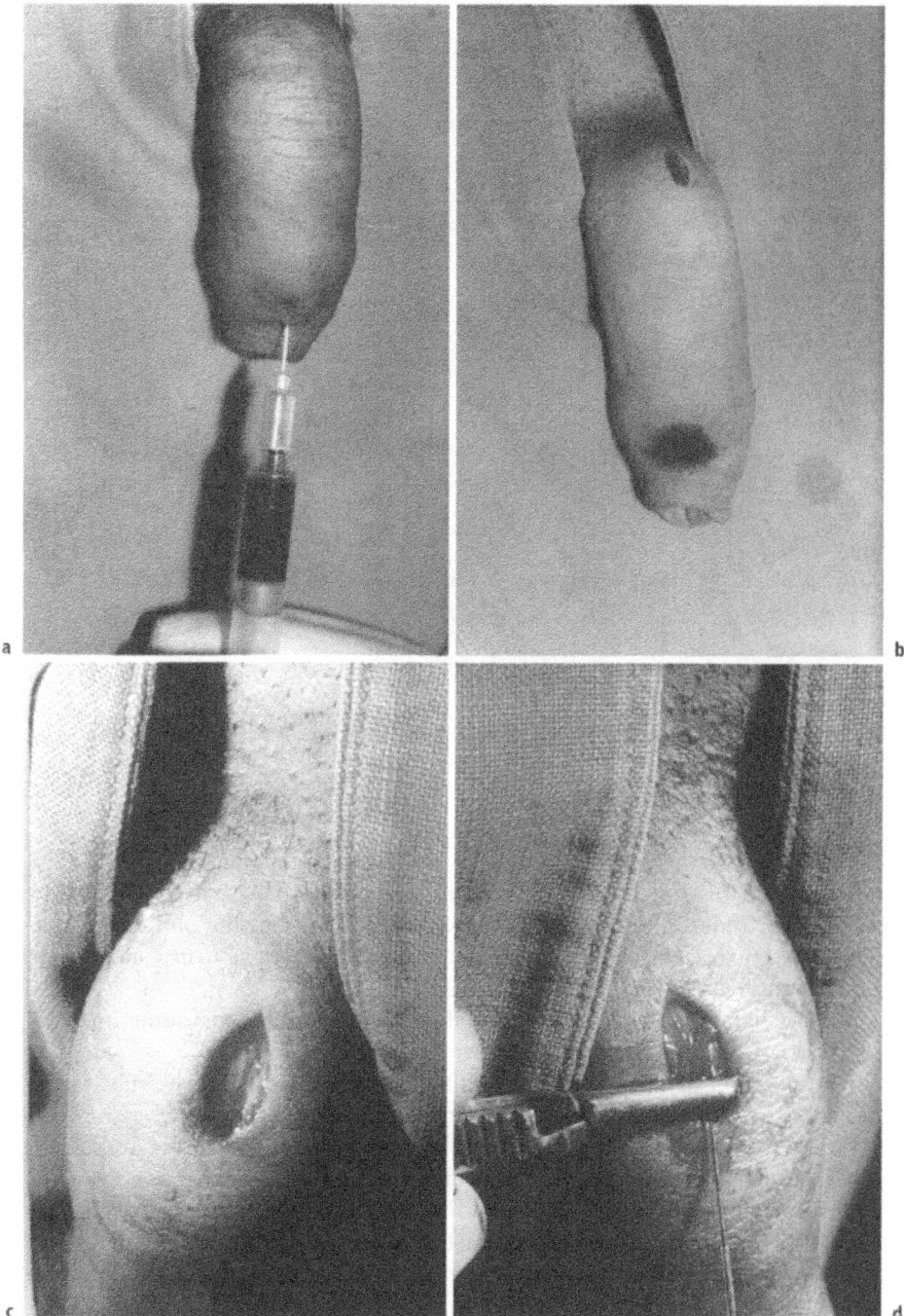

Fig. 8. a Injection of 1% solution of methylene blue (0.5 cc) with 0.5 cc of procaine 1% solution into the dorsal aspect of the prepuce. **b** One cm longitudinal incision is made, that discloses the stained lymph vessel. **c** Identification and isolation of the lymphatic vessel. **d** Cannulation of the Lymphatic vessel

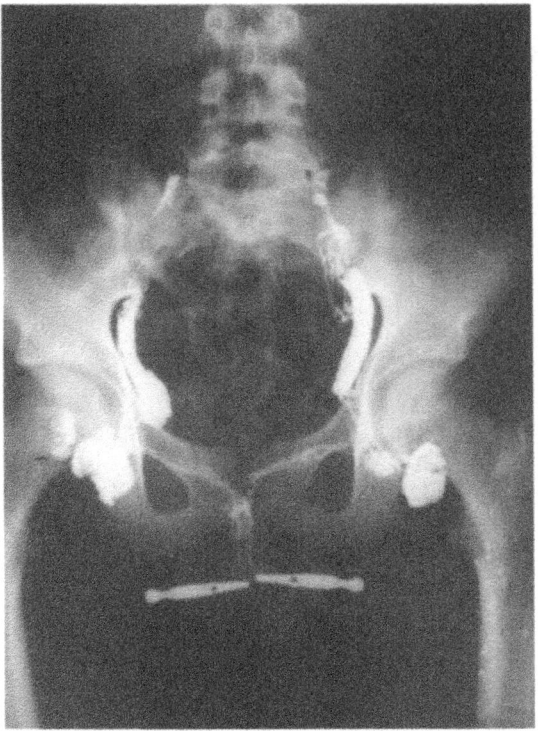

Fig. 9. Lymphangiograms taken at the end of the injection shows the draining lymphatic system of the penis

Cervix carcinoma metastasized to the "principal" lymph node (SLN) located close to the obturator nerve in the minor pelvis, as described by Leveuf and Godard, is adjacent to the external border of the obliterated umbilical artery, in front of the origin of the uterine artery, and in contact with the obturator nerve (Fig. 6) [3, 10, 18, 24].

Lucas Championniere has described a small lymph node sometimes located close to the cervix and the ureter [25].

The injection of methylene blue into the wall of the stomach (subserosal) indicates the blue lymph node of the area (Fig. 7).

If the LAG is carried out via dorsal lymph vessels of the penis, the drainage is into a lymph node frequently located in the anterior or medial aspect of the superficial epigastric vein, corresponding to the superficial epigastric group located medial to and above the epigastric-saphenous junction (Fig. 8 A–D).

The contrast medium after opacifying this lymph center fills the deep inguinal and iliac nodes (Fig. 9) [3–5].

It was found that the SLN in the radiographic antero-posterior view is projected over the junction of the femoral head and the ascending ramus of the pubis (Fig. 10).

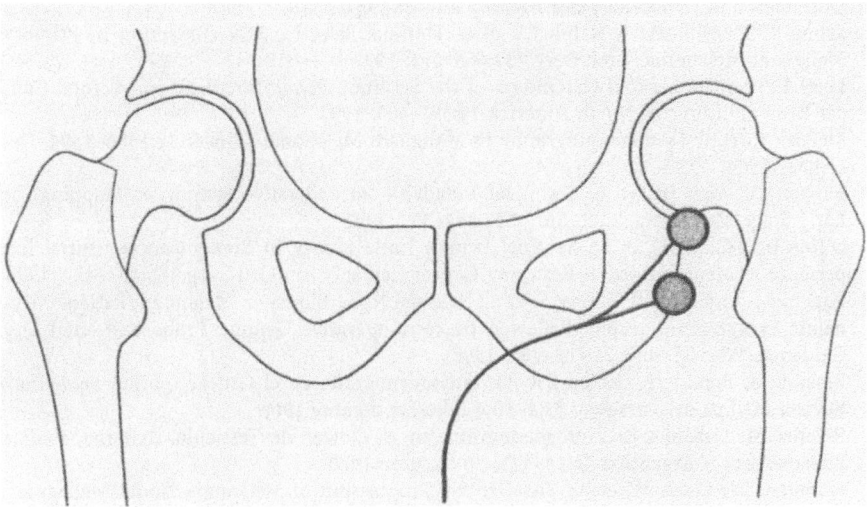

Fig. 10. Illustration of A.P. radiographic location of SLN

In all of our patients with penile carcinoma who had metastases, this SLN was found to contain metastases. Thus, the SLN was the first filter in the penile lymphatic pathway. Injection of Ethyodol into a single dorsal penile lymphatic vessel opacified the lymph nodes on both sides in 12% of the cases.

References

1. Alex J. Krag DN: Gamma Probe Guided Localization of Lymph Nodes. Surg Oncol 2:137–144, 1993
2. Borgstein PJ, Pijpers R, Comans E, Vandiest PJ, Boom RP, Meijer S: Sentinel Lymph Node Biopsy in Breast Cancer: Guidelines and Pitfalls of Lymphoscintigraphy and Gamma Probe Detection. J Am Coll Surg 3:186, 275–283, March 1998
3. Cabanas RM: Thesis: Valoracion Quirurgica de la Linfoadenografia Facultad de Ciencias Medicas. Asuncion, Paraguay, 1969
4. Cabanas RM: An Approach for the Treatment of Penile Carcinoma. Cancer 39:456–466, 1977
5. Cabanas RM: Anatomy and Biopsy of Sentinel Lymph Nodes. Penile, Urethral and Scrotal Cancer. Urologic Clinic of North America 19:267–276, 1992
6. Chiappa S, et al: Combined Testicular and Foot Lymphangiography in Testicular Carcinoma. Surgery, Gynecology, and Obstetrics 123:10–14, July 1966
7. Giuliano AE, Jones RC, et al: Sentinel Lymphadenectomy in Breast Cancer. J Clin Oncol 15:2345–2350, 1997
8. Krag DN, Meijer SJ, et al: Minimal Access Surgery for Staging of Malignant Melanoma. Arch Surg 130:654–658, 1995
9. Krag DN, Weaver D, et al: The Sentinel Node in Breast Cancer, A Multicenter Validation Study. The New England Journal of Medicine 399:941–946, October 1998
10. Leveuf, Godard: Presse Medicale, March 1934

11. Levenback C, Burke TW, et al: Intra-operative Lymphatic Mapping for Vulvar Cancer. Obstetrics and Gynecology 84:163–167, August 1994
12. Leong SPL, Steinmetz I, Habib FA, et al: Optimal Selective SLN Dissection in Primary Malignant Melanoma. Arch Surg 132:666–673, 1997
13. Lowe FC: Squamous-Cell Carcinoma of the Scrotum. Penile, Urethral, and Scrotal Cancer Urologic Clinic of North America 19:397–405, 1992
14. McPeak C, et al: Lymphangiography in Malignant Melanoma. Cancer 12:1586–1594, December 1964
15. Morton DI, Wen JH, et al: Technical Details of Intraoperative Lymphatic Mapping for Early Stage Melanoma. Arch Surg 127:394–399, 1992
16. O'Hea BJ, Hill ADK, et al: Sentinel Lymph Node Biopsy in Breast Cancer: Initial Experience at Memorial Sloan-Kettering Cancer Center. J Am Coll Surg 186:432–427, 1998
17. Pijpers R, Borgstein PJ, Meijer S, et al: Sentinel Node Biopsy in Melanoma Patients: Dynamic Lymphoscintigraphy Followed by Intra-operative Gamma Probe and Vital Dye Guidance. World J Surg 21:788–793, 1997
18. Riveros M, Fresco H, Cabanas R: La Linfoadenografia en el Cancer Genital Femenino. Revista Medica del Paraguay 3:84–100, Julio/Septiembre 1968
19. Riveros M, Cabanas R: Linfoadenografia en el Cancer de Testiculo. Tribuna Medica Buenos Aires – Argentina 4:118–125, 26 Octubre 1970
20. Reintgen DS, Cruse W, et al: The Orderly Progression of Melanoma Nodal Metastases. Ann Surg 220:759–767, 1994
21. Reuhl T, Kaisers H, et al: Radical Axillary Node Resection in Node-Negative Breast Cancer: Can its Indication Be Individualized by Examining the (Primary Tumor – Draining) Sentinel Node? Dtsch-Med-Wochenschr (123) 19:583–587, 08 May 1998
22. Sayeg E, et al: Lymphangiography of the Retroperitoneal Lymph Node through the Inguinal Routes. Journal of Urology 95:102–107, January 1966
23. Testut L, Jacob O: Anatomia Topografica 8th edition. Salvat Editors SA Volume 2:658
24. Testut L, Jacob O: Anatomia Topografica 8th edition. Salvat Editors SA Volume 2:547
25. Tailhefer A, Pilleron JP: La Colpohisterectomia Ampliada con Vaciamiento de los Ganglios de la Cadena de la Pelvis Menor. Cancer – Problemas Clinicos Terapeuticos. Editor Riveros M, Editorial Universitaria Buenos Aires – Argentina 1957
26. Turner R, Ollila D, Krasne D, Giuliano A: Histopathologic Validation of the SLN Hypothesis for Breast Carcinoma. Ann Surg 226:271–276, 1997
27. Veronesi U, Paganelli G, et al: Sentinel-Node Biopsy to Avoid Axillary Dissection in Breast Cancer with Clinically Negative Lymph Nodes. Lancet 349:1864–1867, 1997
28. Van der Veen H, Hoesktra O, et al: Gamma Probe Guided Sentinel Node Biopsy to Select Patients with Melanoma for Lymphadenectomy. Br J Surg 81:1796–1770, 1994

Sentinel Node Localization by Lymphoscintigraphy: A Reliable Technique with Widespread Applications

G. Paganelli, C. De Cicco, and M. Chinol

Division of Nuclear Medicine, European Institute of Oncology, Milan, Italy

Abstract

The concept of the sentinel lymph node (SN) represents an important contribution to guide appropriate surgery of cancer. Diagnostic non-invasive or minimally invasive procedures that provide accurate preoperative staging of the lymph node status are badly needed. The technique of SN biopsy, first developed with the purpose to select melanoma patients for regional node dissection, has been extended to other malignancies. Initial studies in breast carcinoma, conducted with vital blue dye, showed that the SN concept was biologically valid, although SN was missed in up to 30%–40% of cases. If a radioactive tracer is injected close to the tumor, then the SN can be identified by lymphoscintigraphy (LS), and a gamma ray detecting probe (GDP) can be used to locate the skin projection of SN and assist biopsy. These techniques are already used successfully in melanoma and breast carcinoma where the various parameters involved, such as the size of the radioactive particles, the injection site and injection volume, have recently been optimized. In a large series of breast cancer patients, the overall predictive value of the SNs biopsy guided by LS and GDP was 96.8%; in patients with small carcinomas (<1.2 cm diameter), the concordance between SN and axillary status was 98.6%. In patients with melanoma, LS combined with GDP showed itself to be superior to the blue dye mapping. LS associated with GDP allowed the detection of SN in 98% of cases and 72 SNs in 54 basins were localized. Using blue dye instead, SN was stained only in 80% of patients (50 SNs in 40 basins). Lymphoscintigraphic techniques have shown promising results also in tumors such as vulva and tongue. In conclusion, LS is a simple nuclear medicine technique, relatively inexpensive and well accepted by patients. SN biopsy guided by a GDP is becoming widely adopted for a variety of neoplasms, contributing significantly to the search for less aggressive treatments in patients with early stages of cancer.

Recent Results in Cancer Research, Vol. 157
© Springer-Verlag Berlin · Heidelberg 2000

Introduction

A major aim of modern cancer surgery is to employ less aggressive approaches while maintaining oncological radicality. The development of imaging techniques and more sophisticated screening examinations has made it possible to identify malignant lesions at earlier stages, so new cancers are more often of small size and may often be treated less aggressively. This is especially true in breast cancer, where clinically occult lesions are diagnosed with increasing frequency. For such cancers the likelihood of axillary involvement is low [1, 2].

Apart from these considerations, in the absence of non invasive methods to establish the presence of disease in the axilla, the dissection of the axillary lymph nodes continues to be a necessary procedure, not only for therapeutic purposes but mainly as tumor staging [3].

If it were possible to reliably determine whether or not the axilla is involved without complete axillary dissection, this would enable a less aggressive surgical approach to the diseased breast. The technique of sentinel node (SN) biopsy was conceived for this purpose [4, 5].

In this context the concept of the "sentinel node biopsy" was developed many years ago. The idea is simple and has been previously developed by Morton et al. [6, 7] to select melanoma patients for regional node dissection. Assuming that lymphogenic metastasis precedes hematogenic metastasis, they demonstrated that early metastasis of melanoma can be localized in the first draining lymph node (sentinel node). If we apply this concept to the breast and we remove and examine the first lymph node which receives the lymph from the site where the primary carcinoma is located, it is likely that the cancer cells which may have detached from the primary tumor will follow the same route. The logical consequence is that, if a careful examination of the sentinel node does not show the presence of cancer cells, the other axillary nodes should also be free of disease.

Studies conducted using blue vital dye would indicate that this concept can be successfully applied to the management of breast cancer [8]. However, with blue dye the SN can be missed in up to the 30%–40% of cases. Intradermal blue dye injection is a tedious and time consuming technique; moreover substantial experience is required to improve the success rate. In the original procedures reported by Giuliano et al. [8] for breast carcinoma, a vital blue dye was injected just prior to the operation. In our opinion, the use of blue dye has an important drawback: that axillary tissue must be dissected blindly until the blue node is located. This node can be difficult to find since it can be several centimeters from the incision. A nuclear medicine technique such as lymphoscintigraphy (LS) can overcome this problem.

If a radioactive tracer is injected close to the tumor, then the SN can be identified by LS, and a gamma ray detecting probe (GDP) can be used to locate the skin projection of SN and assist biopsy [9].

Lymphoscintigraphy is easy to perform and its use along with a GDP has been successfully applied in melanoma patients [10] and recently in breast cancer patients [5, 9, 11] and to other tumors such as vulva and tongue. The advantage of lymphoscintigraphic imaging technique is that it locates the node and indicates exactly where skin incision should be made. The small hand-held probe guides the dissection itself which is therefore quick and consistently successful. This advantage is sufficient to justify the slightly greater cost of LS compared to the blue dye method.

Carcinoma of the Breast

At the European Institute of Oncology in Milan, radioguided resection of sentinel nodes in breast cancer proved to be simple and effective in a large series of 382 consecutive patients [12].

A recent report thoroughly investigated various parameters such as radioactive particle size, injection site, and injection volume involved in LS of the sentinel node in breast cancer in order to optimize the technique [13].

Two-hundred and fifty patients were studied, divided in subgroups according to the type of colloid administered and mode of injection. Three kinds of ^{99m}Tc colloids were used: (a) antimony sulfide colloid (particle size <50 nm), (b) colloid particles of human albumin (particle size <80 nm), (c) colloid particles of human albumin (particle size in the range 200–1000 nm) administered either subdermally or peritumorally in a volume ranging from 0.2 to 3 ml.

The conclusions of the study were that SN identification is more reliable when large-size radiolabeled colloids are injected subdermally in a relatively small injection volume (0.4 ml). Moreover, the use of GDP greatly facilitates accurate pinpointing and rapid removal of the SN.

In fact, an incision of 2–3 cm is sufficient for the surgeon to remove the SN, and this process is greatly facilitated by use of the probe during dissection.

At present, in a series of 382 cases, the overall predictive value of the SNs biopsy guided by LS and GDP is 96.8%; in patients with small carcinomas (<1.2 cm diameter), the concordance between SN and axillary status is 98.6% [14].

However, this is a sufficiently high value to conclude that axillary dissection is unnecessary in cases where the sentinel node is negative.

We observed false-negative SN in 3.2% of all cases. In two of these cases the primary carcinoma was multifocal. Multifocal tumors which are likely to involve more than one lymphatic trunk from the mammary gland to the axillary nodes, may reduce the accuracy of SN biopsy in predicting the status of the axilla.

We would therefore suggest that the sentinel node method should not be applied to cases of extensive multifocality.

In 371 out of 382 cases at least one axillary SN was removed. The SN was positive for metastases in 168 out of 371 cases (45.3%). In 73 of 168 patients (40.6%), the SN was the only metastatic node; this is an important element in favor of sentinel node biopsy as it indicates the sentinel concept is biologically valid.

In 203 out of 371 patients (55%), the SN did not show metastatic involvement; in 191 of these cases, the axilla was free of disease, while in 12 patients, other axillary nodes were involved (nine cases of the first level, two cases at levels I and II, and one case at levels I, II, and III) [14].

Sentinel node biopsy guided by a GDP can identify a negative axilla with good accuracy, so that women with a negative sentinel node could be spared axillary dissection, and all the risks that the operation entails. Since the technique is also easy to apply we expect that, after further confirmatory studies and a longer follow-up, it will become widely adopted for most cases of breast cancer with clinically negative nodes. The risk of false negative results is low and may be further reduced if multicentric and multifocal cases are excluded. Furthermore, since the predictive value of the technique in our patients with small carcinomas (<1.2 cm) was 98.6%, we believe that the procedure may be implementable immediately in such cases, to substitute axillary dissection [12].

A second factor associated to false negative results was a histopathological condition known as peritumoral vascular invasion (PVI) which was present in 8 cases. We presume that the presence of PVI may make it more likely that more than one pathway of lymphatic spread to the axilla occurs, increasing the risk of metastases skipping the sentinel node. No other variables appeared related to the predictive value of the sentinel node biopsy.

Sentinel node biopsy represents a significant step forward in the search for less aggressive treatments for patients with breast cancer and a great saving in cost due to the reduction in the number of the elective axillary dissections.

Melanoma

After many years of debate about the guidelines to follow when a patient has been diagnosed for a primary melanoma with clinically uninvolved nodes, Morton has probably proposed the best compromise to solve this issue suggesting the possibility of performing elective lymph node dissection only on those patients with histologically positive nodes. The techniques of LS and SN biopsy are aimed at identifying this patient population.

However, the use of the original patent blue dye (PBD) technique to identify SN has shown several drawbacks, mainly low accuracy: in Morton's overall experience, the SN has been identified only in 82% of lymphadenectomy specimens [7]. This low rate of identification has been confirmed in other studies using only the PBD [15, 16].

Several authors have demonstrated that LS associated with GPD is a more sensitive and accurate method in order to identify SN in melanoma [17].

Usually, the day before surgery, LS is performed to study the drainage of lymphatic flow from melanoma skin site to the lymph node basin(s) and to locate the SN(s). ^{99m}Tc radiolabeled colloidal aspecific particles with a diameter ranging from 200–1000 nm, in a volume ranging from 0.2–0.5 ml, are injected with a 27-gauge needle surrounding the primary lesion when still present or the biopsy wound.

Then dynamic images are acquired, for the first 5 min after injection, to visualize the flowing of the tracer in the lymphatic stream towards the lymph node basin until the SN.

Subsequently, planar images in both anterior and posterior view of the involved basins are acquired with a large field of view gamma camera equipped with a high resolution collimator. Moreover, static acquisitions are carried out 10, 15, 30, 60, and 120 min after administration and then after 16-18 h, just before surgical procedures.

In addition to the standard images, oblique views of 30-45° may be obtained whenever the radioactivity of the injection site obscures the SN hot spot.

During acquisition, a cobalt-67 source is used in order to mark the skin with a permanent dye pen corresponding to the first lymph node revealed by the gamma camera, in order to make easier gamma probe detection during surgery procedures.

A recent study [18] reported that the lymphoscintigraphic visualization of SN was possible in 50/50 patients (100%) and that GPD allowed the detection of SN in 49/50 patients (98%) and 72 SNs in 54 basins were localized. Instead using PBD, SN was stained only in 40/50 patients (50 SNs in 40 basins).

The conclusions of the study were that LS combined with GPD is a safe method for detecting SN and more sensitive than the PBD technique.

The LS technique, especially in patients with multiple and unclear drainage sites, offers clear advantages with respect to PBD, so that multiple and unnecessary biopsies can be spared. In conclusion, we may affirm that the PBD technique, due to its low sensitivity, can be considered, nowadays, as a secondary method in SN detection.

In the case of truncal melanoma the lymphatic mapping could be technically problematic, due to unpredictable and variable drainage patterns. Two techniques to locate the SN, GPD after LS and intraoperative PBD mapping, have been recently compared in seventy patients with documented cutaneous melanoma of the trunk. Also in this patient population LS, combined with GPD, proved to be more sensitive than traditional PBD (100% vs. 73%) for detecting SNs especially when axillary basins were involved.

Vulvar Cancer

Vulvar cancer is a rare tumor, accounting for 0.5% of all malignancies; the most frequent histologic type is squamous cell carcinoma, which affects predominantly elderly women.

From 1940 radical vulvectomy with bilateral inguino-femoral lymphadenectomy has been the standard treatment for these patients. This operation entails complete removal of the vulva, mons pubis, inguino-femoral nodes, and sometimes pelvic nodes. Lymphadenectomy involves a high morbidity, with wound breakdown, wound infection occurring in up to 85% of the cases and chronic lymphedema reported in 15%–20% of the patients [19].

In the last 10 years the surgical procedure has become more conservative [20, 21] and in patients with early cancer a modified radical vulvectomy or a wide excision of the tumor has shown to be adequate to eradicate the local vulvar lesion. However, although groin dissection is considered necessary in patients with clinically positive nodes, the procedure seems to be an over-treatment when inguinal nodes are free of disease.

In order to reduce non-useful lymphadenectomies in patients with early stages of vulvar cancer, sentinel node biopsy has been applied in vulvar cancer using both blue dye technique and LS associated with GDP [22, 23].

Our experience begun in 1996: from May 1996 through September 1998, we studied 37 consecutive patients with T1–T2 squamous-cell vulvar cancer and clinically negative groin nodes.

Nineteen patients presented unilateral lesions and 18 patients had midline lesions. Lymphoscintigraphy was performed the day before surgery to establish lymphatic drainage and to define the location of the SNs. ^{99m}Tc-colloidal particles of human serum albumin, with a size of ≤80 nm, were administered around the tumor (2–4 injections in a volume of 0.1 ml).

Planar scans of the vulvar and inguinal areas in anterior and lateral projections were obtained at 5–30 min (early) and 3 h (late) after radiotracer injection and SNs marked on the skin. An intraoperative GDP was used to identify SNs during surgery. A complete inguinofemoral node dissection was then performed. Sentinel nodes were submitted separately to pathologic evaluation. Lymphoscintigraphy was successful in all cases. The mean number of nodes localized was 1.7 in unilateral lesions; in 18 patients with midline lesion an average of 3.3 SNs were detected (1.7 per groin). In 13 out of the 18 patients with midline lesions the SN was identified in both groins. In five patients no contralateral lymphatic drainage was documented. In most cases (33/37, 89%) the SN was visualized in less than 30 min and in four cases in the late images; in two of these patients delayed images were required. The mean number of SN surgically detected with the GDP per groin was 1.4 (range 0–4). The total number of nodes removed was 736 (mean 13; range 9–23).

Eight out of 37 cases had positive nodes; the SN was the only positive node in six cases; in the remainder three, in one case two SNs and one non-SN were positive; in one patient the SN was one of two positive nodes, while in the last case two SNs and other five non-SN were found to have metastases. Twenty-nine patients showed negative SN: all of them resulted negative for lymph node metastasis after complete inguino-femoral node dissection. In five out of 18 patients with midline lesion, in which only one groin showed lymphatic drainage, contralateral lymphadenectomy did not show metastatic nodes.

Sensitivity and predictive value in evaluating inguino-femoral lymphonode status in this series of patients were 100%.

The technique is simple and is ideally suited to be used in large multicenter studies to test the predictivity of sentinel-node biopsy in early vulvar cancer.

If we are successful in staging groin lymph nodes by a simple biopsy, we could eliminate the risk of complications associated with a complete inguino-femoral dissection for most patients and we could achieve great progress in the direction of less aggressive treatments in patients with vulvar cancer.

Carcinoma of the Tongue

The tongue is the commonest site of primary squamous cell carcinoma (SCC) of the oral cavity [24]. The main diagnostic challenge is the detection of nodal micrometastases (cN0 pN1) which are found in up to 50% of cN0 SCCs of the tongue submitted to a neck dissection [25, 26]. Up to now neither clinical staging modalities nor biological markers have yet been identified that can betray cN0 pN1 presence [27].

Search and biopsy of SN in cN0 patients may have a role in deciding whether or not to perform a neck dissection. In particular, a histologically negative SN would indicate that it is safe to avoid neck dissection, while micrometastases would mandate surgical intervention and direct the choice towards additional therapy.

In a pilot study conducted at the European Institute of Oncology in Milan, 11 patients, with lateral T1–T2, N0, M0 SCC of the tongue, underwent LS the day before neck dissection to search for SN. SNs were identified and removed separately with the aid of an intraoperative GDP. SNs were visualized in all cases (8 homolateral to the tumor and 3 contralateral) and sensitivity was 100% in the 8 removed nodes (5 true negative and 3 true positive). Three patients showed metastatic nodes. These preliminary results encourage further investigations in this area in order to better understand the lymphatic drainage from the tongue to the neck and to verify the wisdom of performing selective neck dissection according to the location and size of the tumor.

Conclusions

Lymphoscintigraphy is a simple nuclear medicine technique, relatively inexpensive and well accepted by patients. Sentinel node biopsy guided by a gamma probe is becoming widely adopted for a variety of neoplasms, contributing significantly to the search for less aggressive treatments in patients with early stages of cancer.

References

1. Veronesi U, Rilke F, Luini A, et al. (1986) Distribution of axillary node metastases by level of invasion: an analysis of 539 cases. Cancer 59: 682–687
2. Fisher B, Wolmark N, Bauer M, et al. (1981) The accuracy of clinical nodal staging and of limited axillary dissection as a determinant of histologic nodal status in carcinoma of the breast. Surg Gynecol Obstet 152: 765–772
3. Veronesi U, Luini A, Galimberti V, et al. (1990) Extent of metastatic axillary involvement in 1446 cases of breast cancer. Eur J Surg Oncol 16: 127–133
4. Giuliano AE, Dale PS, Turner RR, et al. (1995) Improved axillary staging of breast cancer with sentinel lymphadenectomy Ann. Surg. 222: 394–401
5. Krag DN, Weaver DL, Alex JC, et al. (1993) Surgical resection and radiolocalization of the sentinel lymph node in breast cancer using a gamma probe. Surg. Oncol. 2: 335–340
6. Morton DL, Wen DR, Cochran A. (1992) Management of early-stage melanoma by intraoperative lymphatic mapping and selective lymphadenectomy: an alternative to routine elective lymphadenectomy or "watch and wait". Surg Oncol Clin North Am 1: 247–259
7. Morton DL, Wen DR, Wong JH, et al. (1992) Technical details of intraoperative lymphatic mapping for early stage melanoma. Arch Surg 127: 392–399
8. Giuliano AE, Dale PS, Turner RR, et al. (1995) Improved axillary staging of breast cancer with sentinel lymphadenectomy. Ann Surg 222: 394–401
9. Albertini JJ, Lyman GH, Cox C, et al. (1996) Lymphatic mapping and sentinel node biopsy in the patient with breast cancer. JAMA 276: 1818–1822
10. Van der Veen H, Hoekstra OS, Paul MA, et al. (1994) Gamma probe-guided sentinel node biopsy to select patients with melanoma for lymphadenoctomy. Br J Sur 81: 1769–1770
11. Veronesi U, Paganelli G, Galimberti V, et al. (1997) Sentinel-node biopsy to avoid axillary dissection in breast cancer with clinically negative lymph-nodes. Lancet 349: 1864–1867
12. Veronesi U, Paganelli G, Viale G, et al. (1999) Sentinel lymph node biopsy and axillary dissection in breast cancer: results in a large series. J Natl Cancer I 91: 368
13. De Cicco C, Cremonesi M, Luini A, et al. (1998) Lymphoscintigraphy and radioguided biopsy of the sentinel axillary node in breast cancer. J Nucl Med 39: 2080–2084
14. De Cicco C, Chinol M, Paganelli G. (1998) Intraoperative localization of the sentinel node in breast cancer: technical aspects of lymphoscintigraphic methods. Semin Surg Oncol 15: 268–271
15. Lingam MK, Mackie RM, Mackay AJ. (1994) Intraoperative lymphatic mapping using patent blue V dye to identify nodal micrometastases in malignant melanoma. Reg Cancer Treat 7: 144–146
16. Godellas CV, Berman CG, Lyman G, et al. (1995) The identification and mapping of melanoma regional nodal metastases: minimally invasive surgery for the diagnosis of nodal metastases. Am Surgeon 61: 97–101
17. Kapteijn BAE, Nieweg OE, Liem IH, et al. (1996) Localizing the sentinel node in cutaneous melanoma: gamma probe detection versus blue dye. Ann Surg Onc 4(2): 156–160
18. Bartolomei M, Testori A, Chinol M, et al. (1998) Sentinel node localization in cutaneous melanoma: lymphoscintigraphy with colloids and antibody fragments versus blue dye mapping. Eur J Nucl Med 25: 1489–1494
19. Podratz KC, Symmonds RE, Taylor F. (1982) Carcinoma of the vulva: analysis of treatment failures. Am J Obstet Gynaecol 143: 340–351
20. Sutton GP, Miser MR, Stehman FB, et al. (1991) Trends in operative management of invasive squamous carcinoma of the vulva at Indiana University, 1974 to 1988. Am J Obstet Gynaecol 164: 1472
21. Cavanagh D. (1997) Vulvar cancer: Continuing evolution in management. Gynaecol Oncol 66: 362–67

22. Levenback C, Burke TW, Morris M, et al. (1995) Potential applications of intraoperative lymphatic mapping in vulvar cancer. Gynaecol Oncol 59: 216
23. Barton DPJ, Berman C, Cavanagh D, et al. (1992) Lymphoscintigraphy in vulvar cancer: a pilot study. Gynaecol Oncol 46: 341–344
24. Shah JP. (1996) Head and neck surgery. 2nd ed. Mosby-Wolfe, pp 167–234
25. Jones AS, Phillips DE, Helliwell TR et al. (1993) Occult node metastases in head and neck squamous carcinoma. Eur Arch Otorhinolaryngol 250: 446–449
26. Kowalski LP, Medina JE. (1998) Nodal metastases; predictive factors. Otolaryngol Clin North Am 31: 621–637
27. Chiesa F, Tradati N, Mauri S et al. (1998) Prognostic factors in head and neck oncology: a critical appraisal for use in clinical practice. Antic Res 18: 4769–4776

Vital Dye and Radiolabelled Colloids – Complement or Alternative?

R. Pijpers[1], P.J. Borgstein[2], G.J.J. Teule[1], and S. Meijer[2]

[1] Department of Nuclear Medicine, Academic Hospital of the Vrije Universiteit, Amsterdam, The Netherlands
[2] Department of Surgical Oncology, Academic Hospital of the Vrije Universiteit, Amsterdam, The Netherlands

Abstract

Several different protocols for retrieval of the sentinel node (SN) have been described: gamma probe (GP) and/or dye guided biopsy, preceded by lymphoscintigraphy or not. Especially in American studies, predominantly executed by surgeons, dye or GP guidance only is used with good results. The disadvantages of applying dye only are: an extensive learning curve, lower retrieval rate of the SN and, especially in the learning phase, a higher rate of false negative biopsies. If only GP guidance is applied, the technique seems more simple to master. A recent multicentre study, however, revealed an unacceptably high false negative rate. It must be considered that most published studies were executed by highly experienced surgeons. In most European studies, scintigraphy is a standard part of the procedure. Lymphoscintigraphy provides the surgeon with a "road map", revealing the number and approximate location of the SNs in the lymphatic basin(s). Scintigraphy proves useful especially if an SN is situated close to the injection site (breast cancer), or if SNs are situated at unexpected locations (head-and-neck or trunk melanoma). A combination of all three available steps results in the highest number of successful procedures with the lowest false negative rate. This may prove to be especially important for general hospitals where the number of biopsy procedures is often smaller compared to specialized centres.

Introduction

This chapter deals with the choices that have to be made when the sentinel node (SN) biopsy is implemented in clinical practice. High success rates, applying dye or gamma probe (GP) guidance only, have been reported by Morton, Krag and Giuliano [1–3]. It has to be born in mind that these are dedicated surgeons with extensive experience in this field of surgery. Reports of later studies show less favourable results [4-8]. However, for the SN procedure to become generally accepted it must have the same accuracy in the hands of surgeons who perform 50 biopsies, or even less, per year. In our opinion, high accuracy not only depends on technical skills, but also on close co-operation between the nuclear medicine physician, surgeon, and pathologist. Therefore, we consider the SN procedure a three-step procedure: scintigraphy followed by GP and dye guided biopsy.

Melanoma

For two reasons, less emphasis is put on melanoma. First, its incidence is considerably lower as compared to breast cancer. Second, SN biopsy in melanoma is still considered to be experimental [9]. It has not been proven yet whether patients with a positive SN biopsy will actually show better survival following a "therapeutic" lymph node dissection (LND). However, if there is one subset of patients that may benefit from a regional LND, it will probably be the subset with proven lymphatic metastases. Third, it has to be established which subset of patients is most eligible for the SN biopsy, to combine the highest yield of positive biopsies at the lowest expense in terms of morbidity and money. Since the publications of Balch in 1979 and 1980 [10, 11], patients with melanomas of an intermediate Breslow thickness (between 0.76 and 4.0 mm) were often considered to be candidates for elective LND [11]. Without setting limits we feel that the Breslow thickness range for patients to be eligible for SN biopsy has to be reconsidered.

Scintigraphy in Melanoma

In the head-and-neck and trunk, drainage to several lymphatic basins can be seen in a large percentage of the patients [13-16]. Dynamic imaging, directly following injection of the tracer, helps to differentiate between multiple SNs and early spill to secondary lymph nodes. In the groin, branching of lymphatics occurs in a considerable number of patients [14]. Directly following the dynamic study, the approximate site of the SN should be marked on the skin to provide the surgeon with a "road map" for the biopsy procedure. Especially if the biopsy is performed under local anaesthesia this may prove useful since this requires the smallest possible invasiveness.

Imaging in other directions can reveal, sometimes unexpected, drainage to additional lymphatic stations (Fig. 1). Static imaging several hours after injection serves to demonstrate late spill to secondary lymph nodes (if any) and interval lymph nodes that were hidden by lymphatic channels during the dynamic study.

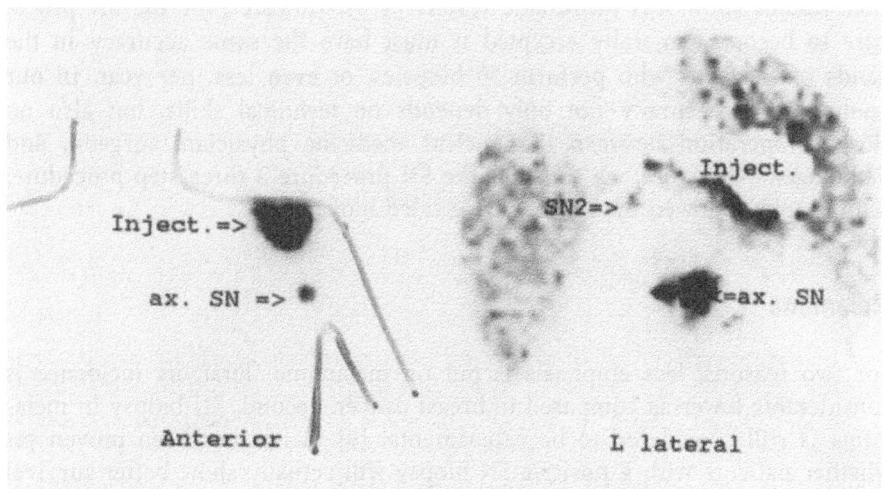

Fig. 1. Patient with a melanoma on the left scapula. In the anterior projection the injection site (shining through the patient) can be seen as well as an axillary sentinel node. The left lateral projection reveals a second sentinel node (⇒) in the anterior triangle of the neck

Gamma Probe Guidance in Melanoma

Skin marks that have been made during scintigraphy, except for the groin, are often not exactly above the SN due to different positioning of the patient during the biopsy procedure [17]. Still, they facilitate the procedure since they roughly indicate the site of the SN and facilitate initial search with the GP. In most cases the SN can be localized externally with help of the GP and the surgeon can use the GP to find the most optimal site for the incision. However, only GP guidance would have been of little help to the surgeon in finding the unexpected SN shown in Fig. 1 due to scattered radiation from the injection site.

In the axilla the GP serves to find the SN, often deeply seated within the fatty tissue [14, 16]. In the head-and-neck area, where injections of dye are not desirable for cosmetic reasons [18], GP guidance has to be used as the solitary guidance tool.

Dye Guidance in Melanoma

If used without scintigraphy and GP guidance, the technique has several disadvantages: a considerable learning curve, a lower identification rate of the SN, and more extensive surgery due to the fact that the surgeon does not know where to look for the SN. Especially in the neck and the axilla, identification rates are compromised [1]. However, in combination with GP guidance it proves to be a useful adjunct for the final visualization of the, often small, lymph nodes within the fatty tissue [14].

Breast Cancer

In breast cancer the SN procedure will obviate the need for axillary lymph node dissections (ALND), introduced by Halsted as part of the therapy. In the last decades, ALND became more and more a staging procedure, excluding lymphatic metastases at the price of considerable short and long-term morbidity. This especially holds for the increasing number of patients with small tumours [19]. Except for being less invasive, there are other reasons to choose this diagnostic strategy in breast cancer staging. Sensitivity to detecting micro-metastatic disease increases, since only one or several nodes have to be evaluated [20, 21]. Second, it may cause cost reduction as consequence of a shorter hospital stay and shortening of the period of incapacity for work in the case of a tumour negative SN biopsy.

Scintigraphy in Breast Cancer

Like in melanoma, scintigraphy is used to provide the surgeon with a road map (Fig. 2). In most patients, scintigraphy provides information about the localization of the SN within the axilla. It tells the surgeon whether he/she has to look for one, two or (rarely) three lymph nodes [21]. Visualization of parasternal or ectopic lymph nodes opens the door to a new field of lymph

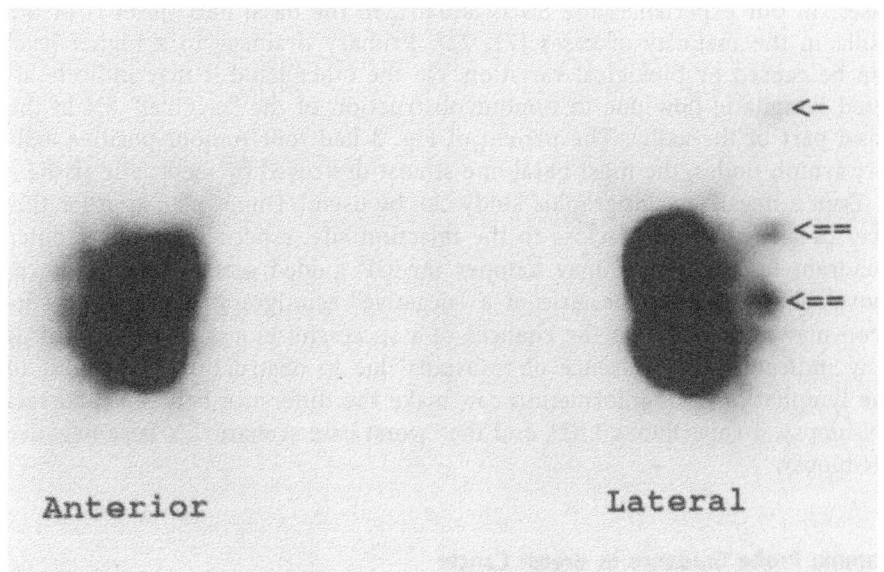

Fig. 2. An anterior image in a patient with left sided breast cancer shows no evidence of tracer transport. The lateral image shows two sentinel nodes (⇐) close to the injection side and a faint secondary node (←). The sentinel nodes could not be localized externally with the gamma probe

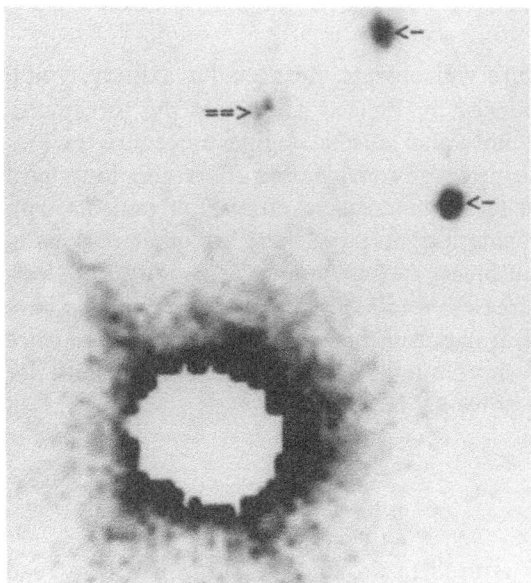

Fig. 3. Patient with a tumour in the lateral quadrant of the right breast. Focal tracer uptake can be seen in two parasternal nodes (←) and (faintly) in a level III lymph node (⟹)

node staging. Drainage to parasternal lymph nodes only, as can be seen in medially localized tumours, will make axillary biopsy superfluous in selected cases. In our experience, the SN is situated in the basal part (level I) of the axilla in the majority of cases [21, 22]. Primary drainage to a higher level can be caused by biological variation. On the other hand it may indicate altered lymphatic flow due to tumour obstruction of the "original" SN in the basal part of the axilla. The patient of Fig. 3 had four tumour-positive axillary lymph nodes, the most basal one almost destroyed by metastatic tissue.

Even a negative scintigraphic study can be useful. One explanation for this may be an SN localized close to the injection site, especially in upper outer quadrant lesions, which may hamper the GP guided search, even after removal of the tumour. Because of a "negative" scintigraphic result, the surgeon may anticipate that the chances of a successful biopsy are decreased. It may indicate a total absence of transport due to obstruction by tumour of the lymphatics. This information can make the difference between a correct SN biopsy, a superfluous LND, and the "worst case scenario", a false negative SN biopsy.

Gamma Probe Guidance in Breast Cancer

Without aid of the GP, interest in the SN procedure would not have gained the position it has now. It makes it possible for a surgeon to master the SN biopsy technique within a reasonable number of training sessions [23]. In most studies, the SN detection rate is over 90% [3, 21, 22, 24, 25]. More importantly, the false negative rate in these studies is less than 5%. In a recent multicentre study, however, where only GP guidance was applied, the localization rate of the SN differed between 79% and 98% [6]. The false negative rate was between 0% and 28%. Addition of preoperative scintigraphy and intraoperative dye guidance might have improved the results. Another reason to suggest caution for is the low number of training procedures: five might have been too few [23].

Dye Guidance in Breast Cancer

If used as a solitary technique, dye guided SN biopsy suffers from the same problems as in melanoma. The SN detection rate in the "learning phase" is between 66% and 77% [4, 5, 26] with a considerable false negative rate [4, 5, 26]. Giuliano has proven that high success rates can be achieved by dye guidance only [3]. However, it will take years for the "average" surgeon to get this experience. Ectopic and parasternal SNs will often be missed, resulting in superfluous lymph node dissections with consecutive morbidity.

As in melanoma, we feel that the addition of dye guidance is a useful tool in the final stage of the biopsy procedure [27]. If several lymph nodes are shown to be labelled by tracer, the dye can be used by the surgeon to verify whether he has indeed biopsied the first one. In the case of a short distance between the injection site and SN (Fig. 2), which hampers GP guidance, the surgeon can use dye as an alternative. Because of skin marks applied during the scintigraphic study, he knows roughly where to give the incision and start the search. Following preparation along blue lymphatic channels the surgeon can often terminate the SN biopsy with the aid of the GP. This is made possible by the fact that scattered radiation from the injection site will cause less noise in the signal from the SN, as the surgeon approaches this SN. Finally, the GP can be used to verify whether the excised lymph node is indeed radioactive, i.e., the SN.

We have chosen not to start with the tumorectomy for three reasons. First, a frozen section can be performed on the SN during the tumorectomy, which saves time. Second, the radioactivity remaining after tumorectomy will often hamper GP guidance in the case of upper outer quadrant tumours. Third, as our surgeons inject the dye intracutaneously [27], primary tumorectomy would result in cutting the lymphatics.

Differences in Results

The different opinions between "dye-party" members [3], "gamma probe-party" members [6] and "scintigraphy-party" members [21, 22, 24, 28] are to a certain extent related to their respective professional background. Most studies performed by surgeons lack the use of scintigraphy. For them it may be less attractive to wait for a scintigraphy to be obtained [2, 6] or even to use tracer guidance [3–5].

Most European studies however, often performed in close co-operation between nuclear medicine physicians and surgeons, have shown that combining all techniques results in the highest SN detection rates with low false negative rates from the start [21, 22, 28, 34]. At the end of the day it may be more economic to combine all three tools instead of failing to use all the potential information.

Conclusions

Each method, scintigraphy, gamma probe and dye guidance, has its own specific advantages and disadvantages. As it is virtually impossible to know beforehand which technique can be skipped in which patient, we feel that a combination of all three will give the individual patient the best treatment at the lowest morbidity. This will not only hold for specialized centres, but perhaps even more for general hospitals.

References

1. Morton DL, Wen DR, Wong JH, et al. Technical details of intraoperative lymphatic mapping for early stage melanoma. Arch Surg 1992;127:392–399
2. Krag DN, Meijer S, Weaver DL, et al. Minimal-access surgery for staging of malignant melanoma. Arch Surg 1995;130:654–658
3. Giuliano AE, Jones RC, Brennan M, et al. Sentinel lymphadenectomy in breast cancer. J Clin Oncol 1997;15:2345–2350
4. Rodier JF, Janser JC. Surgical technical details improving sentinel node identification in breast cancer. Oncol Reports 1997;4:281–283
5. Guenther JM, Krishnamoorthy M, Tan LR. Sentinel lymphadenectomy for breast cancer in a community managed care setting. Cancer J Sci Am 1997;3:336–340
6. Krag DN, Weaver D, Ashikaga T, et al. The sentinel node in breast cancer. N Engl J Med 1998;339:941–946
7. Crossin JA, Johnson AC, Stewart PB, et al. Gamma probe guided resection of the sentinel lymph node in breast cancer. Am Surg 1998;64:666–668
8. Reuhl T, Kaisers H, Markwardt J, et al. Axillary node removal in clinical node-negative breast carcinoma. Can its indication be individualized by sentinel node detection? Dtsch Med Wochenschr 1998;123:583–587
9. Nieweg OE, Kapteijn BAE, Thompson JF, et al. Lymphatic mapping and selective lymphadenectomy for melanoma: not yet standard therapy (review editorial). Eur J Surg Oncol 1997;23:397–398
10. Balch CM, Murad TM, Soong S, et al. Tumor thickness as a guide to surgical management of clinical stage I melanoma patients. Cancer 1979;43:883–888
11. Balch CM. Surgical management of regional lymph nodes in cutaneous melanoma. J Am Acad Dermatol 1980;3:511–524
12. Balch CM, Soong S, Bartolucci AA, et al. Efficacy of an ELND of 1 to 4 mm thick melanomas for patients 60 years of age and younger. Ann Surg 1996;3:255–266

13. Uren RF, Howman-Giles R, Shaw HM, et al. Lymphoscintigraphy in high risk melanoma of the trunk: predicting draining node groups, defining lymphatic channels and locating the sentinel node. J Nucl Med 1993;34:1435–1440
14. Pijpers R, Collet GJ, Meijer S, Hoekstra OS. The impact of dynamic lymphoscintigraphy and gamma probe guidance on sentinel node biopsy in melanoma. Eur J Nucl Med 1995;22:1238–1241
15. O'Brien CJ, Uren RF, Thompson JF, et al. Prediction of potential metastatic sites in cutaneous head and neck melanoma using lymphoscintigraphy. Am J Surg 1995; 170:461–466
16. Pijpers R, Borgstein PJ, Meijer S, et al. Sentinel node biopsy in melanoma patients: Dynamic lymphoscintigraphy followed by Intraoperative gamma probe and vital dye guidance. World J Surg 1997;31:788–793
17. Krag DN, Meijer S, Weaver DL, et al. Minimal-access surgery for staging of malignant melanoma. Arch Surg 1995;130:654–658
18. Ross MI. Lymphatic mapping and sentinel node biopsy for early stage melanoma: how we do it at the M.D. Andersen Cancer Center. J Surg Oncol 1997;66:273–276
19. Silverstein MJ, Gierson ED, Waisman JR, et al. Axillary lymph node dissection for T1a breast carcinoma. Cancer 1994;73:664–667
20. Giuliano AE, Dale PS, Turner RR, et al. Improved axillary staging of breast cancer with sentinel lymphadenectomy. Ann Surg 1995;222:394–401
21. Borgstein PJ, Pijpers R, Comans EFI, et al. Sentinel lymph node biopsy in breast cancer: guidelines and pitfalls of lymphoscintigraphy and gamma probe detection. J Am Coll Surg 1998;186:275–283
22. Pijpers R, Meijer S, Hoekstra OS, et al. Impact of lymphoscintigraphy on sentinel node identification with Tc-99 m colloidal albumin in breast cancer. J Nucl Med 1997;38:366–368
23. Reintgen D, Cox C, Haddad, et al. The role of lymphoscintigraphy in lymphatic mapping for melanoma and breast cancer. J Nucl Med 1998 (December);12:22N–36N
24. Veronesi U, Paganelli G, Galimberti V, et al. Sentinel node biopsy to avoid axillary dissection in breast cancer with clinically negative lymph nodes. Lancet 1997;349:1864–1867
25. Albertini JJ, Lyman GH, Cox C, et al. Lymphatic mapping and sentinel node biopsy in the patient with breast cancer. JAMA 1996;276:1818–1822
26. Giuliano AE, Kirgan DM, Guenther JM, et al. Lymphatic mapping and sentinel lymphadenectomy for breast cancer. Ann Surg 1994;220:391–401
27. Borgstein PJ, Meijer S, Pijpers R. Intradermal blue dye to identify the sentinel lymph node in breast cancer. Lancet 1997;349:1668–1669
28. Paganelli G, De Cicco C, Cremonesi M, et al. Optimized sentinel node scintigraphy in breast cancer. Q J Nucl Med 1998;42:49–53

IV. Sentinel Node Detection in Urogenital Cancer

Application of the Sentinel Node Concept in Urogenital Cancer

R. M. Cabanas

Attending Surgeon, Victory Memorial Hospital, Beth Israel Hospital North Division, Long Island Medical College Hospital, 1725 York Ave. 33 F. N.Y.N.Y. 10128 USA

Abstract

Pre and intra-operative lymphatic mapping and SLN biopsy is readily available in the armamentarium of Urologic Surgical Oncology. The concept of the SLN should be considered for diagnosis and therapy. Ongoing studies are investigating the impact of SLN biopsy on survival as well as the prognostic significance of micro-metastasis founded by histopathology and immunohistological techniques. The concept is simple, the operatory technique is easy, and the blue dye and radioactive agents are available anywhere. The validation in penile carcinoma has demonstrated, based on experience, that metastasis does not occur in other lymph nodes if the SLN is free of metastasis. Its applicability in other areas of urology is still awaiting the enthusiasm of investigators.

Application of the Sentinel Node Concept in Urogenital Cancer

When performing radical ilioinguinal lymphoadenectomy, retroperitoneal lymph node dissection, and pelvic lymph node dissection there is a high likelihood of morbidity. When these procedures are carried out in patients clinically positive but pathologically negative, these procedures are considered unnecessary. The SLN concept has shown that it is the most likely lymph node to harbor metastasis. The patient with histologically negative SLN may be spared a full regional lymph node dissection. As a consequence, the SLN concept can be applied in any human solid cancer.

In the field of urogenital cancer where the concept of the SLN can be applied are penile, scrotal, prostate, and testicular carcinomas. It is obvious that the status of metastasis in SLN in patients with early human cancer has a clear predicted value for survival.

Pelvic lymph node metastasis in the patient with clinically localized prostate carcinoma is a sign of systematic disease. Over five hundred patients with clinically localized prostate cancer who underwent pelvic lymph node dissection and irradiation therapy, found that a single microscopically positive lymph node conferred a likelihood of disease progression and a ten year mortality rate, similar to that of patients with multiple microscopically positive nodes or grossly positive nodes [5]. The potential benefits of intra or peri-prostatic gland injection of radiolabeled colloid, and an injection of 1% isosulfan blue or patent blue V, followed by laparoscopic pelvic SLN identification using an intraoperative surgical gamma probe and its subsequent biopsy, is a protocol still awaiting the enthusiasm of urologist investigators. The evasive pelvic obturator lymph nodes could be well identified and removed surgically (SLN biopsy) to carry out the protocol of pathology and immunohistochemical studies useful in another area.

Squamous cell carcinoma of the scrotum has a poor prognosis unless locally confined. The basic treatment still depends on wide local excision of the primary lesion following by SLN biopsy to establish the needs for a formal ilioinguinal lymphoadenectomy [7].

In testicular carcinoma if the albuginea of the affected testis is injected with radioactive material and Evans blue or 1% methylene blue, the SLN could be identified and removed, and again the protocol can be fully investigated (pathology and immunohistochemical reaction).

In 1977, I proposed an approach for the treatment of penile carcinoma, after I carried out a study to assess whether or not a simple lymph node (SLN) exists, which receives malignant cells from the primary site and whether a clear or negative SLN reliably predicts a disease free lymphatic system (Fig. 1A, B) [2–4].

I concluded that the SLN is visualized radiographically, on the antero-posterior view, at the junction of the femoral head and the ascending ramus of the pubis. Anatomically, the SLN is part of the lymphatic system around the superficial epigastric vein. Forty-six SLN biopsies were performed with fifteen patients positive for metastatic disease. In these fifteen patients, an inguinofemoroiliac dissection was performed; in twelve cases there was no involvement of other lymph nodes. Lymphatic channels draining into the iliac lymph nodes without first draining into the sentinel lymph node were never demonstrated, nor were the inguinal-femoral lymph nodes involved in the absence of SLN involvement. On this basis, we recommend preliminary bilateral SLN biopsy to be followed by inguinofemoroiliac dissection when biopsy of the SLN is positive. When biopsy of the SLN is negative for metastatic disease, no further surgical therapy is immediately indicated. With negative SLN, 5-year survival was 90%. When SLN alone was involved, 5-year survival was 70%. Five-year survival was 50% with both SLN and other inguinal nodes involved. When iliac metastases were also present, 3-year survival was 20%. The technique of SLN described was using anatomical parameters. The procedure is performed without the use of methylene blue or radioactive tracers. A 5 cm incision is made parallel to the inguinal ligament, two fingerbreadths (4.5 cm) lateral and two fingerbreadths distal to the pubic tubercle. This point lies over the saphenofemoral junction. By inserting the finger un-

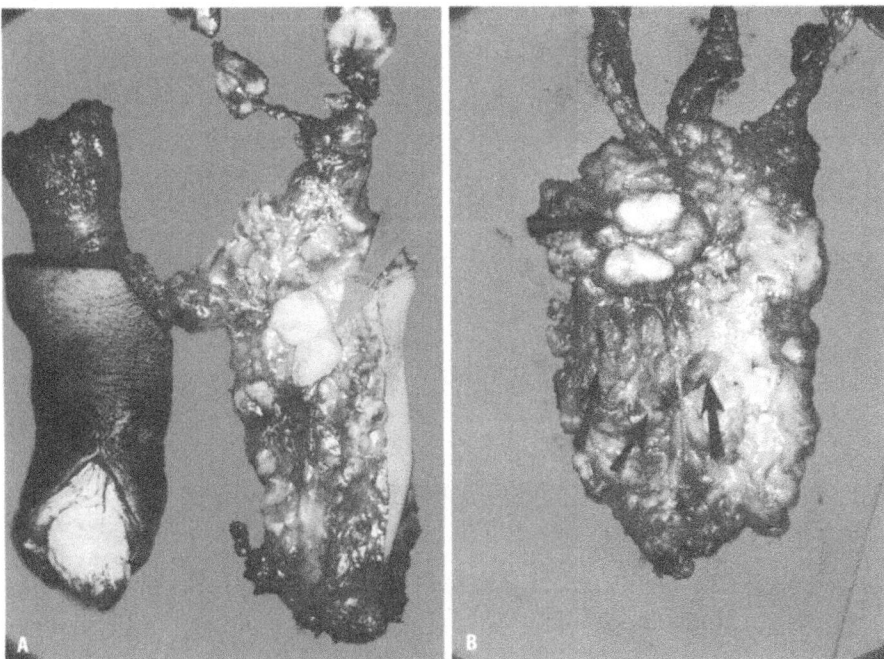

Fig. 1A. Surgical specimen. Penile amputation – Radical Ilioinguinal Lymphoadenectomy. Arrow indicates SLN, the only node that harbors metastasis

Fig. 1B. Surgical specimen. Radical Ilioinguinal Lymphoadenectomy. Superior arrow indicates SLN, the only node that harbors metastasis

der the upper flap toward the pubic tubercle, the sentinel lymph node is encountered.

The sentinel lymph node corresponds to the lymph nodes associated with the superficial epigastric vein. The position of the sentinel lymph node in relation to this vein may vary but never by a distance greater than 1 cm. The superficial epigastric vein is absent in only 1.4% of cases. In some cases, there is more than one lymph node in the superficial epigastric group. In this situation, all (two or three) lymph nodes should be removed, but the true sentinel lymph node is always the larger and more medially situated.

It is well established that the lymphatics of the penis drain to the lymph node located in the superficial inguinal nodes of the medial group and particularly in the superomedial nodes. This is exactly the same lymph center that we first opacified when we formed lymphangiography via the dorsal lymphatics of the penis [3, 4]. There is persisting uncertainty regarding the optimal management of the inguinal lymph nodes in patients with penile cancer, and in consequence, the concept of the sentinel lymph node and its clinical application are matters of controversy.

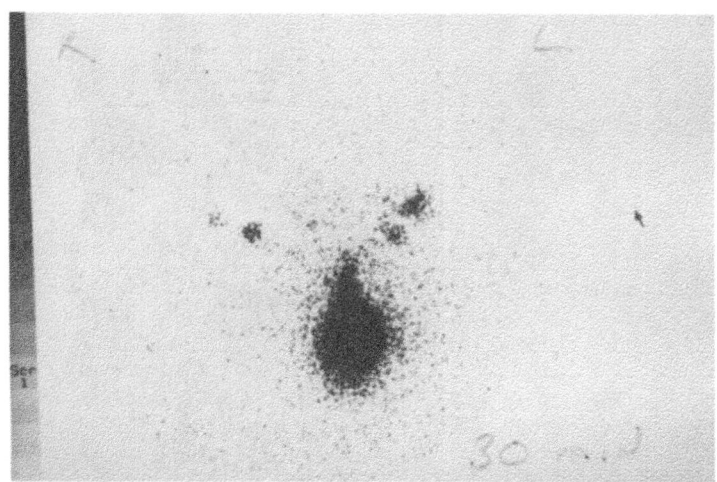

Fig. 2 A. Patient A

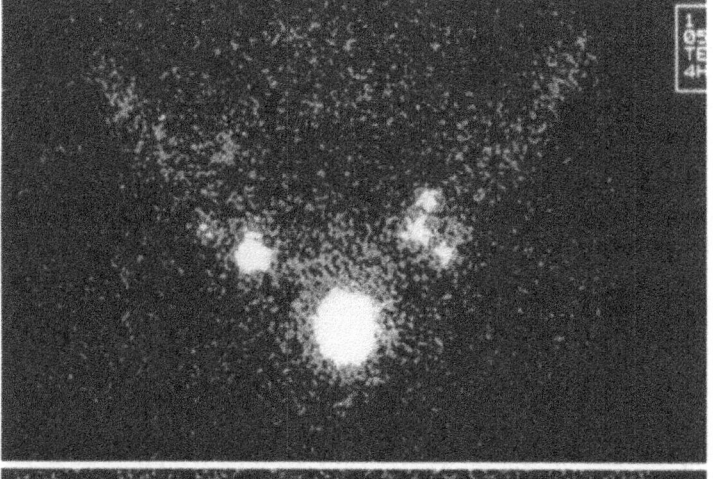

Fig. 2 B. Patient B

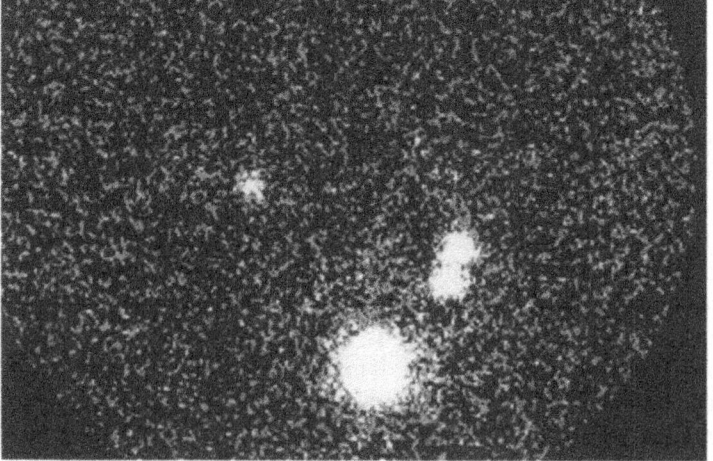

Fig. 2 C. Patient C

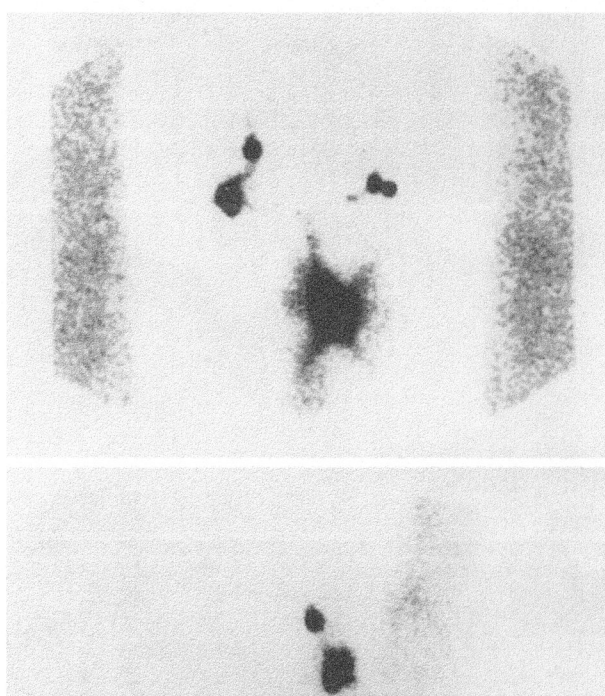

Fig. 3 A. A. P. View

Fig. 3 B. Lateral View

Actually, the biopsy of the SLN has been improved, being accurate, minimally invasive, and easy to identify. We welcome the procedure of Morton and associates using intradermal injection of "blue dye" at the primary tumor site in malignant melanomas [8]. We also welcome the technique of Alex and Krag, injecting radio-colloid at the level of the lesion, and using a manual gamma-probe as a guide to identify the SLN (radiolabeled) for excisional biopsy [1].

Modern techniques of the SLN biopsy include: injection of unfiltered technetium-99 m (Tc 99 m) sulfur colloid, a dose of 0.3 mCi in 4 ml of normal saline injected in the foreskin of the penis or proximal and close to the lesion. After thirty minutes, the image of SLN visualizes (Fig. 2 A–C). European investigators are using radiolabeled serum albumin (Nanocoll) for SLN biopsy (Fig. 3 A, B) [9]. Using the manual gamma probe we count the amount of radioactivity at the level of injection (Fig. 4 A). A focal area of

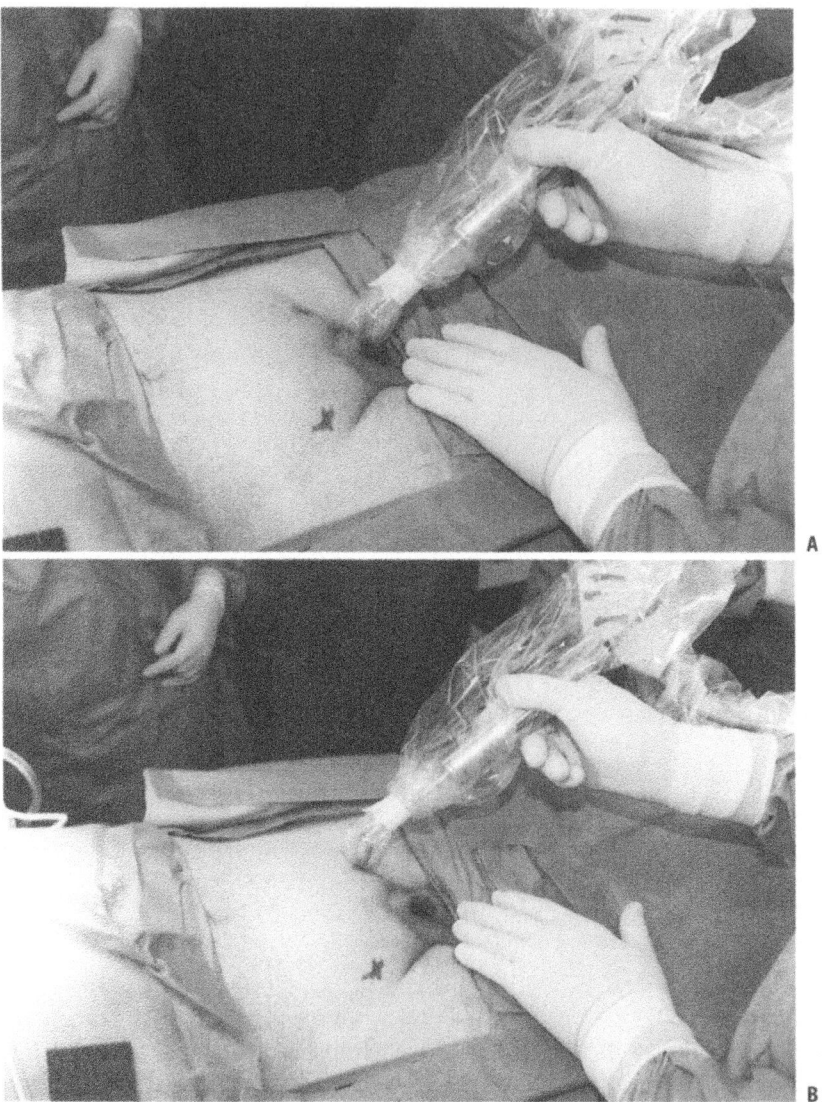

Fig. 4A. Counting the amount of radioactivity at the level of injection (lesion) using the manual gamma probe

Fig. 4B. The point of maximal emissions identifies the SLN

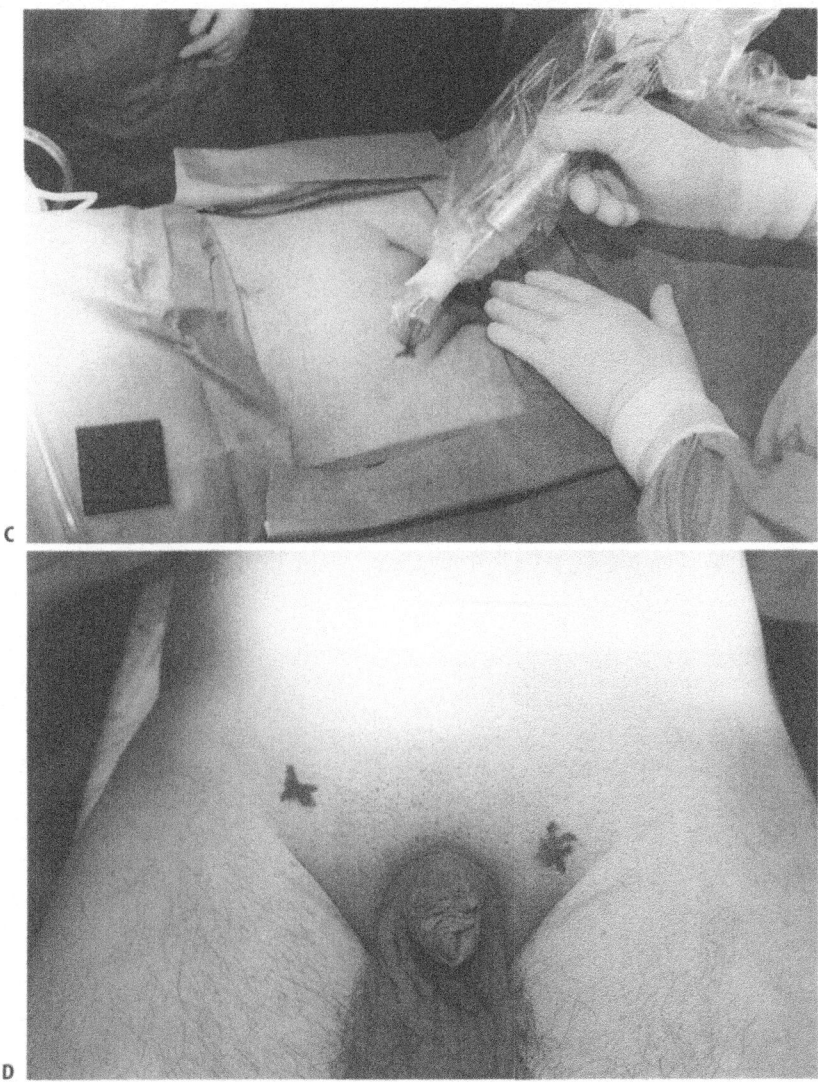

Fig. 4 C. The point of maximal emissions identifies the SLN on the opposite side

Fig. 4 D. Identification of the point of maximal emission with marker

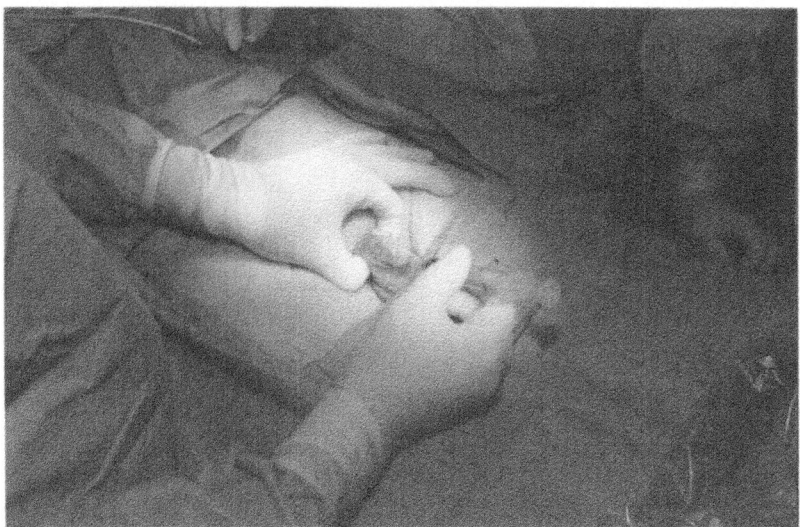

Fig. 5. Injection of the blue dye at the level of the lesion

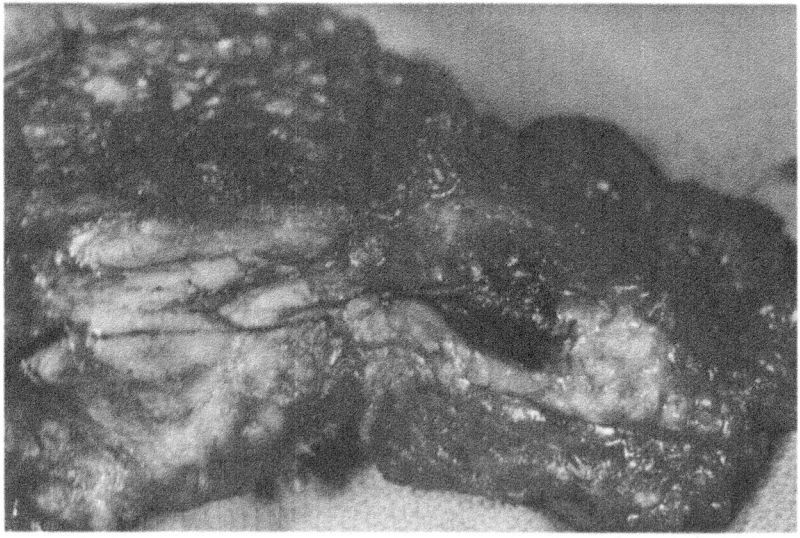

Fig. 6. The blue dye identifies the lymphatic duct draining into the SLN

radionuclide accumulations is readily discerned by listening to the audio signal, which increases pitch as the emission levels increase.

The point of maximal emission identifies the SLN (Fig. 4B, C). We identify this spot in the patient with a pen marker (Fig. 4D). With the same technique we identify the opposite SLN.

The time between injections of the technetium-99 sulfur colloid, lympho-scintigraphy, identification of the SLN and surgery must be at least two hours (two to four hours).

At the operation 5 ml (0.5 cc) off patent blue dye or Evans blue or 1% methylene blue or isosulfan blue dye is injected close to the tumor. A gentle massage at the level of the injection is advised in order to feel the lymphatic ducts with the blue dye injected (Fig. 5A).

Following the same surgical steps described here and elsewhere about the technique of the SLN biopsy, incision of the skin is made, this point correlating well with the "hot spot".

The dissection guided by the hand-held gamma detector was carried straight down to the level of radiolabeled SLN. Simultaneously we can be guided by the "blue" color of the lymphatics draining into the SLN (Fig. 6).

References

1. Alex J, Krag DN (1993) Gamma Probe Guided Localization of Lymph Nodes. Surg Oncol 2:137–144
2. Cabanas RM (1969) Thesis: Valoracion Quirurgica de la Linfoadenografia Facultad de Ciencias Medicas. Asuncion, Paraguay
3. Cabanas RM (1977) An Approach for the Treatment of Penile Carcinoma. Cancer 39:456–466
4. Cabanas RM (1992) Anatomy and Biopsy of Sentinel Lymph Nodes. Penile, Urethral and Scrotal Cancer. Urologic Clinic of North America 19:267–276
5. Gervasi LA, Mata J, et al (1989) Prognostic Significance of Lymph Node Metastases in Prostate Cancer. J Urol 142:332
6. Horenblas S, Jansin L, et al: Detection of Occult Metastases in Squamous Cell Carcinoma of the Penis Using a Dynamic Sentinel Node Procedure. To be published.
7. Lowe FC (1992) Squamous-Cell Carcinoma of the Scrotum. Penile, Urethral, and Scrotal Cancer Urologic Clinic of North America 19:397–405
8. Morton DI, Wen JH, et al (1992) Technical Details of Intraoperative Lymphatic Mapping for Early Stage Melanoma. Arch Surg 127:394–399
9. Valdes-Olmos RA: Personal Communication. Amsterdam, The Netherlands

Intraoperative Lymphatic Mapping and Sentinel Node Identification: Gynecologic Applications

C. Levenback

Department of Gynecologic Oncology, The University of Texas M.D. Anderson Cancer Center, 1515 Holcombe Blvd., Box 67, Houston, TX 77030, USA

Abstract

The status of regional lymph nodes is a powerful predictor of survival in patients with early cancers of the vulva, cervix, and uterus. Radical resection of vulvar and cervix cancers along with extensive lymphadenectomy remains the standard of care for these cancers. Intraoperative lymphatic mapping and sentinel node identification has the potential to improve the treatment of patients with gynecologic cancer with improved detection of lymph node metastases and reduced morbidity. This chapter will focus primarily on vulvar cancer and include a review of previous innovations in treatment and current experience with intraoperative lymphatic mapping in these patients.

Introduction

Intraoperative lymphatic mapping with sentinel node identification which is already changing the surgical management of cancers at several disease sites, is doing the same for gynecologic cancers. This historical review will show how this technique has developed and how it is improving the way gynecologic cancers, especially those of the vulva, are treated.

Intraoperative Lymphatic Mapping of the Vulva

The fascinating surgical history of vulvar cancer, full as it is of failures, is also full of many innovations that have improved the care of women with this disease. Among the innovations, and one with growing potential, is lymphatic mapping of the vulva.

Recent Results in Cancer Research, Vol. 157
© Springer-Verlag Berlin · Heidelberg 2000

Pathogenesis of Vulvar Cancer

Vulvar cancer is a relatively rare disease. In the United States just over 3000 new cases of vulvar cancer occur each year compared with over 175 000 new cases of breast cancer [1]. Over 90% of vulvar cancer patients have a squamous cancer; the rest have a melanoma, adenocarcinoma, or basal cell carcinoma. Two etiologic categories of squamous vulvar cancer have been proposed. In the first, which is related to infection with human papillomavirus (HPV), patients are typically young smokers who present with an invasive cancer within a larger carcinoma in situ. In the second, which is not related to HPV infection, patients are generally older and have no other lower genital tract lesions [2]. Factors leading to chronic irritation of the vulva, including vulvar dystrophy, and exposure to perfumes and chemicals, have been implicated in the development of the non-HPV-related vulvar cancers. The incidence of vulvar cancer continues to increase with age and does not plateau or decline like some other gynecologic cancers.

Radical Vulvectomy and Bilateral Inguinal Femoral Lymphadenectomy

At the turn of the 20th century, vulvar cancer was considered incurable. Topical therapies, cautery, and local excision all proved inadequate. Furthermore, the social and sexual standards of the time made it difficult for patients and physicians to discuss vulvar complaints openly. Moreover, as one contemporary account put it:

"Death from carcinoma of the vulva is particularly revolting ... If untreated, the disease progresses slowly and remorselessly and often is extremely painful ... Micturition and defaecation become agony. Later the urethra and vagina and anus are destroyed ... The groin nodes ulcerate and become infected and discharge pus until finally the patient expires ... This process may take two years and ... is sometimes shortened by the inguinal nodes eroding the femoral artery with a consequent sudden and fatal haemorrhage ... In one case this occurred whilst the district nurse was dressing the groin. About three pints of blood poured from the wound in a fountain, covering the nurse, the patient and one of her relatives, as well as the floor and one wall of the room. The ensuing chaos beggars all description." [3]

To treat this horrible disease, radical vulvectomy and bilateral inguinal femoral lymphadenectomy were combined utilizing one continuous incision and their use was popularized by pioneers including Kehrer, Basset, Taussig, Way, and Twombly [4]. In 1971, Plentl and Friedman in their widely respected and quoted *Lymphatic System of the Female Genitalia*, [5] summarized the conventional wisdom of proponents of radical vulvectomy: (1) continuity of the lymphatics of the vulva made location of the primary irrelevant, (2) partial vulvectomy was always inadequate, (3) procedures that allowed primary closure were inadequate, and (4) results obtained with radiation were poor. These concepts led to the surgical principle of removing the tumor along with all of the skin and lymphatic channels of the vulva and the lymph nodes of the groin and pelvic nodes at risk.

Needless to say, radical vulvectomy was terribly morbid, with early series marked by frequent wound breakdown and lymphedema (over half of all cases). The impact on body image and sexual function was also devastating. Yet, because it was very effective, the combination of radical vulvectomy and bilateral inguinal, femoral, and pelvic lymphadenectomy quickly became and remained the treatment of choice for vulvar cancer.

Reducing the Radicality of Surgery for Vulvar Cancer

As early as the 1940s, however, several changes in practice made vulvar cancer surgery less morbid and fatal. The result of evolutionary thinking in cancer surgery at other sites, such as the breast, as well as in medicine and society in general, made it easier for patients and physicians to discuss vulvar complaints and for physicians to approach vulvar cancer as a treatable disease. Patients now arrived at referral centers with smaller tumors and a lower risk of lymph node metastasis.

One of the first efforts at making surgery for vulvar cancer less radical was the so-called "triple incision" technique. In this approach, the groin incisions were made separately from the vulvectomy incision, leaving a bridge of skin between the groin and vulva. In 1977, Morris suggested hemivulvectomy for patients with unilateral lesions [7]. Several investigators suggested abandoning pelvic node dissection since pelvic nodes were never positive if the femoral nodes were negative. This move was finally validated by a randomized Gynecologic Oncology Group (GOG) study reported by Homelsy in 1986 [6].

In the 1960s and 1970s interest shifted to defining "microinvasive" vulvar cancer. At this time, it was becoming clear that some patients with minimally invasive cervix cancer had essentially no risk of lymph node metastasis. Some authors thus made the logical leap to vulvar cancer by suggesting that patients with superficially invasive vulvar cancers could be treated "conservatively" with vulvectomy that omitted the groin dissection [8]. This concept proved to be incorrect. A large clinical pathologic study by the GOG showed that patients with as little as 1 mm of invasion could have lymph node metastases [9]. Consequently, virtually all authors now advocate lymph node assessment for all patients with deeper than 1 mm invasion.

History of Lymphatic Mapping of the Vulva

Most early anatomists studied the lymphatics of cutaneous structures in cadavers. They injected various materials under pressure to help visualize these fine structures. The lymphatic channels of the skin form a fragile low-pressure system in which lymph fluid can easily change course and direction when obstructed. Such studies shed little light on the in vivo behavior of the lymphatic system and led to errors in anatomic description of vulvar lymphatics.

Hudack and McMaster [10] in 1933 used several blue dyes in vivo with hyaluronidase to study the lymphatic anatomy of the skin. But being primarily interested in the microanatomy of the skin, they did not describe the location of lymph nodes in relation to the injection sites. In the early 1950s, Eichner [11] directly injected the dye Sky Blue into the ovary, cervix, uterus, and the vulva of some of his patients and then systematically described the results. In the case of the vulva, Eichner preoperatively injected the dye into the deep subcutaneous tissues although it is not clear how long this was prior to exploratory laparotomy. In addition, Eichner did not identify afferent lymphatic channels. Eichner reported finding blue staining along the major vessels of the pelvis but never in the inguinal area. Eichner thus concluded that the "labial and vulvar drainage does not go directly into the inguinal nodes ..." [12]

In 1963, Parry-Jones published *Lymphatics of the Vulva,* [13] in which he described his attempts to, first, determine if the vulvar lymphatics crossed the labial crural fold as classically described from cadaver studies and, second, reveal the path of lymphatic drainage from the vulva directly to the pelvis. Thinking that Eichner had made his injections too deep and following the example of Kinmonth, [14] Parry-Jones approached his first goal by injecting Patent Blue into the vulvar dermis. In this way, he was able to show that no matter where the vulva was injected, the dye, and thus the lymphatic channels, never crossed the labial crural fold. Consequently, Parry-Jones recommended modifying the vulvar incisions during radical vulvectomy so as to spare the skin of the inner thigh and allow primary wound closure.

Reaching his second objective was not so easy, however. In none of his injected patients could Parry-Jones trace the drainage of Patent Blue into the pelvis. In fact, in a series of patients undergoing radical vulvectomy, he found that the dye was arrested in the groin and did not reach the pelvis. Unfortunately, Parry-Jones thus concluded that he had chosen the wrong dye, even though the lymphatic mapping concept as we currently know it was at his fingertips. So he began using Imferon, an iron-containing compound and deeper injection sites. Histologic analysis of pelvic lymph nodes revealed microscopic evidence of iron particles in the pelvic nodes, leading him to conclude incorrectly that there was direct lymphatic drainage from the vulva to the pelvis. Although iron-containing compounds are now being studied as magnetic resonance lymphography agents, [15] they are not suitable as a mapping agent. Direct lymphatic drainage from the vulva to the pelvis has never been convincingly demonstrated.

The Sentinel Node Concept in Patients with Vulvar Cancer

In 1977, Ramon Cabanas first reported the identification of sentinel nodes by lymphography in patients with penile cancer [16]. In this study, contrast material injected into a cannulated dorsal lymphatic of the penis identified a specific lymph node or nodes in the groin, which would be the initial site of metastases. He referred to these as "sentinel" nodes. Cabanas importantly noted that inguinal lymphatic channels were never seen to drain to the pelvis without first draining to these sentinel nodes and that other inguinofemoral nodes were not involved if the sentinel nodes were negative. On the basis of these results, Cabanas therefore recommended sentinel node biopsy, to be followed by inguinofemoral lymph node dissection only if the sentinel nodes were positive.

In 1979, DiSaia et al., published *An Alternate Approach to Early Cancer of the Vulva*, [17] which emphasized the devastating and long-overlooked impact of radical vulvectomy on body image and sexual function. DiSaia et al., challenged the concept that radical vulvectomy was conservative and suggested that radical local excision with superficial inguinal lymphadenectomy was adequate treatment for patients with small vulvar cancers. They described how, in 79 cases, they never observed positive femoral nodes below the cribriform fascia if inguinal nodes above the cribriform fascia were negative. In describing this phenomenon, they cited the work of Cabanas and borrowed his term "sentinel nodes". DiSaia's sentinel nodes comprised the 8–10 inguinal nodes above the cribriform fascia and did not involve any mapping procedures as opposed to Cabanas's one or two nodes that directly drained the primary tumor demonstrated by lymphography. It would take another 20 years for lymphatic mapping to be tried in patients with vulvar cancer. In the meantime, the opinions of DiSaia et al., on how to treat vulvar cancers would be put to the test.

Groin Dissection in Patients with Vulvar Cancer

The response by gynecologic oncologists to the concepts formulated by DiSaia et al., was intense interest mixed with concern that the efficacy of radical vulvectomy and inguinal femoral lymphadenectomy not be compromised. The GOG in particular responded by treating stage I vulvar cancer with ipsilateral superficial inguinal lymphadenectomy and modified radical hemivulvectomy and reporting its results in 1992 [18]. The nine groin recurrences seen in 121 patients with negative ipsilateral groin dissections (7.5%, six on the ipsilateral side and three on the contralateral side) led the GOG to conclude that DiSaia's concept of sentinel nodes could not be supported.

Meanwhile, in the 13 years between the work of DiSaia et al., and the GOG's, many clinicians, including most at The University of Texas M. D. Anderson Cancer Center, performed superficial inguinal lymphadenectomy on patients with vulvar cancer [19]. We found 6% of patients with negative superficial inguinal lymphadenectomy recurred in the groin. Although the last report by DiSaia et al., on this subject in 1989 [20] reported no such failures, the gynecologic oncology community has since then been moving away from superficial inguinal lymphadenectomy. Borgno and colleagues have helped us understand groin anatomy better with the observation that all femoral nodes occur medial to the femoral vein, [21] a concept elegantly supported by the embryological studies of Micheletti [22]. These authors recommend removing the nodes above and below the cribriform fascia while sparing the fascia lata and avoiding transposition of the sartorius muscle. Superficial inguinal and medial femoral lymphadenectomy should be the standard for patients undergoing full groin dissection for invasive vulvar cancer [23].

Sentinel Node Identification with Blue Dye in Vulvar Cancer

M. D. Anderson's experience with intraoperative lymphatic mapping to identify sentinel nodes in vulvar cancer began in earnest in 1993, when a 40-year-old patient arrived at M. D. Anderson with a small cutaneous melanoma of the right thigh. Attending physician, Paul Mansfield directed her to the cancer screening clinic, where a small squamous carcinoma of the cervix was discovered and she was referred to me. In planning our joint surgical approach, Mansfield described to me a new concept in the management of cutaneous melanoma, intraoperative lymphatic mapping, which he was planning to use on the patient. Still, on the day of the surgery, I was amazed to see the afferent lymphatic channel and sentinel node clearly appear following the injection of blue dye and skin incision. The sentinel node was negative and a groin dissection averted. The application of this approach as described by Morton et al., [24] being clear, our group therefore launched a pilot study that ultimately confirmed the feasibility of the technique in a small series of nine patients with vulvar cancer [25]. In 1996, we further solidified this in a series of 21 patients [26]. In that latter study, we also emphasized that lymphatic mapping may hold the key to understanding recurrences in node-negative groins following superficial inguinal lymphadenectomy, and we identified sentinel nodes in a variety of locations within the groin and, in one case, below the cribriform fascia.

Preliminary Data on Lymphatic Mapping of the Vulva with Blue Dye

All told, in the last 5 years we have performed intraoperative lymphatic mapping of the vulva with Lymphazurin Blue in just over 40 patients. In all these cases, mapping was done even when lymph nodes appeared grossly suspicious. The most common groin procedure has been superficial inguinal lymphadenectomy, followed by radiation therapy when positive nodes have been found. This has allowed us to identify the sentinel node in approximately 90% of the patients. In the roughly half of patients who had midline tumors and therefore underwent bilateral groin dissections, the sentinel node was found in approximately 75% of the groins. The location of the primary tumor strongly influences sentinel node identification: the sentinel node was identified in all but one patient with a labial primary tumor, in about 75% of groins in patients with clitoral tumors, and in only about 50% of groins in patients with perineal tumors. On the other hand, in no case have we seen a false-negative sentinel node [27]. Together, our data suggest that lymphoscintigraphy may play a useful role in the lymphatic mapping of vulvar cancer, particularly in patients with midline tumors.

Combined Intraoperative Lymphatic Mapping of the Vulva

While blue dye has been the agent of choice in mapping vulvar cancers, some groups have experimented with combining a dye with a radioactive tracer. For example, in several small series, patients have undergone combined intraoperative lymphatic mapping with a blue dye and a radionucleotide [28, 29] with results similar to those at other disease sites. Radiolocalization with preoperative and intraoperative lymphoscintigraphy increased the chance of finding the sentinel node to over 95%. This technique requires additional resources and training, however, these early results appear to show real benefits. These results have prompted the GOG to open in the near future a study of the combined technique in a large group of patients.

Intraoperative Lymphatic Mapping of the Uterus

While the use of intraoperative lymphatic mapping in the vulva is gaining wider acceptance, controversy still exists regarding the indications for pelvic and paraaortic lymphadenectomy or lymph node sampling in patients with endometrial cancer. Endometrial cancer is the most common gynecologic cancer with 33000 new cases each year. Consequently, to understand better the lymphatic drainage in such cancers, Burke injected the dye isosulfan blue into the fundus and anterior and posterior myometrium in a series of patients with endometrial cancer [30]. As hoped, the blue dye was seen to travel to multiple pelvic nodes. More important, however, was that the dye always revealed the sentinel paraaortic nodes to be above the origin of the inferior mesenteric artery near the renal vessels, which suggests that an adequate lymph node assessment in patients with endometrial cancer must reach as high as the renal vessels.

Intraoperative Lymphatic Mapping of the Cervix

As for intraoperative lymphatic mapping of the cervix, we have performed circumferential cervical injection of blue dye in a small group of patients and located sentinel nodes along the external iliac arteries, common iliac arteries, precaval area, and left paraaortic areas [31]. We have, however, had difficulty timing the injection of dye in relation to the retroperitoneal dissection and have not yet developed an ideal mapping strategy for cervix cancer. Nevertheless, the high morbidity of total pelvic lymphadenectomy, the low rate of nodal positivity in patients with small tumors, and the efficacy of chemoradiation [32] in controlling regional metastases make cervix cancer an attractive target for lymphatic mapping.

Conclusion

The next step in the continued evolution of the surgical treatment of vulvar cancer is intraoperative lymphatic mapping with sentinel node identification. Future studies will determine the role of sentinel node identification in the clinical management of patients with vulvar cancer and possibly in patients with other gynecologic cancers as well.

References

1. Landis SH, Murray T, Bolden S, et al (1999) Cancer Statistics, 1999. Cancer J Clin 49:8–31
2. Bloss JD, Ligo SY, Wilczynski SP, et al (1991) Clinical and histologic features of vulvar carcinomas analyzed for human papilloma virus status: evidence that squamous carcinoma of the vulva has more than one etiology. Hum Pathol 22:7–11
3. Way S (1951) Carcinoma of the Vulva. In Way S (ed) Malignant Disease of the Female Genital Tract. The Blakiston Co, Philadelphia, pp 27–28
4. Twombly GH (1953) The technique of Radical Vulvectomy for Carcinoma of the Vulva. Cancer 6:516–530
5. Plentl AA, Friedman EA (1971) Clinical Significance of Vulvar Lymphatics. In Plentl AA, Friedman EA (eds) Lymphatic System of the Female Genitalia. WB Saunders, Philadelphia, pp 27–43
6. Morris JM (1977) A formula for selective lymphadenectomy. Obstet Gynecol 50:152–158
7. Homesley HD, Bundy BN, Sedlis A, et al (1986) Radiation therapy versus pelvic node resection for carcinoma of the vulva with positive groin nodes. Obstet Gynecol 68:733–740
8. Wharton JT, Gallager S, and Rutledge FN (1974) Microinvasive carcinoma of the vulva. Am J Obstet Gynecol 118:159–162
9. Sedlis A, Homesley H, Bundy BN, et al (1987) Positive groin lymph nodes in superficial squamous cell vulvar cancer. A Gynecologic Oncology Group study. Am J Obstet & Gynecol 156(5):1159–1164
10. Hudak SS, McMaster PD (1933) The Lymphatic Participation in Human Cutaneous Phenomena: A Study of the Minute Lymphatics of the Living Skin. J Exp Med 57:751–774, plates 46–49
11. Eichner E, Goldberg I, and Bove ER (1954) In vivo studies with direct Sky Blue of the lymphatic drainage of the internal genitals of women. Am J Obstet & Gynecol 67(6):1277–1287
12. Eichner E, Mallin LP, and Angell ML (1955) Further experiences with direct Sky Blue in the in vivo study of gynecic lymphatics. Am J Obstet & Gynecol 69(5):1019–1026
13. Parry-Jones E (1963) Lymphatics of the vulva. J Obstet Gynecol Br Cwlth 70:751–765
14. Kinmonth JB (1952) Lymphangiography in man. Clinical Science 11:13–20
15. Hamm B, Taupitz M, Hussmann P, et al (1992) MR lymphography with iron oxide particles: Dose-response studies and pulse sequence optimization in rabbits. Am J Research 158:183–190
16. Cabanas RM (1977) An approach to treatment of penile carcinoma. Cancer 39:456–466
17. DiSaia PJ, Creasman WT, and Rich WM (1979) An alternative approach to early cancer of the vulva. Am J Obstet Gynecol 133:825–832

18. Stehman FB, Bundy BN, Dvoretsky PM, et al (1992) Early stage I carcinoma of the vulva treated with Ipsilateral superficial inguinal lymphadenectomy and modified radical hemivulvectomy: A prospective study of the gynecologic oncology group. Obstet Gynecol 79:490–497

19. Burke TW, Levenback C, Coleman RL, et al (1995) Surgical therapy of T1 and T2 vulvar carcinoma: Further experience with radical wide excision and selective inguinal lymphadenectomy. Gynecol Oncol 57:215–220

20. Berman ML, Soper JT, Creasman WT, et al (1989) Conservative surgical management of superficially invasive stage I vulvar carcinoma. Gynecol Oncol 35:352–357

21. Borgno G, Micheletti L, Barbero M, et al (1990) Topographic distribution of groin lymph nodes: A study of 50 female cadavers. J Reprod Med 35:1127–1129

22. Micheletti L, Levi AC, and Bogliatto F (1998) Anatomosurgical implications derived from an embryological study of the Scarpa's Triangle with particular reference to groin lymphadenectomy. Gynecol Oncol 70:358–364

23. Levenback C, Morris M, Burke TW, et al (1996) Groin dissection practices among gynecologic oncologists treating early vulvar cancer. Gynecol Oncol 62:73–77

24. Morton DL, Wen D-R, Wong JH, et al (1992) Technical details of intraoperative lymphatic mapping for early stage melanoma. Arch Surg 127:392–399

25. Levenback C, Burke TW, Gershenson DM, et al (1994) Intraoperative lymphatic mapping for vulvar cancer. Obstet Gynecol 84:163–167

26. Levenback C, Burke TW, Morris M, et al (1995) Potential applications of intraoperative lymphatic mapping in vulvar cancer. Gynecol Oncol 59:216–220

27. Levenback C, unpublished data.

28. de Hullu JA, Doting E, Piers DA, et al (1998) Sentinel lymph node identification with Technetiu-99m-labeled nanocolloid in squamous cell cancer of the vulva. J Nuclear Med 39(8):1381–1385

29. Terada KY, Coel MN, Ko P, et al (1998) Combined use of intraoperative lymphatic mapping and lymphoscintigraphy in the management of squamous cell cancer of the vulva. Gynecol Oncol 70:65–69

30. Burke TW, Levenback C, Tornos C, et al (1996) Intraabdominal lymphatic mapping to direct selective pelvic and paraaortic lymphadenectomy in women with high-risk endometrial cancer: results of a pilot study. Gynecol Oncol 62(2):169–173

31. Levenback C, unpublished data.

32. Morris M, Eifel PJ, Lu J, Grigsby PW, Levenback C, Stevens RE, Rotman M, Gershenson DM, Mutch DG (1999) Pelvic Radiation with concurrent chemotherapy compared with pelvic and para-aortic radiation for high-risk cervical cancer. NEJM 340:1137–1143

V. Sentinel Node Detection in Malignant Melanoma

Sentinel Node Detection in Malignant Melanoma

A. D. Chan and D. L. Morton

John Wayne Cancer Institute, 2200 Santa Monica Boulevard, Santa Monica,
CA 90404-2302, USA

Abstract

The initial application of intraoperative lymphatic mapping and sentinel lymphadenectomy followed by selective complete lymphadenectomy (LM/SL/
SCLND) was in melanoma. This arose as a solution to the ongoing debate
concerning immediate vs. delayed lymph node dissection. Acceptance of the
concept and advances in nuclear medicine, surgery, and pathology aspects of
the sentinel node procedure have brought it into widespread use for melanoma and have expanded its application for other solid tumors that progress
through the lymphatic route. Although the diagnostic accuracy of the procedure has been demonstrated in multicenter trials, caution should be exercised regarding therapeutic aspects until definitive benefit can be shown
from well-designed clinical trials. Current issues of active discussion and debate are reviewed including ideal nomenclature, clinical significance of occult
metastatic disease, quality assurance, and the role of LM/SL/SCLND outside
high-volume melanoma centers.

Concept, Scientific Basis, and Development

The initial application of intraoperative lymphatic mapping and sentinel lymphadenectomy followed by selective complete lymphadenectomy (LM/SL/
SCLND) was in melanoma. The concept evolved from the need for a better
alternative to either routine immediate lymph node dissection or delayed
lymph node dissection and from the need for more sensitive methods for detection of melanoma tumor cells in the regional lymph nodes [1].

Dr. Chan is currently affiliated with the Naval Medical Center, San Diego, CA, and the Uniformed Services University of the Health Sciences, Bethesda, MD. The views expressed herein are those of the authors and do not necessarily reflect the views of the Uniformed Services University of the Health Sciences, US Navy, US Army, or the Department of Defense.

The most important prognostic factor for most solid neoplasms including melanoma is the status of the regional lymph nodes draining the primary neoplasm. The relative 5-year survival rates for 4570 AJCC (American Joint Committee on Cancer) stage II patients versus 3341 stage III patients were 77% versus 50% in the National Cancer Database from the Commission on Cancer of the American College of Surgeons and the American Cancer Society [2]. The relative survival rate adjusts the observed survival rate for the risks of dying from causes other than melanoma [3]. The incidence of regional lymph node and distant metastasis increases with thickness of the primary [4–6]. Thus the incidence of synchronous lymph node metastasis is low in patients with primary tumors <0.76 mm but increases to 20–25% for patients with tumors 1–4 mm in thickness, and up to 60% in patients with tumors >4 mm. Similarly, the low incidence of synchronous distant metastasis in patients with primary tumors 1–4 mm in thickness increases to 72% when the thickness of the primary tumor exceeds 4 mm [4–6]. In the past, the only method to identify occult regional lymph node metastasis was complete lymphadenectomy (LND) and pathological examination of a cross-section of each excised node using hematoxylin and eosin staining. This technique sampled only a small portion of the total lymph node volume and therefore severely underestimated the frequency of nodal involvement.

Despite its shortcomings as a staging procedure, the routine use of complete LND was rationalized by its potential therapeutic value in patients who have a stepwise progression of metastases from the primary site to the regional lymph nodes before transit to distant sites. Others argued that routine LND subjected the patient to the risk of operative morbidity without realized benefit. Several randomized trials have investigated the potential survival benefit of routine elective (immediate) LND (ELND) [7–13]. The World Health Organization trial concluded that delayed LND is just as effective as ELND if the patient can be closely followed [7, 8]. The Mayo Clinic study showed no improvement in overall or disease-free survival with routine ELND [9–12]. Although the interim analysis of the Intergroup Melanoma Surgical Program showed no overall 5-year or 10-year survival difference between ELND and observation [13, 14], the Intergroup trial identified a statistically significant survival advantage for ELND in patients younger than 60 years of age with nonulcerative melanoma and/or primary tumors 1 to 2 mm in thickness.

Major criticisms of these trials have included the nonroutine use of lymphoscintigraphy to identify all basins at risk, the inadequate statistical power to eliminate a false-negative result, and the use of post hoc analysis to identify significant subgroups. Therefore, no prospective randomized trial has demonstrated conclusively that there is a survival benefit from ELND. Its routine use exposes patients to the morbidity of lymphedema and nerve injury [15, 16], in most cases without the possibility of therapeutic benefit since only about 20% of patients with intermediate-thickness primaries are expected to have metastases in the regional lymph nodes [17, 18]. Moreover, the cost of ELND is at least 5-fold that of wide local excision alone [19].

Our lymphatic studies leading to the sentinel node (SN) hypothesis and the selective approach to lymphadenectomy were initiated over 20 years ago. At that time, ELND was avoided for truncal melanomas located in ambiguous sites such as the midline of the back or close to the umbilicus or shoulder, because these tumors can drain to two or more lymphatic basins. In 1977, we described the use of cutaneous lymphoscintigraphy to identify the lymph basins at risk for metastasis from truncal primary melanomas, and introduced the concept of selective lymphadenectomy of the deep iliac/ obturator lymph nodes directed by the pathologic status of Cloquet's node and the superficial inguinal nodes [20]. Our mapping studies with various radiopharmaceuticals were the impetus for the intraoperative use of vital dyes to identify the first (sentinel) lymph node within the lymphatic basin reached by lymph draining the primary lesion.

Interestingly, although we were not aware of his work, at around the same time we were mapping the lymphatics, Cabanas [21] used the term "sentinel node" in penile cancer to indicate a node detected by lymphangiography in an anatomic location fixed adjacent to the inferior epigastric vein. Although Cabanas proposed this node as the most likely regional site of any tumor cells metastasizing from the primary lesion, its fixed anatomic site contradicted our SN concept. Cabanas' observations were not confirmed by other investigators. Because our studies showed great variability in the lymphatic drainage patterns, we assumed that the location of the first (sentinel) lymph node draining melanoma, breast cancer, and other solid tumors depended on the pathway of its lymphatics and could only be determined by developing accurate methods to identify regional lymphatic patterns.

Our technique of intraoperative lymphatic mapping and sentinel lymphadenectomy (LM/SL) was initially developed using vital dyes to identify the sentinel node for surgical excision. In 1991 our group reported using a feline model to compare several dyes for lymphatic mapping [22]. Isosulfan or patent blue dye injected intradermally resulted in coloration of the afferent lymphatic channel and staining of the SN. Dye-directed LM/SL was first presented at the Society of Surgical Oncology meeting [17] in 1990 and first reported in the literature [18] in 1992. LM/SL was undertaken in 237 lymphatic basins of 223 patients, all of whom subsequently underwent LND. An SN was identified in 194 (82%) lymphatic basins. Forty patients (21%) had tumor-positive SNs. Only two lymphatic basins had tumor-negative SNs in the presence of tumor-positive nonsentinel nodes, a false-negative rate of 1.0%.

We developed LM/SL/SCLND to more accurately stage the regional lymph node basin using a less morbid technique and to avoid the need for lymph node dissection in the 80% of patients with tumor-negative lymph nodes. This approach also allows an alternative to routine superficial parotidectomy for cutaneous melanomas involving the head region [23]. When the SN contains occult tumor cells, the incidence of additional tumor in the lymph node basin is significant [24, 25]. The melanoma database at the John Wayne Cancer Institute, which contains data for over 8700 patients, shows that 36% of nonsentinel lymph nodes contain tumor when the SN contains tumor. The incidence of tumor-containing SNs increases with increasing thickness of the primary tumor [26]. For primaries with thicknesses ≤1.50 mm, 1.51–4.00 mm, and ≥4.01 mm, the incidence of tumor-containing SNs is 4.8%, 19.2%, and 34.4%, respectively. Several studies have confirmed the SN hypothesis in melanoma and breast cancer [27–34]. The tumor status of the SN has been identified as a significant prognostic factor in disease-free and disease-specific survival by univariate and multiple covariate analyses [26, 35].

Using preoperative dynamic lymphoscintigraphy to identify the drainage basin has increased the accuracy of the technique. Several radiopharmaceutical agents have been used for lymphoscintigraphy – initially colloidal gold [20, 36, 37] and later other substances including ^{99m}Tc antimony trisulfide colloid [38], colloidal albumin [39, 40], ^{99m}Tc-human serum albumin [41–44], and ^{99m}Tc sulfur colloid [38, 45]. Currently, the only commercially available products in the United States are ^{99m}Tc-HSA and ^{99m}Tc-SC [46]. ^{99m}Tc-nanocolloidal albumin is widely used in Europe [47] and ^{99m}Tc antimony trisulfide colloid is commonly used in Australia [48].

Radioisotopes are used in both the preoperative identification of the drainage basin and the intraoperative identification of the SN(s) in that basin. In 1993, Alex et al. [49] used technetium-99m labeled colloid and a gamma probe to label and detect the SN in animals and then in ten melanoma patients. Since then, there have been several clinical trials of LM/SL in melanoma using dye and/or radiopharmaceutical (Table 1) [18, 24, 26, 33–35, 50–54]. The reported overall identification rate has ranged from 82% to 100%. SNs have been tumor-positive in 15–26% of patients, with a false-negative rate of 0–2%. These multiple studies have validated LM/SL as a safe, accurate, and reproducible method of identifying melanoma patients with lymph

Table 1. Summary of clinical trials of LM/SL for melanoma

Senior author	No. of patients	No. of basins	Routine LND	SN Identification rate*			Tumor status of nodes		
				Overall	Dye	Probe	SN pos	NSN pos	SN false neg
Morton [18]	223	237	Yes	82%	82%	N/A	22%	37%	1.0%
Reintgen [51]	42	42	Yes	100%	100%	N/A	19%	12%	0%
Krag [34]	121	140	No	98%	91%	98%	12%	N/R	N/A
Thompson [52]	118	120	Yes	87%	87%	N/A	21%	18%	1.7%
Albertini [33]	106	129	No	96%	80%	N/R	15%	N/R	N/A
Leong [50]	163	189	No	98%	74%	98%	18%	18%	N/A
Lingam [53]	35	35	No	100%	100%	N/A	26%	22%	N/A
Morton [24]	72	79	No	90%	90%	N/A	15%	N/R	N/A
Bostick [54]	87	100	No	98%	94%	92%	17%	24%	N/A
Gershenwald [26]	612	683	No	93%	N/A	N/A	15%	21%	1.3%
Morton [35]	1,135	1,299	No	97%	95%	99%**	19%	N/R	N/A

N/R = Not reported; N/A = not applicable
*Per basin
**Dye plus probe

node metastases, when undertaken by an experienced nuclear medicine/surgical oncology/pathology team.

The SN specimen allows a focused pathological evaluation that is not possible with the much larger LND specimen [55]. This detailed examination of one or two SNs uses serial sectioning and immunohistochemical examination, techniques that would be impractical and costly if applied to the entire lymphatic basin. If metastases are present, they will be found in the SN.

Immunohistochemical techniques have further improved the diagnostic sensitivity of detecting occult tumor cells in the regional lymph node basin. The most common targets of immunohistochemical staining for melanoma are the S-100 protein [56, 57] and HMB-45 antigen [58–61]. Immunohistochemical staining is far more sensitive than conventional hematoxylin and eosin staining, but care must be taken to avoid identifying benign nodal nevi as metastatic disease [62]. The very detailed examination of the SN is much more effective than the superficial examination of multiple nodes.

Since our original description of LM/SL in patients with primary cutaneous melanoma in 1990, there has been tremendous interest in the SN concept. Investigators have applied LM/SL to vulvar tumors [63], breast carcinoma [27], thyroid carcinoma [64], and other tumor types [65].

Current Issues in Melanoma LM/SL/SCLND

LM/SL has been recommended as an option in the standard therapy of early-stage melanoma [66, 67]. As the use of this technique becomes more widespread in the treatment of melanoma, breast cancer, and other tumors, several areas of active discussion and debate have emerged. These include the ideal nomenclature for the procedure, the definition of a "hot" (radioactive) SN, the clinical significance of occult metastatic disease, quality assurance, and the role of the procedure outside high-volume melanoma centers.

Ideal Nomenclature

Our original term, intraoperative lymphatic mapping and selective lymphadenectomy [17], has been paraphrased in the literature as selective lymphadenectomy [68], sentinel lymph node dissection [50], sentinel lymphadenectomy [69], sentinel node biopsy [68, 70], sentinel node harvest [71], minimal-access surgery [34], and gamma probe-guided lymph node localization [49]. None of these more recent terms is wrong, but we believe the most accurate description of the identification and excision of the sentinel lymph node is "intraoperative lymphatic mapping and sentinel lymphadenectomy" (LM/SL). This combined with "selective complete lymphadenectomy" (SCLND) best describes the selective approach to complete lymphadenectomy used in patients with tumor-positive lymph nodes.

Definition of an SN by Its Radioactive Count

When LM/SL is performed with a radiocolloid and hand-held gamma probe, the definition of a hot lymph node varies widely. Probe-directed LM/SL is based on the identification of hot lymph nodes that have taken up the radio-colloid. Hot nodes are usually identified by comparing lymph node radioactivity with background radioactivity. The radioactivity of the identified lymph node has been reported as in vivo or ex vivo [33, 72]. The background has been defined as the radioactivity of the nonsentinel nodes, the surrounding lymph node basin, or an area of the body outside the lymph node basin [33, 72]. The node:background count ratio has been defined as 2:1, 3:1, or even 10:1 [33, 49, 73–75]. Other definitions of a hot SN include a radioactive count of ≥15 in 10 s [34], a count of 300–3000 in 10 s [76], an in vivo node:background count ratio of ≥2 or 3 [74], and an ex vivo sentinel:nonsentinel node count ratio of >10 [33]. The multiple definitions and methodologies make evaluation of the literature more complex. Accurate uniform terminology would do much to provide a standard for discussion in the medical literature and forums.

Adding to the confusion are variations in technique. The number of hot lymph nodes will depend on the radiocolloid agent used and the time interval between its injection and the surgical procedure. As the radiolabeled colloid flows along the lymphatic chain, the SN should be the first draining lymph node and the only hot node *if* the mapping procedure is performed within 20–30 min of radiocolloid injection. However, as additional time elapses, the radiolabeled colloid flows up the chain of nodes and additional nodes become hot; therefore, not all hot nodes are SNs (Fig. 1). The hottest node is usually, but not always, the SN. Therefore, the surgeon using radio-colloid alone may not be able to determine the true SN. In contrast, the blue dye rapidly dilutes out and rarely stains any node but the SN, as shown in Fig. 1. To address these technical issues, our procedure has been described in detail [77, 78].

Clinical Significance of Occult Tumor Cells in the SNs

Thus far, no prospective trial has examined the clinical significance of micro-metastatic melanoma in the regional lymph nodes. However, two prospective studies have examined the outcome of therapeutic interventions in patients whose regional lymph nodes were clinically tumor-negative but pathologically tumor-positive. Kirkwood et al. [79] in 1996 reported a significant disease-free and overall survival advantage in patients treated postoperatively with interferon a-2b (IFNa-2b) or observed without postoperative treatment. Among patients who were observed following pathologic evidence of lymph node metastases, those whose lymph nodes had been clinically normal (n = 14) appeared to have a slightly better relapse-free survival rate than

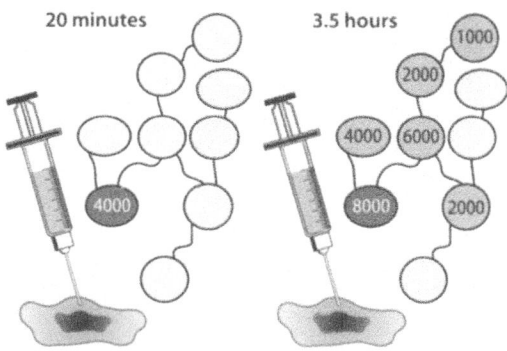

Fig. 1. Shortly after its injection, the radiocolloid flows through the lymphatics to the sentinel node; after 20–30 min, radioactivity will be localized only in the sentinel node. However, after several hours, radiolabeled colloid has progressed along the lymphatic chain to mark additional nodes. Therefore, not all hot (radioactive) nodes are sentinel nodes. In contrast, blue dye rapidly dilutes out and rarely stains any node but the sentinel node blue. *Numbers* indicate radioactivity in counts/unit time. Reprinted with permission from Morton and Chan [105]

those whose lymph nodes had been clinically involved (n = 87) (Fig. 2). Unfortunately, the results of confirmatory trial EST-1690 showed no overall survival benefit in patients receiving high-dose IFNa-2b [80]. Therefore, LM/SL can no longer be proposed for the sole purpose of selecting patients for adjuvant therapy since at the present time no postsurgical therapy for high-risk melanoma is effective in prolonging survival.

Cascinelli et al. [7] in 1998 reported results from the World Health Organization Melanoma Programme trial, which randomized patients with a truncal melanoma ≥1.5 mm in thickness to either immediate or delayed regional LND. There was no overall survival advantage for either treatment arm. In patients with occult metastases, the 5-year survival rate was 48% with immediate LND vs. 27% with delayed LND. The apparent survival advantage of immediate LND in this group (Fig. 3) must be viewed with caution because it was based on a post-hoc subset analysis.

Retrospective matched-pair analysis has demonstrated equivalent rates of 5-year overall survival following LM/SL/SCLND versus ELND (88% versus 86%), but LM/SL/SCLND was more effective in identifying occult nodal metastases in patients with intermediate-thickness (0.75–4.0 mm) melanomas (24% vs. 12%) [81].

Quality Control

As with any evolving surgical technique, ensuring quality is of the utmost importance. However, quality control and credentialing in LM/SL is problematic because of the multidisciplinary expertise required from nuclear medicine, surgery, and pathology.

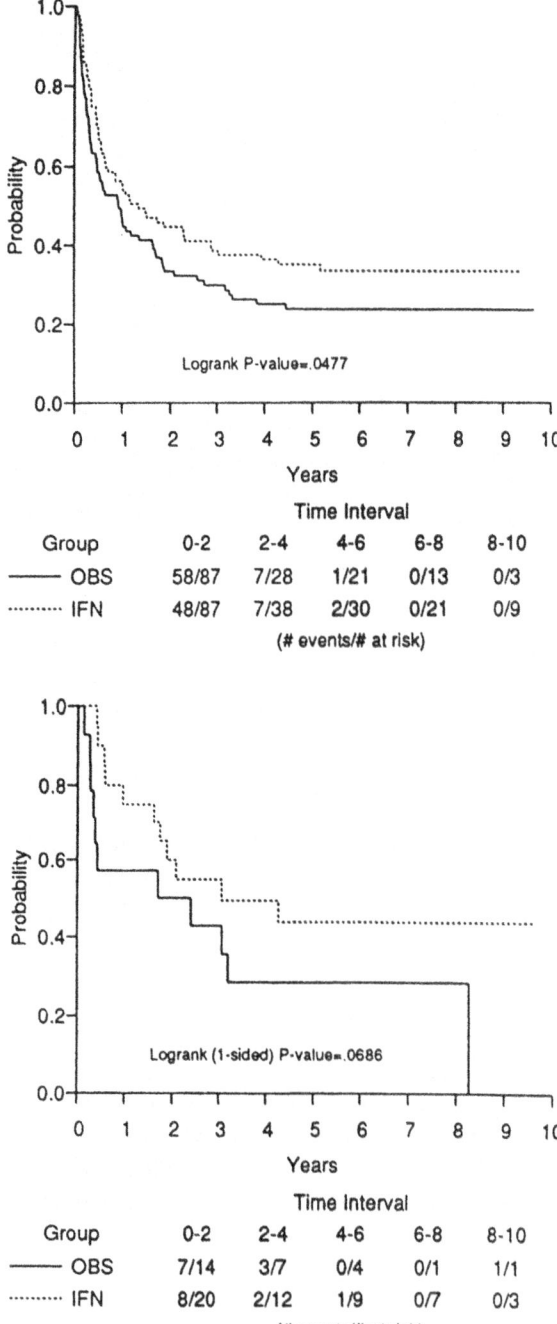

Group   Time Interval

Group	0-2	2-4	4-6	6-8	8-10
—— OBS	58/87	7/28	1/21	0/13	0/3
········ IFN	48/87	7/38	2/30	0/21	0/9

(# events/# at risk)

Group	0-2	2-4	4-6	6-8	8-10
—— OBS	7/14	3/7	0/4	0/1	1/1
········ IFN	8/20	2/12	1/9	0/7	0/3

(# events/# at risk)

Fig. 2. Relapse-free survival following excision of clinically positive, pathologically positive lymph nodes (*top*) or clinically negative, pathologically positive lymph nodes (*bottom*). The observation (OBS) arm of the clinically negative group seems to show a slight relapse-free survival advantage over the OBS arm of the clinically positive group. *IFN*=postoperative adjuvant treatment with interferon. Reprinted with permission from Kirkwood et al. [79]

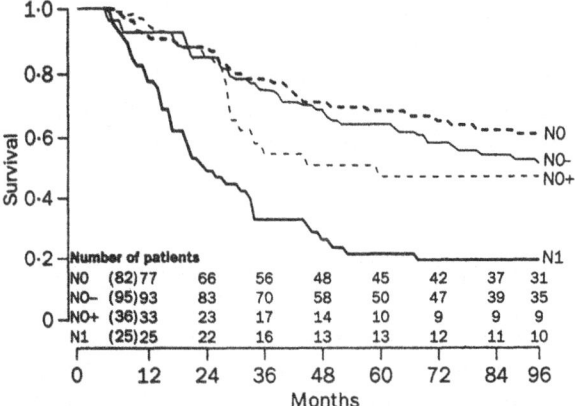

Fig. 3. Following wide excision and immediate or delayed lymph node dissection, patients with clinically and histologically tumor-negative regional lymph nodes seemed to have a higher rate of survival than patients with clinically negative but histologically tumor-positive nodes. N0 = patients who never developed node metastases after wide excision of primary. N0− = patients with clinically and histologically negative nodes at elective node dissection. N0+ = patients with clinically negative and histologically positive nodes at elective node dissection. N1 = patients who developed node metastases during follow-up and underwent delayed regional node dissection. Reprinted with permission from Cascinelli et al. [7]

The role of the nuclear medicine physician is important in identifying the nodal basins at risk and accurately marking the cutaneous location overlying the lymph node, to direct the surgeon properly. The nuclear medicine physician must be familiar with the common lymphatic drainage patterns from the many different areas of the body, in addition to the many aberrant routes that lymphatics may travel and the correspondingly aberrant locations of the SN [75, 76, 82–87]. Imaging must be timed to avoid missing any true SNs or incorrectly identifying nonsentinel nodes as SNs [40, 46].

Recent advances in pathological analysis have improved the accuracy of tumor detection in the lymph node. Because only a very small portion of an individual lymph node is sampled for pathological analysis, the use of immunohistochemical techniques has reduced the incidence of nodes pathologically negative for tumor. Gershenwald et al. [88] in 1998 reported that ten of 243 patients with AJCC stage I or II melanoma developed a first recurrence in a previously mapped negative nodal basin. Re-evaluation of the SNs using immunohistochemical staining with anti-S100 and anti-HMB45 antibodies demonstrated occult metastatic disease in seven of the ten patients. Unfortunately this study did not attempt an equal sampling of SNs from patients who did not recur, to determine how often they would also contain tumor cells. Use of RT-PCR for tyrosinase [89–92], MART-1(melanoma-antigen recognized by T-cells) [93], GalNAc-T [94], and other markers [95, 96] may further upstage patients whose SNs are tumor-free by hematoxylin and eosin staining (H & E) and immunohistochemical techniques. Shivers et al. [91] used nested PCR and ethidium-bromide agarose gel electrophoresis to study H&E-negative SNs from 114 patients. At a mean follow-up of 28 months, the recurrence rate was lower for patients whose SNs were RT-PCR negative for tyrosinase (2%) vs. RT-PCR positive (61%). Bostick et al. [97] used a multimarker RT-PCR approach to identify metastases in the SN and found it to be a more powerful predictor of regional and distant recurrence than H & E or immunohistochemistry. Another interesting means of ultrastaging is the use of cell culture to increase the detection of tumor cells in lymph nodes [98, 99].

Role of LM/SL/SCLND Outside High-Volume Melanoma Centers

Although LM/SL is now recommended as an option in the standard treatment of melanoma by expert consensus [66, 67, 100], the procedure itself is undergoing randomized clinical trials to validate its therapeutic efficacy using survival endpoints [77, 101, 102]. A multinational randomized trial was initiated in 1994 at the John Wayne Cancer Institute to compare survival after wide excision plus LM/SL/SCLND versus wide excision alone (Fig. 4) [35, 77, 101, 102]. More than 1550 patients thus far have been accrued; the accrual goal is 1600. The results from this study will definitively determine the validity of LM/SL in the management of the melanoma patient [35]. In another prospective study, the pathology results of WLE with LM/SL/SCLND are being studied (Fig. 5) [103, 104]. Until these trials are complete, LM/SL, as with any new technique, should be undertaken only under the auspices of a clinical trial [105].

Experienced investigators at many centers have achieved high rates of SN identification and accurate pathological validation. However, each surgeon must climb his or her own learning curve of technical expertise. Although one-day training workshops in LM/SL have been described [34], many re-

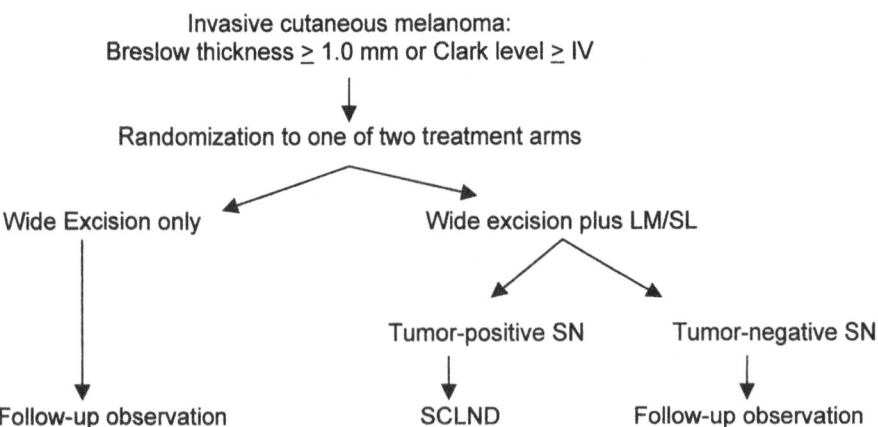

Fig. 4. The phase III randomized multinational trial initiated in 1994 at the John Wayne Cancer Institute is examining survival after wide excision plus LM/SL/SCLND versus wide excision alone. More than 1550 patients thus far have been accrued; the accrual goal is 1600. The results from this study will definitively determine the validity of LM/SL/SCLND in the management of the melanoma patient

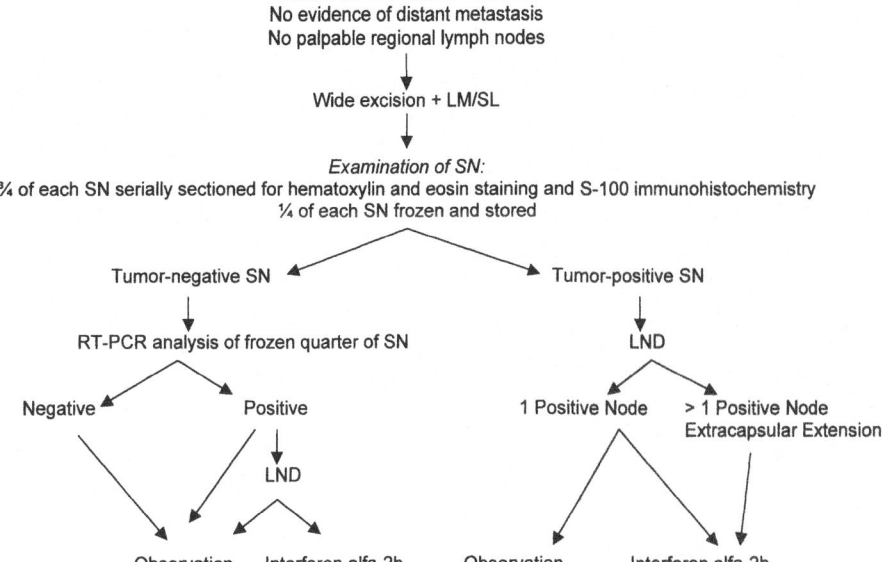

Cutaneous melanoma > 1.0 mm
No evidence of distant metastasis
No palpable regional lymph nodes

Wide excision + LM/SL

Examination of SN:
¾ of each SN serially sectioned for hematoxylin and eosin staining and S-100 immunohistochemistry
¼ of each SN frozen and stored

Tumor-negative SN ← → Tumor-positive SN

RT-PCR analysis of frozen quarter of SN   LND

Negative   Positive   1 Positive Node   > 1 Positive Node
                                                        Extracapsular Extension

LND

Observation   Interferon alfa-2b   Observation   Interferon alfa-2b

Fig. 5. The Sunbelt Melanoma Trial was established to prospectively study the pathology results of sentinel nodes examined by hematoxylin and eosin staining, immunohistochemistry, and reverse transcriptase-polymerase chain reaction (RT-PCR) with tyrosinase. It also is examining the efficacy of SCLND and adjuvant interferon α-2b

ports show that LM/SL has a shallow learning curve that requires many cases to attain an acceptable level of skill (at least 90% accuracy) in identifying the SN. This level of expertise probably requires 30 to 50 cases for melanoma [35, 106, 107], which exceeds the usual caseload of most community-based surgeons.

The experience at the John Wayne Cancer Institute and other cancer centers clearly shows that successful LM/SL is directly related to the surgeon's experience. We have found that the rate of SN identification is highest for a surgeon's most recent cases and for the surgeon performing the most mapping procedures [18, 24]. Accurate results for SN identification have been duplicated worldwide by participants in the phase III multinational randomized trial of LM/SL/SCLND, after successful completion of a learning phase of ≥30 consecutive cases [35]. While ascending the learning curve, the surgeon *must* perform a complete lymphadenectomy after LM/SL to monitor the rate of false-negative SNs identified by dye, probe, or dye plus probe (our preference). Unless each surgeon can validate his or her own accuracy, the patient is at risk of undergoing an expensive procedure that may not accurately reflect the true tumor status of the SN.

Conclusions

The technique of LM/SL shows much promise in the management of the patient with melanoma. The SN hypothesis has been validated in animal and clinical studies. The technical details of preoperative localization and surgical identification have been refined. Pathologic detection of occult tumor cells has been improved by application of immunohistochemical and molecular detection techniques. However, determination of the therapeutic utility of LM/SL/SCLND awaits results of a randomized multicenter clinical trial.

A more uniform nomenclature and definition of the SN will facilitate reporting and discussion. LM/SL/SCLND eventually should be utilized in the community setting, but before then it must be validated within the confines of a clinical trial conducted by academic centers. Except at centers that have validated results for the identification of the SN and for pathologic accuracy, LM/SL should be considered a pathologic adjunct to be followed by complete lymphadenectomy. Even though it has been recommended as an option in standard therapy by expert consensus, extreme caution should be exercised by ensuring multidisciplinary quality and validating results.

Acknowledgements. Supported by grant CA29605 from the National Cancer Institute and by funding from the Wrather Family Foundation (Los Angeles).

References

1. Morton D, Chan A. The concept of sentinel node localization: how it started. Semin Nucl Med 2000;30:4–10
2. American Joint Committee on Cancer. AJCC Cancer Staging Handbook. 5th ed. Philadelphia: Lippincott-Raven; 1998
3. Ederer F, Axtell L, Cutler S. The relative survival rate: a statistical methodology. Natl Cancer Inst Monogr 1961;6:101–121
4. Breslow A. Thickness, cross-sectional areas and depth of invasion in the prognosis of cutaneous melanoma. Ann Surg 1970;172:902–8
5. Balch CM, Murad TM, Soong SJ, Ingalls AL, Richards PC, Maddox WA. Tumor thickness as a guide to surgical management of clinical stage I melanoma patients. Cancer 1979;43:883–8
6. Schneebaum S, Briele HA, Walker MJ, Greager J, Wood DK, Ronan SG, et al. Cutaneous thick melanoma. Prognosis and treatment. Arch Surg 1987;122:707–11
7. Cascinelli N, Morabito A, Santinami M, MacKie RM, Belli F. Immediate or delayed dissection of regional nodes in patients with melanoma of the trunk: a randomised trial. WHO Melanoma Programme. Lancet 1998;351:793–6
8. Veronesi U, Adamus J, Bandiera DC, Brennhovd O, Caceres E, Cascinelli N, et al. Delayed regional lymph node dissection in stage I melanoma of the skin of the lower extremities. Cancer 1982;49:2420–30
9. Sim FH, Nelson TE, Pritchard DJ. Malignant melanoma: Mayo Clinic experience. Mayo Clin Proc 1997;72:565–9
10. Sim FH, Taylor WF, Pritchard DJ, Soule EH. Lymphadenectomy in the management of stage I malignant melanoma: a prospective randomized study. Mayo Clin Proc 1986;61:697–705

11. Sim FH, Taylor WF, Ivins JC, Pritchard DJ, Soule EH. A prospective randomized study of the efficacy of routine elective lymphadenectomy in management of malignant melanoma. Preliminary results. Cancer 1978;41:948-56

12. Pritchard DJ, Sim FH. Surgical management of malignant melanoma of the trunk and extremities. Mayo Clin Proc 1989;64:846-51

13. Balch CM, Soong SJ, Bartolucci AA, Urist MM, Karakousis CP, Smith TJ, et al. Efficacy of an elective regional lymph node dissection of 1 to 4 mm thick melanomas for patients 60 years of age and younger. Ann Surg 1996;224:255-63

14. Balch C, Ross M, Soong S, Harrison R. Long-term results of a prospective, randomized trial involving elective regional lymph node dissection in patients with intermediate thickness melanomas. Presented at the Annual Meeting of the Society of Surgical Oncology, Orlando, Florida, March 4-7, 1999

15. Urist MM, Maddox WA, Kennedy JE, Balch CM. Patient risk factors and surgical morbidity after regional lymphadenectomy in 204 melanoma patients. Cancer 1983; 51:2152-6

16. Karakousis CP, Driscoll DL. Groin dissection in malignant melanoma. Br J Surg 1994;81:1771-4

17. Morton D, Cagle L, Wong J, et al. Intraoperative lymphatic mapping and selective lymphadenectomy: technical details of a new procedure for clinical stage I melanoma. Presented at the Annual Meeting of the Society of Surgical Oncology, Washington DC, 1990

18. Morton DL, Wen DR, Wong JH, Economou JS, Cagle LA, Storm FK, et al. Technical details of intraoperative lymphatic mapping for early stage melanoma. Arch Surg 1992;127:392-9

19. Essner R, Conforti A, Kelley M, et al. Cost-conscious management of the inguinal nodes in early-stage melanoma. Melanoma Res 1997;7(suppl 1):S29

20. Holmes EC, Moseley HS, Morton DL, Clark W, Robinson D, Urist MM. A rational approach to the surgical management of melanoma. Ann Surg 1977;186:481-90

21. Cabanas RM: An approach for the treatment of penile carcinoma. Cancer 1977; 39:456-466

22. Wong JH, Cagle LA, Morton DL. Lymphatic drainage of skin to a sentinel lymph node in a feline model. Ann Surg 1991;214:637-41

23. Ollila DW, Foshag LJ, Essner R, Stern SL, Morton DL. Parotid region lymphatic mapping and sentinel lymphadenectomy for cutaneous melanoma. Ann Surg Oncol 1999; 6:150-4

24. Morton DL, Wen DR, Foshag LJ, Essner R, Cochran A. Intraoperative lymphatic mapping and selective cervical lymphadenectomy for early-stage melanomas of the head and neck. J Clin Oncol 1993;11:1751-6

25. Cochran AJ, Wen DR, Morton DL. Management of the regional lymph nodes in patients with cutaneous malignant melanoma. World J Surg 1992;16:214-21

26. Gershenwald JE, Thompson W, Mansfield PF, Lee JE, Colome MI, Tseng CH, et al. Multi-institutional melanoma lymphatic mapping experience: the prognostic value of sentinel lymph node status in 612 stage I or II melanoma patients. J Clin Oncol 1999; 17:976-83

27. Giuliano AE, Kirgan DM, Guenther JM, Morton DL. Lymphatic mapping and sentinel lymphadenectomy for breast cancer. Ann Surg 1994;220:391-8

28. Giuliano AE, Dale PS, Turner RR, Morton DL, Evans SW, Krasne DL. Improved axillary staging of breast cancer with sentinel lymphadenectomy. Ann Surg 1995;222:394-9

29. Turner RR, Ollila DW, Krasne DL, Giuliano AE. Histopathologic validation of the sentinel lymph node hypothesis for breast carcinoma. Ann Surg 1997;226:271-6

30. Krag DN, Weaver DL, Alex JC, Fairbank JT. Surgical resection and radiolocalization of the sentinel lymph node in breast cancer using a gamma probe. Surg Oncol 1993; 2:335-9

31. Albertini JJ, Lyman GH, Cox C, Yeatman T, Balducci L, Ku N, et al. Lymphatic mapping and sentinel node biopsy in the patient with breast cancer. JAMA 1996;276:1818-22

32. McCarthy W, Thompson J, Uren R. Invited commentary. Arch Surg 1995;130:659-660

33. Albertini JJ, Cruse CW, Rapaport D, Wells K, Ross M, DeConti R, et al. Intraoperative radio-lympho-scintigraphy improves sentinel lymph node identification for patients with melanoma. Ann Surg 1996;223:217–24

34. Krag DN, Meijer SJ, Weaver DL, Loggie BW, Harlow SP, Tanabe KK, et al. Minimal-access surgery for staging of malignant melanoma. Arch Surg 1995;130:654–8

35. Morton DL, Thompson JF, Essner R, Elashoff R, Stern SL, Nieweg OE, et al. Validation of the accuracy of intraoperative lymphatic mapping and sentinel lymphadenectomy for early-stage melanoma: a multicenter trial. Multicenter Selective Lymphadenectomy Trial Group. Ann Surg 1999;230:453–63

36. Robinson DS, Sample WF, Fee HJ, Holmes C, Morton DL. Regional lymphatic drainage in primary malignant melanoma of the trunk determined by colloidal gold scanning. Surg Forum 1977;28:147–8

37. Fee HJ, Robinson DS, Sample WF, Graham LS, Holmes EC, Morton DL. The determination of lymph shed by colloidal gold scanning in patients with malignant melanoma: a preliminary study. Surgery 1978;84:626–32

38. Strand SE, Persson BR. Quantitative lymphoscintigraphy I: Basic concepts for optimal uptake of radiocolloids in the parasternal lymph nodes of rabbits. J Nucl Med 1979;20:1038–46

39. Saha G, Feiglin D, O'Donnell J, Go R, Karam P, MacIntyre W. Experience with technetium-99 m albumin colloid kit for reticuloendothelial system imaging. J Nucl Med Technol 1986;14:149–151

40. Pijpers R, Collet GJ, Meijer S, Hoekstra OS. The impact of dynamic lymphoscintigraphy and gamma probe guidance on sentinel node biopsy in melanoma. Eur J Nucl Med 1995;22:1238–41

41. Lamki L, Haynie T, Balch C, Bhadkamkar V, Podoloff D, Kim E. Lymphoscintigraphy in the surgical management of patients with truncal melanoma: comparison of technetium sulfur colloid with technetium human serum albumin [abstract]. J Nucl Med 1989;30:844

42. McNeill GC, Witte MH, Witte CL, Williams WH, Hall JN, Patton DD, et al. Whole-body lymphangioscintigraphy: preferred method for initial assessment of the peripheral lymphatic system. Radiology 1989;172:495–502

43. Kataoka M, Kawamura M, Hamada K, Itoh H, Nishiyama Y, Hamamoto K. Quantitative lymphoscintigraphy using ^{99m}Tc human serum albumin in patients with previously treated uterine cancer. Br J Radiol 1991;64:1119–21

44. Esato K, Ohara M, Seyama A, Akimoto F, Kuga T, Takenaka H, et al. ^{99m}Tc-HSA lymphoscintigraphy and leg edema following arterial reconstruction. J Cardiovasc Surg (Torino) 1991;32:741–6

45. Bertil R, Persson R, Naversten Y. Technetium-99 m sulfide colloid preparation for scintigraphy of the reticuloendothelial system. Acta Radiol Ther Phys Biol 1970;9:567–76

46. Glass EC, Essner R, Morton DL. Kinetics of three lymphoscintigraphic agents in patients with cutaneous melanoma. J Nucl Med 1998;39:1185–90

47. Wilhelm AJ, Mijnhout GS, Franssen EJ. Radiopharmaceuticals in sentinel lymph-node detection – an overview. Eur J Nucl Med 1999;26:S36–42

48. Thompson JF, Uren RF, Shaw HM, McCarthy WH, Quinn MJ, O'Brien CJ, et al. Location of sentinel lymph nodes in patients with cutaneous melanoma: new insights into lymphatic anatomy. J Am Coll Surg 1999;189:195–204

49. Alex JC, Weaver DL, Fairbank JT, Rankin BS, Krag DN. Gamma-probe-guided lymph node localization in malignant melanoma. Surg Oncol 1993;2:303–8

50. Leong SP, Steinmetz I, Habib FA, McMillan A, Gans JZ, Allen RE Jr, et al. Optimal selective sentinel lymph node dissection in primary malignant melanoma. Arch Surg 1997;132:666–72

51. Reintgen D, Cruse CW, Wells K, Berman C, Fenske N, Glass F, et al. The orderly progression of melanoma nodal metastases. Ann Surg 1994;220:759–67

52. Thompson JF, McCarthy WH, Bosch CM, O'Brien CJ, Quinn MJ, Paramaesvaran S, et al. Sentinel lymph node status as an indicator of the presence of metastatic melanoma in regional lymph nodes. Melanoma Res 1995;5:255–60

53. Lingam MK, Mackie RM, McKay AJ. Intraoperative identification of sentinel lymph node in patients with malignant melanoma. Br J Cancer 1997;75:1505-8

54. Bostick P, Essner R, Glass E, Kelley M, Sarantou T, Foshag LJ, et al. Comparison of blue dye and probe-assisted intraoperative lymphatic mapping in melanoma to identify sentinel nodes in 100 lymphatic basins. Arch Surg 1999;134:43-9

55. Cochran AJ, Wen DR, Morton DL. Occult tumor cells in the lymph nodes of patients with pathological stage I malignant melanoma. An immunohistological study. Am J Surg Pathol 1988;12:612-8

56. Gaynor R, Herschman HR, Irie R, Jones P, Morton D, Cochran A. S100 protein: a marker for human malignant melanomas? Lancet 1981;1:869-71

57. Cochran AJ, Lu HF, Li PX, Saxton R, Wen DR. S-100 protein remains a practical marker for melanocytic and other tumours. Melanoma Res 1993;3:325-30

58. Ordonez NG, Ji XL, Hickey RC. Comparison of HMB-45 monoclonal antibody and S-100 protein in the immunohistochemical diagnosis of melanoma. Am J Clin Pathol 1988;90:385-90

59. Ordonez NG, Sneige N, Hickey RC, Brooks TE. Use of monoclonal antibody HMB-45 in the cytologic diagnosis of melanoma. Acta Cytol 1988;32:684-8

60. Walts AE, Said JW, Shintaku IP. Cytodiagnosis of malignant melanoma. Immunoperoxidase staining with HMB-45 antibody as an aid to diagnosis. Am J Clin Pathol 1988; 90:77-80

61. Fernando SS, Johnson S, Bate J. Immunohistochemical analysis of cutaneous malignant melanoma: comparison of S-100 protein, HMB-45 monoclonal antibody and NKI/C3 monoclonal antibody. Pathology 1994;26:16-9

62. Carson KF, Wen DR, Li PX, Lana AM, Bailly C, Morton DL, et al. Nodal nevi and cutaneous melanomas. Am J Surg Pathol 1996;20:834-40

63. Levenback C, Burke TW, Gershenson DM, Morris M, Malpica A, Ross MI. Intraoperative lymphatic mapping for vulvar cancer. Obstet Gynecol 1994;84:163-7

64. Kelemen PR, Van Herle AJ, Giuliano AE. Sentinel lymphadenectomy in thyroid malignant neoplasms. Arch Surg 1998;133:288-92

65. Bilchik AJ, Giuliano A, Essner R, Bostick P, Kelemen P, Foshag LJ, et al. Universal application of intraoperative lymphatic mapping and sentinel lymphadenectomy in solid neoplasms. Cancer J Sci Am 1998;4:351-8

66. Houghton A, Coit D, Bloomer W, Buzaid A, Chu D, Eisenburgh B, et al. NCCN melanoma practice guidelines. National Comprehensive Cancer Network. Oncology (Huntingt) 1998;12:153-77

67. Coit D, Wallack M, Balch C. Society of Surgical Oncology practice guidelines. Melanoma surgical practice guidelines. Oncology (Huntingt) 1997;11:1317-23

68. Ross MI, Reintgen D, Balch CM. Selective lymphadenectomy: emerging role for lymphatic mapping and sentinel node biopsy in the management of early stage melanoma. Semin Surg Oncol 1993;9:219-23

69. Bachter D, Balda BR, Vogt H, Buchels H. Primary therapy of malignant melanomas: sentinel lymphadenectomy. Int J Dermatol 1998;37:278-82

70. van der Veen H, Hoekstra OS, Paul MA, Cuesta MA, Meijer S. Gamma probe-guided sentinel node biopsy to select patients with melanoma for lymphadenectomy. Br J Surg 1994;81:1769-70

71. Reintgen D. Lymphatic mapping and sentinel node harvest for malignant melanoma. J Surg Oncol 1997;66:277-81

72. Kapteijn BA, Nieweg OE, Muller SH, Liem IH, Hoefnagel CA, Rutgers EJ, et al. Validation of gamma probe detection of the sentinel node in melanoma. J Nucl Med 1997; 38:362-6

73. Brobeil A, Kamath D, Cruse CW, Rapaport DP, Wells KE, Shons AR, et al. The clinical relevance of sentinel lymph nodes identified with radiolymphoscintigraphy. J Fla Med Assoc 1997;84:157-60

74. Glass LF, Messina JL, Cruse W, Wells K, Rapaport D, Miliotes G, et al. The use of intraoperative radiolymphoscintigraphy for sentinel node biopsy in patients with malignant melanoma. Dermatol Surg 1996;22:715-20

75. Bostick P, Essner R, Sarantou T, Kelley M, Glass E, Foshag L, et al. Intraoperative lymphatic mapping for early-stage melanoma of the head and neck. Am J Surg 1997;174:536–9

76. Mudun A, Murray DR, Herda SC, Eshima D, Shattuck LA, Vansant JP, et al. Early stage melanoma: lymphoscintigraphy, reproducibility of sentinel node detection, and effectiveness of the intraoperative gamma probe. Radiology 1996;199:171–5

77. Kelley MC, Ollila DW, Morton DL. Lymphatic mapping and sentinel lymphadenectomy for melanoma. Semin Surg Oncol 1998;14:283–90

78. Morton DL, Bostick PJ. Will the true sentinel node please stand? [editorial]. Ann Surg Oncol 1999;6:12–4

79. Kirkwood JM, Strawderman MH, Ernstoff MS, Smith TJ, Borden EC, Blum RH. Interferon a-2b adjuvant therapy of high-risk resected cutaneous melanoma: the Eastern Cooperative Oncology Group Trial EST 1684. J Clin Oncol 1996;14:7–17

80. Kirkwood J, Ibrahim J, Sondak V, Ernstoff M, Flaherty L, Smith T, et al. Role of high-dose IFN in high-risk melanoma: preliminary results of the E1690/S9111/C9190 US Intergroup postoperative adjuvant trial of high and low-dose IFNa2b (HDI and LDI) in resected high-risk primary or regionally lymph node metastatic melanoma in relation to 10-year updated results of E1684. Presented at the Symposium on Advances in Biology and Treatment of Cutaneous Melanoma, Boston, November 7, 1998

81. Essner R, Conforti A, Kelley MC, Wanek L, Stern S, Glass E, et al. Efficacy of lymphatic mapping, sentinel lymphadenectomy, and selective complete lymph node dissection as a therapeutic procedure for early-stage melanoma. Ann Surg Oncol 1999;6:442–9

82. Dale PS, Foshag LJ, Wanek LA, Morton DL. Metastasis of primary melanoma to two separate lymph node basins: prognostic significance. Ann Surg Oncol 1997;4:13–8

83. O'Brien CJ, Uren RF, Thompson JF, Howman-Giles RB, Petersen-Schaefer K, Shaw HM, et al. Prediction of potential metastatic sites in cutaneous head and neck melanoma using lymphoscintigraphy. Am J Surg 1995;170:461–6

84. Wong JH, Truelove K, Ko P, Coel MN. Localization and resection of an in transit sentinel lymph node by use of lymphoscintigraphy, intraoperative lymphatic mapping, and a hand-held gamma probe. Surgery 1996;120:114–6

85. Taylor A, Jr, Murray D, Herda S, Vansant J, Alazraki N. Dynamic lymphoscintigraphy to identify the sentinel and satellite nodes. Clin Nucl Med 1996;21:755–8

86. Alazraki NP, Eshima D, Eshima LA, Herda SC, Murray DR, Vansant JP, et al. Lymphoscintigraphy, the sentinel node concept, and the intraoperative gamma probe in melanoma, breast cancer, and other potential cancers. Semin Nucl Med 1997;27:55–67

87. Lieber KA, Standiford SB, Kuvshinoff BW, Ota DM. Surgical management of aberrant sentinel lymph node drainage in cutaneous melanoma. Surgery 1998;124:757–61

88. Gershenwald JE, Colome MI, Lee JE, Mansfield PF, Tseng C, Lee JJ, et al. Patterns of recurrence following a negative sentinel lymph node biopsy in 243 patients with stage I or II melanoma. J Clin Oncol 1998;16:2253–60

89. Van der Velde-Zimmermann D, Roijers JF, Bouwens-Rombouts A, De Weger RA, De Graaf PW, Tilanus MG, et al. Molecular test for the detection of tumor cells in blood and sentinel nodes of melanoma patients. Am J Pathol 1996;149:759–64

90. Joseph E, Messina J, Glass FL, Cruse CW, Rapaport DP, Berman C, et al. Radioguided surgery for the ultrastaging of the patient with melanoma. Cancer J Sci Am 1997;3:341–5

91. Shivers SC, Wang X, Li W, Joseph E, Messina J, Glass LF, et al. Molecular staging of malignant melanoma: correlation with clinical outcome. JAMA 1998;280:1410–5

92. Wang X, Heller R, VanVoorhis N, Cruse CW, Glass F, Fenske N, et al. Detection of submicroscopic lymph node metastases with polymerase chain reaction in patients with malignant melanoma. Ann Surg 1994;220:768–74

93. Goydos JS, Ravikumar TS, Germino FJ, Yudd A, Bancila E. Minimally invasive staging of patients with melanoma: sentinel lymphadenectomy and detection of the melanoma-specific proteins MART-1 and tyrosinase by reverse transcriptase polymerase chain reaction. J Am Coll Surg 1998;187:182–8

94. Kuo CT, Bostick PJ, Irie RF, Morton DL, Conrad AJ, Hoon DS. Assessment of messenger RNA of β-1 → 4-N-acetylgalactosaminyl-transferase as a molecular marker for metastatic melanoma. Clin Cancer Res 1998;4:411–8

95. Doi F, Chi DD, Charuworn BB, Conrad AJ, Russell J, Morton DL, et al. Detection of β-human chorionic gonadotropin mRNA as a marker for cutaneous malignant melanoma. Int J Cancer 1996;65:454–9

96. Sarantou T, Chi DD, Garrison DA, Conrad AJ, Schmid P, Morton DL, et al. Melanoma-associated antigens as messenger RNA detection markers for melanoma. Cancer Res 1997;57:1371–6

97. Bostick PJ, Morton DL, Turner RR, Huynh KT, Wang HJ, Elashoff R, et al. Prognostic significance of occult metastases detected by sentinel lymphadenectomy and reverse transcriptase-polymerase chain reaction in early-stage melanoma patients. J Clin Oncol 1999;17:3238–3244

98. Heller R, King B, Baekey P, Cruse W, Reintgen D. Identification of submicroscopic lymph node metastases in patients with malignant melanoma. Semin Surg Oncol 1993; 9:285–9

99. Heller R, Becker J, Wasselle J, Baekey P, Cruse W, Wells K, et al. Detection of submicroscopic lymph node metastases in patients with melanoma. Arch Surg 1991; 126:1455–9

100. Kroon BB, Bergman W, Coebergh JW, Ruiter DJ. Consensus on the management of malignant melanoma of the skin in The Netherlands. Dutch Melanoma Working Party. Melanoma Res 1999;9:207–12

101. Essner R. The role of lymphoscintigraphy and sentinel node mapping in assessing patient risk in melanoma. Semin Oncol 1997;24:S8–10

102. Morton DL. Sentinel lymphadenectomy for patients with clinical stage I melanoma. J Surg Oncol 1997;66:267–9

103. Edwards MJ, Martin KD, McMasters KM. Lymphatic mapping and sentinel lymph node biopsy in the staging of melanoma. Surg Oncol 1998;7:51–7

104. McMasters KM, Sondak VK, Lotze MT, Ross MI. Recent advances in melanoma staging and therapy. Ann Surg Oncol 1999;6:467–75

105. Morton DL, Chan AD. Current status of intraoperative lymphatic mapping and sentinel lymphadenectomy for melanoma: is it standard of care? J Am Coll Surg 1999; 189:214–23

106. Morton DL. Intraoperative lymphatic mapping and sentinel lymphadenectomy: community standard care or clinical investigation? Cancer J Sci Am 1997;3:328–30

107. Morton DL, Giuliano AE, Reintgen DS, Roses DF, Ross MI, Thompson JF. Symposium: Lymphatic mapping and sentinel node biopsy in patients with breast cancer and melanoma. Contemporary Surg 1998;53:353–361

Adjuvant Therapy of Malignant Melanoma and the Role of Sentinel Node Mapping

A. M. M. Eggermont

Erasmus Medical Center Rotterdam, Department of Surgical Oncology,
University Hospital Rotterdam–Daniel Den Hoed Cancer Center,
301 Groene Hilledijk, 3075 EA Rotterdam, The Netherlands

Abstract

Background: Controversy still exists about standard management of a primary melanoma. Over the last decades randomized phase III trials have addressed questions about the width of margin in relation to the Breslow thickness of the primary lesion, the role of prophylactic isolated limb perfusion, and the role of elective lymph node dissection. Overall these trials have demonstrated that less extensive surgery is as good as more extensive surgery. Wide excision margins, prophylactic isolated limb perfusions, or the elective lymph node dissection did not improve overall survival significantly in any of the phase III trials conducted.

Adjuvant Therapy in High Risk Melanoma: No standard systemic adjuvant therapy with confirmed impact on overall survival has been identified thus far for clinically node negative stage I–II (TxN0M0) patients after excision of the primary, nor for clinically node positive stage III (TxN1–2M0) patients after lymph node dissection for metastasic regional node involvement.

Poor Staging in the Past. One of the main problems associated with the trials assessing systemic adjuvant treatments in management of high risk primary melanoma is the fact that in general patients were poorly staged. About 25%–30% of patients with primaries thicker than 1.5 mm have micrometastatic disease in the regional lymph nodes and beyond. This population was usually submerged by the other 70%–75% of the patients with excellent prognosis, obscuring the potential benefit of the adjuvant surgical procedure (ELND) or a systemic adjuvant treatment.

Sentinel Lymph Node Mapping: Sentinel lymph node (SLN) mapping is resolving many of the inadequacies of the past and has completely changed the management of primary melanoma. As a small procedure with low morbidity it identifies that part of the population which has microscopic involvement of regional lymph nodes with greater precision than an elective lymph node dissection.

Recent Results in Cancer Research, Vol. 157
© Springer-Verlag Berlin · Heidelberg 2000

SLN-mapping allows for a detailed histopathologic evaluation involving multiple sections, H&E staining in combination with IHC (immunohisto-chemical staining) of the node with the highest chance of containing meta-static foci. Moreover in the near future it is most likely that RT-PCR on neg-ative nodes will complete the diagnostic workup as a promising last step in the procedure to determine whether tumor cells are present in the sentinel node. Sentinel lymph node status has been shown recently to be by far the strongest independent prognostic factor of melanoma stage I–II patients. SLN-status is a much stronger prognostic factor than tumor thickness, which looses its prognostic relevance in SLN-positive patients.

Consequences for Development and/or Allocation of Adjuvant Therapy: Thus we now have a procedure by which the melanoma stage I–II population can be dissected in a group at truly high risk for recurrence and a group with truly low risk of recurrence. The high risk group with a greater than 75% chance for systemic disease can then be selected for trial participation of various systemic adjuvant therapy regimens that may be allowed to be toxic, considering the very high risk for relapse in these patients. The node nega-tive group of patients can be selected for participation in trials evaluating systemic adjuvant treatment of low toxicity considering the low chance for distant metastatic disease.

Adjuvant Therapy of Malignant Melanoma

Adjuvant therapies in the management of primary malignant melanoma can be locoregional or systemic in nature. Locoregional adjuvant therapies are surgical procedures that are performed in addition to the simple excision of the primary melanoma in the absence of clinical evidence of the presence of locoregional disease. These procedures are: (1) reexcision of the excisional biopsy area to obtain wide excision margins; (2) elective lymph node dissec-tion (ELND) of the regional lymph nodes; (3) adjuvant isolated limb perfu-sion (ILP) with cytostatic drug(s). Systemic adjuvant therapies have the goal to eradicate micrometastatic deposits throughout the body after surgical management of primary melanomas with a high risk of systemic dissemina-tion without clinical evidence of the presence of metastatic disease.

Adjuvant Surgical Procedures in the Management of Primary Melanoma

(Re)Resection to Obtain Wide Margin

The dogma of wide excision of ≥5 cm lost its rationale when Breslow demon-strated that prognosis correlated with thickness of the primary melanoma. The concept of the necessity of a 5 cm margin was challenged and evaluated in a number of phase III trials. Three trials were conducted in patients with

Table 1. Surgical margins and outcome in primary melanoma

Study (Reference)	Margin (cm)	No. of patients	NE LR	WE LR	NE OS	WE OS	AT (years)
Melanomas <2 mm							
WHO-10 [3–4]	1 vs. 3	623	2.5%	1.0%	87%	87%	10 yrs
French Trial [1]	2 vs. 5	319	–	–	93%	90%	4 yrs
Scandinavian [2]	2 vs. 5	769	0.8%	1.0%	90%	93%	5 yrs
Melanomas 1–4 mm							
Intergroup Trial [5]	2 vs. 4	486	0.8%	1.7%	80%	82%	6 yrs
Update [6]	2 vs. 4	470	2.1%	2.6%	ns	ns	8 yrs
Melanomas ≥2 mm							
Nonrandomized study [7]	<2 vs. 3–5	278	8%	16%	58%	50%	5 yrs

NE, narrow excision; *WE,* wide excision; *LR,* local recurrence; *OS,* overall survival.

thin melanomas <2 mm. In the French Trial [1] (319 patients) and the Scandinavian Trial [2] (769 patients) patients were randomized to undergo an excision with margins of 2 cm vs. 5 cm, while in the WHO-Melanoma Program Trial #10 [3–4] (623 patients) margins were 1 cm vs. 3 cm. The Intergroup Trial in the USA [5–6] (486 patients) compared different margins (2 cm vs. 4 cm) in the management of thicker melanomas (1–4 mm melanomas). Table 1 demonstrates that all trials had very similar results: local recurrence rates, disease-free survival (DFS) and overall survival (OS) were virtually identical in the narrow excision and the wide excision arm in all 4 trials. The conclusion from these trials is that a 1 cm margin is sufficient for melanomas less than 2 mm and that a margin of 2 cm is adequate for melanomas 1–4 mm. A nonrandomized study based on 278 cases [7] demonstrated a lack of impact of wider than 2 cm excision margins on the local recurrence rate, DFS and OS in patients with melanomas thicker than 2 mm. Taken together it shows that a 2 cm margin can be considered adequate for all melanomas thicker than 2 mm. This means that virtually all melanomas at any site can be treated by excision and primary closure.

Adjuvant Isolated Limb Perfusion

Isolated limb perfusion was believed to have an impact on survival in the treatment of high risk primary melanoma through the mechanism of ridding the extremity of in-transit micrometastases, being in-transit on their way to form regional lymph node metastases and establish in transit metastases in the (sub)cutaneous compartment. Macroscopic in-transit metastases are known to develop in 5%–8% of the patients with a high risk primary melanoma [8].

While retrospective studies suggested that a prophylactic ILP improved outcome in patients with high risk primary melanoma, this was not observed in a large matched-controlled study [9]. Two very small and inadequate phase III trials claimed a benefit for ILP [10–11]. The only valid and definitive trial addressing the question of the value of a prophylactic ILP with melphalan in the management of high risk primary melanoma of the extremity, is the intergroup trial of the EORTC-WHO and NAPG (North American Perfusion Group) conducted in 832 patients which shows not even a hint of a survival benefit [12]. Prophylactic ILP should no longer be performed. It is a harmful procedure with significant morbidity and costs and without any impact on survival.

Elective Lymph Node Dissection

Elective lymph node dissection (ELND) has been practiced widely based on the hypothesis that micrometastases from the primary melanoma disseminate sequentially from the primary tumor to regional lymph nodes and then to distant sites. As in breast cancer, lymphatic and haematogenic spread occur commonly simultaneously and it is therefore unlikely that removal of lymph nodes containing micrometastases changes the prognosis as most often widespread micrometastatic disease is present.

Retrospective studies using historic controls, studies marred by methodologic problems such as understaging of historic controls and selection bias, usually demonstrated a survival benefit in patients treated by excision plus ELND instead of just excision of the primary [13–15]. Three large studies comprising some 10 000 patients – that did not compare results between different time periods, but evaluated results over one period in time comparing outcome in patients that did undergo excision alone versus excision plus ELND – failed to show an overall benefit for ELND [16–18]. Four randomized phase III trials have been conducted. These trials have failed to demonstrate a significant effect of ELND on overall survival. In the first 2 trials, the large WHO-1 Trial [19–20] and in the much smaller Mayo Clinics Trial [21–22] no benefit was observed for ELND. Patients with microscopically involved lymph nodes in the ELND arm did not fare better than the patients who underwent a delayed lymph node dissection for clinically positive nodes. The overall outcome of the USA Intergroup trial in patients with intermediate primaries of 1–4 mm thickness was also negative [23]. No benefit from ELND occurred in the 2–3 mm or 3–4 mm thick melanomas, but only in the patients with relatively thin melanomas of 1–2 mm in thickness was a benefit from ELND was observed. The recently reported WHO-14 trial in patients with truncal melanomas thicker than 1.5 mm also did not show a significant benefit of ELND overall [24]. In this trial, however, patients with micrometastases in the lymph nodes discovered after ELND fared better than the patients who underwent a delayed lymph node dissection for clinically positive nodes. Routine ELND is overtreatment in 80% of the patient population and is even without convincing proof of impact on survival in the remaining 20%. Thus ELND must be abandoned. Sentinel lymph node mapping is the elegant solution to the problem.

Sentinel Lymph Node Mapping

The sentinel node (SN) mapping procedure presents an attractive option to circumvent the problem of overtreatment and of inflicting morbidity on the whole patient population. The method, using blue dye only, was propagated for the management of melanoma by Morton [25]. The methodology has gained much in accuracy by expanding the methodology by using radiolabeled colloid and a hand-held probe for intraoperative SN identification as well as by the preoperative use of lymphoscintigraphy resulting in an almost 100% identification rate of the SN [26–30]. Sentinel lymph node mapping is a small procedure with low morbidity that identifies that part of the population which has microscopic involvement of regional lymph nodes, with greater precision than an elective lymph node dissection.

SLN-mapping allows for a detailed histopathologic evaluation involving multiple sections, H&E staining in combination with IHC (immunohistochemical staining) of the node with the highest chance of containing metastatic foci. The chance to identify microscopic foci by these procedures is considerably higher than by simply bivalving lymph nodes and evaluating a large number of nodes as is done in the evaluation of full ELND-material. It is now clear that missing microscopic disease in the regional lymph nodes by routine histopathologic evaluation of an elective lymph node dissection, explains the observation in the WHO-1 trial that patients who underwent no ELND and remained free of overt metastases to the regional lymph nodes, had a significantly better survival curve than the patients that underwent an ELND and were found to contain no microscopic involvement of the regional lymph nodes. SN-mapping with meticulous histopathologic work-up of just one or a few sentinel nodes will be associated with a much lower rate of false negative diagnosis. Moreover in the near future it is most likely that RT-PCR on negative nodes will complete the diagnostic workup as a promising last step in the procedure to determine whether tumor cells are present in the sentinel node. It is quite clear from the initial reports from the group of Reintgen of the Lee Moffit Cancer Center that the SN-PCR positive rate corresponds most closely to the eventual relapse and death rates in patients, as we know them to correlate with Breslow thickness [31]. Although it is unlikely that selective lymph node dissection (SLND) will improve survival by itself it is an extremely useful procedure as SN-status has been demonstrated to be the best prognostic factor by far [32]. The use of SN mapping divides the heterogeneous groups of patients (stage IIA–IIB) into truly node-positive and truly node-negative populations with very different prognosis: SN-negative patients have a 5-year survival better than 90% while SN-positive patients have one of about 50%. SLN thus will lead to cleaner phase III trials to identify therapeutic systemic regimens in high risk melanoma patients to treat the concomitant systemic micrometastatic disease.

Systemic Adjuvant Therapy
and the Role of Sentinel Lymph Node Mapping

Results of Various Adjuvant Therapy Trials in High Risk Stage II–III Melanoma

Adjuvant therapy of stage IIA–IIB/III malignant melanoma with various agents has been performed. In terms of impact on overall survival, virtually all trials with interferon-α, with the exception of only one or possibly two trials, have been negative. Seventeen negative reports on efficacy or adjuvant therapy with DTIC (CCNU or BCNU) and/or BCG, C. Parvum or Levamisole have been published [33– 46]. Five reports on sizable "active specific immunotherapy" trials with either whole tumor cell vaccines [47–49] or viral lysates of melanoma cells [50–51] have shown no impact on survival by any of these adjuvant regimens. Finally, phase III trials by the SWOG on adjuvant treatment with Vitamin A [52] and yet another SWOG trial on adjuvant therapy with interferon-gamma [53] have been reported, results being negative. One negative report has been made on the use of s.c. IL2 (in combination with IFNalpha) in the adjuvant setting in high risk melanoma [54]. One randomized phase III trial report on the use of GM2-ganglioside has shown that, in a rather small trial, a benefit could be observed in those patients who were seronegative prior to the vaccination and became seropositive after vaccination [55].

Past, Present and Future Adjuvant IFNα Trials

Reported Phase III trials regarding the adjuvant use of IFN-alpha in melanoma patients with intermediate risk for relapse (stage II) or high risk for relapse (stage III) are summarized in Table 2.

Trials in Patient with Intermediate Risk Melanoma Stage IIA–IIB (>1.5 mm; node negative)
and future impact of SN-mapping
The most recent phase III adjuvant trials have investigated the efficacy of various regimens with IFNα. In patients with primary melanomas greater than 1.5 mm, clinically node negative, three trials in Europe have been completed. These three trials are similar in design, all using IFNα2a at low doses of 3 MU for 6 months (Scottish Trial), 12 months (Austrian Trial), or 18 months (French Trial). A preliminary report on the Scottish trial has not demonstrated a benefit in disease-free survival (DFS) or overall survival (OS) [56], whereas its use over 12 months has been reported to result in a significant benefit on relapse rate [57]. The Austrian study has not reached maturity and so far no significant impact on overall survival (OS) has been observed. The French trial has reached maturity and a significantly prolonged DFS was observed in the IFN-arm and a favorable trend for survival [58]. The NCCTG trial which evaluated the impact of high-dose IFN, intramuscularly, tiw for 3 months was negative both for DFS and OS in a mixed popula-

Table 2. Reported IFN-alpha adjuvant therapy phase III trials in patients with intermediate risk for relapse stage (IIA–IIB) – high risk for relapse (Stage III) melanoma

Study	IFN-alpha regimen	Outcome
ECOG EST 1684 $n = 280$IIB–IIIB	20 MU/m^2 i.v. 5 days per week for 4 wks (induction) 10 MU/m^2 s.c. tiw for 48 wks (maintenance) vs. Observation	Significant DFS benefit (5-yr RFS: IFN, 37%; obs, 26%); significant OS benefit (5-yr OS rate: IFN, 46%; Obs, 37%)
NCCTG 83–7052 $n = 262$T>1.7mm N0M0TxN1–2M0	20 MU/m^2 i.m. tiw for 3 months vs. Observation	No significant difference in DFS or OS
WHO-16 $n = 444$TxN1–2M0	3 MU s.c. tiw for 3 years vs. Observation	No significant difference in DFS or OS
EORTC 18871 $n = 830$T>3mm N0M0TxN1–2M0	1 MU IFNα-2b s.c. on alternate days or IFN-gamma s.c. on alternate days or Iscador or Observation	No significant difference in DFS or OS
ECOG EST 1690 $n = 642$ IIB–III	20 MU/m^2 i.v. 5 days per week for 4 weeks then 10 MU/m^2 s.c. tiw for 48 weeks vs. 3 MU s.c. 3 tiw for 104 weeks vs. Observation	Significant DFS benefit with high-dose IFN, not with low-dose IFN; no OS benefit with high or low dose regimen (hazard ratio = 1.0; p = 0.995)
French Cooperative Melanoma Group $n = 499$IIA–IIB	3 MU s.c. 3 times per week for 18 months vs. Observation	Significant DFS benefit: IFN 100 pts; Obs 119 ptsIFNα 2a 43%, observation 51%: trend for OS benefit with IFN (p = 0.06)
Austrian Cooperative Melanoma Group $n = 311$ IIA–IIB	3 MU s.c. daily for first 3 weeks and tiw for 11 months vs. Observation	Significant DFS benefit: IFN 37 pts (24%); observation 57 pts (57%); no OS benefit (too early for analysis)

OS = Overall Survival; DFS = Disease-Free Survival; RFS = Relapse-Free Survival; Obs = observation; wks = weeks; tiw = three times per week; sc = subcutaneously; im = intramuscularly; iv = intravenously.

tion of stage II-III patients [59]. Overall the data on the impact of treatment with IFN-alpha are still unclear, especially whether the treatment will have any sizeable effect on overall survival. The EORTC-melanoma co-operative group has preferred to investigate a treatment option with considerable fewer side-effects in this Stage II patient population which, as a consequence of the increasing use of SN-staging, will be transformed into a population with a much better prognosis and lower risk for relapse, which will no longer justify (even the evaluation of) toxic adjuvant therapy [56]. Hence in trial #18961 in a population of thirteen hundred patients the efficacy of vaccination with the ganlioside vaccine GM2-KLH/QS-21 will be compared to the outcome in patients receiving standard of care (observation).

Very High Risk Melanoma (Stage IIB–III) and the Impact of SN-Staging on Future Trials
In one rather small trial in 280 patients (ECOG 1684) a significant benefit on DFS and OS has been reported after high dose treatment with IFN-2b for

one year [60]. In the NCCTG Trial (262 patients) it was demonstrated that the same high dose when administered intramuscularly, tiw, for only 12 weeks, resulted only in a trend towards prolonged survival in the TxN1M0 melanoma patients [59]. Both regimens were associated with significant toxicity in the range of grade III–IV toxicity in about 75% of the patients, requiring dose reductions and interruptions of the treatment schedules. No DFS or OS benefit was observed in the low dose IFN (3 MU, tiw, for 3 years) WHO-16 trial in 444 stage IIIB patients [61]. Another low dose IFNalpha one-year regimen was evaluated in the EORTC-18871 trial showing no trend toward benefit [62]. Unfortunately the impact on overall survival by high dose IFNalpha therapy was not confirmed by the recently non-blind ECOG 1690 study, in spite of a significant benefit on DFS [63]. Low-dose IFNalpha treatment in the ECOG 1690 trial did not demonstrate a benefit for either DFS of OS, just like in the WHO-16 trial. Overall it can be stated that observations have been inconsistent on the efficacy of IFNalpha in the adjuvant setting for high risk melanoma. Dose intensity as well as duration of treatment are not clearly defined and the efficacy of any regimen has yet to be demonstrated or confirmed by more than one trial. Table 2 summarizes the experience with IFNalpha in adjuvant phase III trials up till 1999.

On the basis of the results with IFN in stage II patients and on the basis of the observation of a rebound in relapse rates in the IFN treated patients in a number of trials (WHO-16 trial in stage III, French trial in stage II) the hypothesis has been raised that IFN needs to be administered for very long periods of time in order to be effective. This hypothesis is also based on the antiangiogenic mode of action of IFN. Therefore the EORTC-Melanoma Cooperative Group will evaluate longterm therapy with IFN to standard of care (observation) in stage III melanoma. Longterm therapy has two prerequisites: low toxicity and easy administration. Therefore a well tolerated dose of the pegylated form of interferon-alpha (Peg-Intron) will be evaluated, as this agent needs only to be administered s.c. one a week, for a total treatment period of 5 years. This trial (EORTC 18991) will be activated spring 2000. Roughly 50% of the total population of about 900 patients will enter the trial as patients with microscopic metastatic involvement of regional lymph node(s) as a consequence of the steady increase in SN-mapping in Europe. The other 50% will be patients with clinically overt (palpable) regional node involvement. Side studies regarding the value of RT-PCR of the SN and other nodes in the regional node basin and of RT-PCR of blood samples will provide further insight into the biologic importance and predictive value of such procedures. The first report on the predictive value for relapse on the basis of RT-PCR on the SN, by the Reintgen group of the Lee Moffit Cancer Center, are very promising and convincing in this respect [32].

Conclusions

Phase III trials have demonstrated that extensive surgical procedures such as margins wider than 2 cm, elective lymph node dissections, and prophylactic isolated limb perfusions, bring no survival benefit in comparison to limiting the surgery of the primary melanoma to an excision with a relatively narrow margin of maximally 2 cm and primary closure. The prognosis of patients with primary melanomas depends on the presence or absence of systemic micrometastatic disease. This cannot be changed by extended locoregional surgical procedures. The sentinel node procedure provides us with the best information regarding the prognosis of the patient. In case of a positive node, full regional lymph node dissection by itself is unlikely to improve the prognosis of the patient significantly. In the absence of a standard adjuvant therapeutic regimen of proven efficacy for lymph node positive patients, the value of the sentinel node procedure is limited to providing us with the best staging system to perform clean phase III trials to discover an effective adjuvant systemic therapy. Unfortunately no standard adjuvant systemic treatment with confirmed activity has been identified thus far in malignant melanoma.

References

1. Banzet P, Thomas A, Vuillemin E, et al: Wide versus narrow surgical excision in thin (<2 mm) stage I primary cutaneous malignant melanoma: long term results of a french multicentric prospective randomized trial on 319 patients. Proc. Am. Assoc. Clin. Oncol. 12:387, 1993
2. Ringborg U, Andersson R, Eldh J, et al: Resection margins of 2 versus 5 cm for cutaneous malignant melanoma with a tumor thickness of 0.8 to 2.0 mm: randomized study by the Swedish Melanoma Study Group. Cancer 77:1809–1814, 1996
3. Veronesi U, Cascinelli N, Adamus J, et al: Thin stage I primary cutaneous malignant melanoma. Comparison of excision with margins of 1 or 3 cm [published erratum appears in N Engl J Med 1991 Jul 25;325(4):292]. N Engl J Med 318:1159–1162, 1988
4. Cascinelli N: Update WHO-10 trial. WHO-program meeting, May 1995, Albany, NY, USA:317–321, 1995
5. Balch CM, Urist MM, Karakousis CP, et al: Efficacy of 2-cm surgical margins for intermediate-thickness melanomas (1 to 4 mm). Results of a multi-institutional randomized surgical trial [see comments]. Ann Surg 218:262–267; discussion 267–269, 1993
6. Karakousis CP, Balch CM, Urist MM, et al: Local recurrence in malignant melanoma: long-term results of the multiinstitutional randomized surgical trial. Ann Surg Oncol 3:446–452, 1996
7. Heaton KM, Sussman JJ, Gershenwald JE, et al: Surgical margins and prognostic factors in patients with thick (>4 mm) primary melanoma. Ann Surg Oncol 5:322–328, 1998
8. Eggermont AMM. Treatment of melanoma in-transit metastasis confined to the limb. Cancer Surveys 1996; 26:335–349
9. Franklin HR, Schraffordt Koops H, Oldhoff J, et al: To perfuse or not to perfuse? A retrospective comparative study to evaluate the effect of adjuvant isolated regional perfusion in patients with stage I extremity melanoma with a thickness of 1.5 mm or greater. J Clin Oncol 6:701–708, 1988
10. Ghussen F, Nagel K, Groth W, et al: A prospective randomized study of regional extremity perfusion in patients with malignant melanoma. Ann Surg 200:764–768, 1984

11. Fenn NJ, Horgan K, Johnson RC, et al: A randomized controlled trial of prophylactic isolated cytotoxic perfusion for poor-prognosis primary melanoma of the lower limb. Eur J Surg Oncol 23:6–9, 1997

12. Schraffordt Koops H, Vaglini M, Suciu S, et al: Prophylactic isolated limb perfusion for localized, high-risk limb melanoma: results of a multicenter randomized phase III trial. European Organization for Research and Treatment of Cancer Malignant Melanoma Cooperative Group Protocol 18832, the World Health Organization Melanoma Program Trial 15, and the North American Perfusion Group Southwest Oncology Group-8593. J Clin Oncol 16:2906–2912, 1998

13. Balch CM, Soong S-J, Milton GW, Shaw HM, McGovern VJ, Murad TM, McCarthy WH, Maddox WA. A comparison of prognostic factors and surgical results in 1,786 patients with localized (stage I) melanoma treated in Alabama USA, and New South Wales. Australia Ann Surg 1982; 196:677

14. Milton GW, Shaw HM, McCarthy WH, Pearson L, Balch CM, Soong S-J. Prophylactic lymph node dissection in clinical stage I cutaneous malignant melanoma: results of surgical treatment in 1319 patients. Br J Surg 1982; 69:108

15. Reintgen DS, Cox EB, McCarthy KS Jr, Vollmer RT, Seigler HF. Efficacy of elective lymph node dissection in patients with intermediate thickness primary melanoma. Ann Surg 1983; 198:379

16. Drepper H, Kohler CO, Bastian B, et al: Benefit of elective lymph node dissection in subgroups of melanoma patients. Results of a multicenter study of 3616 patients. Cancer 72:741–74, 1993

17. Slingluff CL, Jr., Stidham KR, Ricci WR, et al: Surgical management of regional lymph nodes in patients with melanoma. Ann Surg 219:120–130, 1994

18. Coates AS, Ingvar CI, Petersen-Schaefer K, et al: Elective lymph node dissection in patients with primary melanoma of the trunk and limbs treated at the Sydney Melanoma unit from 1960 to 1991 [see comments]. J Am Coll Surg 180:402–409, 1995

19. Veronesi U, Adamus J, Bandiera DC, et al: Inefficacy of immediate node dissection in stage 1 melanoma of the limbs. N Engl J Med 297:627–630, 1977

20. Veronesi U: Delayed regional lymph node dissection in stage I melanoma of the skin of the lower extremities. Cancer 49:2420–2430, 1982

21. Sim FH: A prospective randomized study of the efficacy of routine elective lymphadenopathy in management of malignant melanoma; preliminary results. Cancer 41:948–951, 1985

22. Sim FH: Lymphadenectomy in the management of stage I malignant melanoma: a prospective randomized study. Mayo Clin Proc 61:697–705, 1986

23. Balch CM, Soong SJ, Bartolucci AA, et al: Efficacy of an elective regional lymph node dissection of 1 to 4 mm thick melanomas for patients 60 years of age and younger. Ann Surg 224:255–263; discussion 263–266, 1996

24. Morton DL, Wen D-R, Wong JH, et al. Technical details of intraoperative lymphatic mapping for early stage melanoma. Arch Surgery 1992; 127:392–399

25. Albertini JJ, Cruse W, Berman C, et al. Intraoperative radiolymphoscintigraphy impoves sentinel lymph node identification for patients with melanoma. Ann Surg, 1996; 223:217–224

26. Thompson JF, McCarthy WH, Bosch CMJ, et al. Sentinel lymph node status as an indicator of the presence of metastatic melanoma in regional lymph nodes. Melanoma Res, 1995; 5:255–260

27. Gershenwald JE, Tscheng C-h, Thompson W, et al. Improved sentinel lymph node localization in primary melanoma patients with the use of radiolabeled colloid. Surgery, 1998; 124:203–210

28. Krag DN, Meijer SL, Weaver DL, et al. Minimal-access surgery for staging of melanoma. Arch Surg 1995; 130:654–658

29. Uren RF, Howman-Giles R, Thompson JF, et al. Lymphoscintigraphy to identify sentinel lymph nodes in patients with melanoma. Melanoma Res, 1994; 4:395–399

30. Gershenwald JE, Colomi MI, Thompson W, Mansfield PE, Lee JE, Colome MI, Tcheng C-h, Balch CM, Reintgen DS, Ross MI. Patterns of recurrence following a negative sen-

tinel lymph node biopsy in 243 patients with stage I or II melanoma. J Clin Oncol, 1998; 16:2253-2260

31. Gershenwald JE, Thompson W, Mansfield PE, Lee JE, Colome MI, Tcheng C-h, Balch CM, Reintgen DS, Ross MI. Multi-institutional melanoma lymphatic mapping experience: value of sentinel lymph node status in 612 stage I or stage II melanoma patients. J Clin Oncol, 1999; 17:976-983

32. Shivers SC, Wang X, Li W, Joseph E, Messina J, Glass LF, DeConti R, Cruse CW, Berman C, Fenske NA, Lyman GH, Reintgen DS. Molecular staging of malignant melanoma: correlation with clinical outcome. JAMA 1998; 28(16)1410-1415

33. Hill GJ II, Moss SE, Golomb FM, et al. DTIC and combination therapy for melanoma. Cancer 1981; 47:2556-2562

34. Pinsky CM, Oettgen HF: Surgical adjuvant for malignant melanoma. Surg Clin North Am 1981; 61:1259-1266

35. Veronesi U, Adamus J, Aubert C, et al. A randomized trial of adjuvant chemotherapy and immunotherapy in cutaneous melanoma. N Engl J Med 1982; 307:913-916

36. Quirt IC, DeBoer G, Kersey PA, et al. Randomized controlled trial of adjuvant chemoimmunotherapy with DTIC and BCG after complete excision of primary melanoma with a poor prognosis or melanoma metastases. Can Med Assoc J 1983; 128:929-936

37. Fisher RI, Terry WD, Hodes RJ, et al. Adjuvant immunotherapy or chemotherapy for malignant melanoma: Preliminary report of the National Cancer Institute randomized clinical trial. Surg Clin North Am 1981; 61:1267-1277

38. Loutfi A, Shakr A, Jerry M, et al. Double blind randomized prospective trial of levamisole/placebo in stage I cutaneous malignant melanoma. Clin Invest Med 1987; 10:325-328

39. Tranum BL, Dixon D, Quagliana J, et al. Lack of benefit of adjunctive chemotherapy in stage I malignant melanoma: A Southwest Oncology Group study. Cancer Treat Rep 1987; 71:643-644

40. Czarnetzki BM, Macher E, Suciu S, Thomas D, Steerenberg PA, Rümke Ph. Long-term adjuvant immunotherapy in stage I high risk malignant melanoma, comparing two BCG preparations versus non-treatment in a randomised multicentre study (EORTC PROTOCOL 18781). Eur J Cancer 1993; 29A:1237-1242

41. Lejeune FJ, Macher E, Kleeberg UR et al. An Assessment of DTIC versus Levamisol and placebo in the treatment of high risk stage I patients after removal of a primary melanoma of the skin, A phase III adjuvant study. EORTC PROTOCOL 18761. Eur J Cancer Clin Oncol, 1988; 24:881-890

42. Quirt IC, Shelley WE, Pater JL. et al. Improved survival in patients with poor prognosis malignant melanoma treated with adjuvant levamisole: a phase III study by the national cancer institute of Canada clinical trials group. J Clin Oncol 1991; 9:729-735

43. Spitler LE. A randomized trial of levamisole versus placebo as adjuvant therapy in malignant melanoma. J Clin Oncol 1991; 9:736-740

44. Karakousis CP, Didolkar MS, Lopez R, et al. Chemoimmunotherapy (DTIC and Corynebacterium *parvum*) as adjuvant treatment in malignant melanoma. Cancer Treat Rep 1979; 63:1739-1743

45. Balch CM, Smalley RV, Bartolucci AA et al. A randomized prospective trial of adjuvant C. Parvum immunotherapy in 260 patients with clinically localized melanoma (stage I): progrnostic factors analysis and preliminary results of immnotherapy. Cancer 1982;49:1079-1084

46. Thatcher N, Mene A, Banerjee SS, et al. Randomized study of Corynebacterium *parvum* adjuvant therapy following surgery for (stage II) malignant melanoma. Br J Surg 1986; 73:111-115

47. Morton DL, Holmes EC, Eilber FR, et al. Adjuvant immunotherapy: Results of a randomized trial in patients with lymph node metastases, in Terry WD, Rosenberg SA (eds): Immunotherapy of Human Cancer. New York, NY, Elsevier North Holland, 1982, pp 245-249

48. Terry WD, Hodes RJ, Rosenberg SA, et al. Treatment of stage I and II malignant melanoma with adjuvant immunotherapy or chemotherapy: Preliminary analysis of a pro-

spective randomized trial, in Terry WD, Rosenberg SA (eds): Immunotherapy of Human Cancer. New York, NY, Elsevier North Holland, 1982, pp 252–257

49. Morton DL. Adjuvant immunotherapy of malignant melanoma: Status of clinical trials at UCLA. Int J Immunother 1986; 2:31–36

50. Wallack MK, Sivanandham M, Balch CM, et al. A phase III randomized, double-blind, multiinstitutional trial of vaccinia melanoma oncolysate-active specific immunotherapy for patients with stage II melanoma. *Cancer* 1995; 75:34–42

51. Hersey P, Coates P, Tyndall L. Is adjuvant therapy worthwhile? *Melanoma Res* 1997; 7(Suppl): (abstract) 78

52. Meyskens FL, Liu PY, Tuthill RJ, et al. Randomized trial of vitamin A versus observation as adjuvant therapy in high-risk primary malignant melanoma: a Soutwest Oncology Group Study *J Clin Oncol* 1994; 12:2060–2065

53. Meyskens FL, Kopecky KJ, Taylor CW et al. Randomized trial of adjuvant human Interferon-gamma versus observation in high risk cutaneous melanoma: a Southwest Oncology Group Study. *J Natl Cancer Inst* 1995; 87:1710–1713

54. Hauschild A, Burg G, Dummer R. Prospective randomized multicenter trial on the outpatient use of subcutaneous interleukin 2 and interferon a 2b in high risk melanoma patients. *Melanoma Res* 1997; 7(Suppl 1):(abstract) 401

55. Livingstone PO, Wong GYC, Adluri S, et al. Improved survival in stage III melanoma patients with GM2 antibodies: a randomised trial of adjuvant vaccination with GM2 ganglioside. *J Clin Oncol* 1994; 12: 1036–44

56. Eggemont AMM. The Current Melanoma Cooperative Group adjuvant trial programme on malignant melanoma: prognosis versus efficacy, toxiity and costs. Melanoma Research, 1997; 7(S2)127–131

57. Pehamberger H, Soyer P, Steiner A, Kofler R, Binder M, Mischer P, Pachinger W, Auböck J, Fritsch P, Kerl H, Wolff K. Adjuvant interferon a-2a treatment in resected primary stage II cutaneous melanoma. J Clin Oncol, 1998; 16:1425–1429

58. Grob JJ, Dreno B, Chastang C, Guillot B, Cupissol D, Souteyrand P, Sassolas B, Cesarini JP, Thivolet J, Denoeux JP, Ortonne JP, Thomas T, Beylot C, Truchetet F, Lorette G, Chemaly C, Meynadier J, Amblard P, Thyss P, Avril MF, Prigent F, Bonerandi JJ. Randomised trial of interferon a-2a as adjuvant therapy in resected primary melanoma thicker than 1.5 mm without clinically detectable node metastases. The Lancet, 1998; 351: 1905–1910

59. Creagan ET, Dalton RJ, Ahmann DL, et al. Randomized surgical adjuvant clinical trial or recombinant interferon-alfa-2a in selected patients with malignant melanoma. J Clin Oncol 1995; 13:2776–2783

60. Kirkwood JM, Strawderman MH, Ernstoff MS, Smith TJ, Borden EC, Blum RH. Interferona2b adjuvant therapy of high-risk resected curaneous melanoma: the Eastern Cooperative Oncology Group Trial EST 1684. J Clin Oncol 1996; 14:7–17

61. Cascinelli N: Evaluation of efficacy of adjuvant rIFNa 2 A in regional node metastases. Proc Am Soc Clin Oncol 14:410, 1995 (abstr)

62. Kleeberg U, Broecker EB, Chartier C, et al. EORTC 18871 adjuvant trial in high risk melanoma patients IFNa vs IFNgamma vs Iscador vs Observation. Eur J Cancer 1999: 35(S4):264(abstr)

63. Kirkwood JM, Ibrahim J, Sondak V, et al: Preliminary analysis of the E1690/S9111/C9190 Intergroup Postoperative Adjuvant Trial of High- and Low-Dose IFNalpha2b (HDI and LDI) in High-Risk Primary or Lymph Node Metastatic Melanoma. Proc Am Soc Clin Oncol 1999; 18:2072 (abstr)

VI. Sentinel Node Detection in Neck and Thyroid Cancer

Selective Neck Dissection and Sentinel Node Biopsy in Head and Neck Squamous Cell Carcinomas

G. Mamelle

Département de Chirurgie Cervico-Faciale, Institut Gustave Roussy, Rue Camille Desmoulins, 94805 Villejuif, France

Abstract

The Sentinel Node concept is now well established for HNSCC and gives us a strong basis to treat patients with N0 neck where the rate of occult node metastasis is high. At the present time, the most accurate method for staging N0 neck is pathologic examination of the neck content. In this way, sentinel node dissection (SND) and sentinel node biopsy (SNB) are complementary surgical procedures.

SNB has limited indications in HNSCC because of the inaccessibility of most of the primary sites to local injection of Tc99m colloid. However it seems to be an encouraging approach for small tumors of the oral cavity.

In other primary sites, except for small glottic tumors, patients must undergo an SND.

Supraomohyoid neck dissection which removes levels I, II and III, is performed in oral cavity tumors.

Lateral neck dissection which removes levels II, III and IV, is used by many authors for laryngeal, oropharyngeal and hypopharyngeal tumors. In our experience, SND could be limited to levels II and III for laryngeal and oropharyngeal tumors without more neck failures.

SND is a reliable procedure, we report only 1.5% of skip nodal metastases in 464 patients who had this staging procedure.

Introduction

Lymphatic metastasis is the most important mechanism in the spread of head and neck squamous cell carcinomas (HNSCC). The rate of node metastasis probably reflects the aggressiveness of the primary tumor and is an important prognosticator. The node metastasis rate is strongly correlated with the distant metastasis rate.

The use of sentinel node dissection (SND) in HNSCC is based on anatomic considerations of the lymphatic drainage of these tumors. SND is used as a staging procedure for patients without clinical node to reduce the morbidity of most invasive procedures such as modified neck dissection. Many studies have confirmed the safety of SND as a diagnostic procedure. More recently, sentinel node biopsy (SNB) has been introduced for patients without clinical node involvement in melanomas and breast cancer. This procedure could be used in some restricted indications in HNSCC.

Lymph Node Involvement

We reviewed, at our Institute, 914 patients who underwent a neck dissection between 1980 and 1985 [1]. Patients with prior treatment, multiple primaries, distant metastasis, or unknown primary were excluded from this analysis. The primary sites were 287 oral cavity, 249 hypopharynx, 247 larynx and 131 oropharynx.

Clinical lymph nodes were classified according to the recommendations of the American Joint Committee on Cancer (AJCC). Primary tumors were restaged according to the Union Internationale Contre le Cancer (UICC).

Table 1 shows patients distribution by T-stage and N-stage. Most patients, 53%, were T3 and 51% were N0.

The lymphatic metastasis spread was related to the primary site (Table 2). We observed 45% of node involvement in the larynx, 51% in the oral cavity, 63% in the oropharynx ,and 86% out of 73% of extracapsular spread in the hypopharynx.

Table 1. T-N stage distribution

	T1	T2	T3	T4	Total
N0	33	182	226	23	464
N1	8	71	109	8	196
N2a	7	29	53	4	93
N2b	5	11	44	5	65
N2c	2	13	28	5	48
N3	5	12	29	2	48
Total	60	318	489	47	914

Table 2. Lymph node involvement

Localisation	No. of patients	%N−	%N+ECS−	%N+ECS+
Larynx	247	55.5	18.6	25.9
Oral cavity	287	48.8	26.6	30.7
Oropharynx	131	26.7	24.4	48.9
Hypopharynx	249	14.1	13.3	72.7

Table 3. Occult nodal metastasis rate in negative neck

	Author			
	Shah	Jones	Li	IGR
No. of patients	343	117	161	399
Oral cavity	34%	29%	26%	34%
Oropharynx	31%	25%	32%	45%
Hypopharynx	4/24	50%	50%	53%
Larynx	37%	21%	40%	27%
Global	33%	32%	32%	34%

This node involvement rate has a direct implication on node dissection modalities.

On one hand, it is not necessary to perform a node dissection on small glottic tumors which have a low risk of node metastasis, and it is questionable for T1 of oral cavity which have a risk of less than 20% of node involvement. On the other hand, we must perform a modified neck dissection (MND) for all hypopharyngeal primaries were nodal involvement is high.

For patient with negative neck, the risk of occult nodal metastasis is in the range 21%–53% [2–4]. The risk depends on the size, site and other characteristics of the tumor (Table 3). In many head and neck primaries, not only is the ipsilateral site of the neck at risk but the contralateral site has a significant risk to harbor metastases as well, especially when the primary has grown close to or extends over the midline.

Neck palpation is both easy and inexpensive to assess the nodal status. The low sensitivity of palpation is at risk of harboring occult metastasis. Other modalities of investigation like CT Scan, MR Imaging, ultrasonics, and positron emission tomography can give us a more precise idea of node status [5] but none gives us certitude.

Because of the fallibility of palpation and other modalities of investigation, it is widely accepted to treat the neck electively if the risk of occult metastases is high.

In our experience, we can avoid elective neck dissection and use a wait-and-see policy in T1 of glottic tumors of the larynx and oral cavity tumors. Negative imaging results can be use as an argument to refrain from elective treatment of the neck.

Sentinel Node Levels

Sentinel node (SN) level is a concept that relies on anatomical [6] and clinical considerations [7]. SN level is predicated on the relative risk for metastasis to specified cervical lymphatic basins for a given primary tumor site within the upper respiratory and digestive tracts.

Table 4. Node involvement by level and primary site (IGR)

	No. of patients	Level I	Level II	Level III	Level IV	Level V
Oral cavity	287	25.4%	35.5%	21.6%	8.4%	4.5%
Oropharynx	131	6.1%	65.6%	43.5%	22.9%	13.0%
Hypopharynx	249	0.8%	73.9%	58.6%	41.8%	12.9%
Larynx	247	0.0%	32.0%	27.9%	8.9%	4.9%

They are defined by international node level classification (Table 4). The neck node levels are coded as (I) sub-mandibular and submental, (II) upper jugular from the skull base superior to the hyoid bone or inferior to the carotid bifurcation, (III) middle jugular from the hyoid bone or carotid bifurcation to the cricothyroid membrane or omohyoid muscle inferiorly, (IV) lower jugular from the omohyoid muscle to the clavicle, (V) posterior triangle nodes and (VI) anterior neck compartment comprising the paratracheal and thyroidal basins [8].

Table 4 shows the relative risk of node involvement for each main primary site in our retrospective study.

For oral cavity tumors, main lymph nodes metastases are located in levels I–III with a maximum of 35% in level II. Anatomic dissection has shown direct connecting lymphatic channels between oral cavity tumor and juguloomohyoid nodes (III). Sentinel node levels for oral cavity are located in levels I–III. For tumors of the anterior floor of the mouth and the anterior two-thirds of the tongue, sentinel nodes are located on both sides of the neck.

Main node metastasis of laryngeal tumors are located in levels II and III with respectively 32% and 28% of node involvement (Table 4). We must take into account invaded structures of the larynx.

Supraglottic tumors give more node metastasis than glottic tumors with nearly a rate of 30% in most studies. At the opposite end, the percentage of node involvement in small glottic tumors (T1) is very low, 5%–7%. Tumors of the subglottic area give node metastasis in level VI (lymph nodes along the recurrent laryngeal nerve). SN are located in levels II and III.

For oropharyngeal tumors, node metastasis occurs preferentially in levels II and III, and less in level IV (Table 4). SN are located in levels II and III. Hypopharynx is at highest risk of lymph node metastasis. Levels I–III are at risk with a maximum of 74% for level II. SN are located in level II–IV.

Selective Neck Dissection

SND consists of en bloc removal of SN related to the location of the primary tumor. It is a less radical procedure than MND with associated reduced morbidity, less cosmetic deformity, and less major function impairment of spinal accessory nerve (shoulder drop, shoulder pain, adhesive capsulitis). It must be considered as a diagnostic procedure for patients with negative neck, at risk for early lymph node metastases. In our retrospective study, patients who underwent SND had pathological frozen sections examination of all lymph nodes removed. In case of positive node, an MND is performed and patients had postoperative radiotherapy 50 Gy on the neck with 15 Gy boost on extracapsular spread areas. The liability of SND can be evaluated by the rate of skip nodal metastases which is the rate of positive disease found outside the SN areas without positive node in SN basins.

Supraomohyoid Neck Dissection

The supraomohyoid neck dissection removes nodal regions I–III. This procedure is recommended for oral cavity tumors. SND of contralateral neck is indicated for tumors involving the two anterior thirds of the oral cavity. The rationale for this neck dissection is based on several studies.

The incidence of skip nodal metastasis outside levels I–III was: 1.5% in 192 patients for Shah [9], 3.3% in 270 patients for Byers [10] in level IV, and 1.5% in 201 patients in our own experience.

Manni has observed 7% of nodal failure with local failure in 57 patients with oral cancer who underwent supraomohyoid dissection [11].

Henick [12] found, in 75 patients, a sensitivity of 82%, a negative predictive value of 91%, and an accuracy of 94% to detect cervical metastasis in SND.

Lateral Neck Dissection

Lateral neck dissection removes nodal regions II–IV. This procedure is used for laryngeal, oropharyngeal and hypopharyngeal tumors. For tumors arising or invading midline visceral structures, SND is performed on both sides.

For patients with N0 neck and laryngeal tumors, Shah [2] reported 1.2% of skip nodal metastasis.

In our experience, we removed only levels II and III. We did not observe lymph node metastasis in level IV without nodal disease in level II or III. Only one patient out of 178 (0.6%) developed a nodal recurrence in contraleral level V.

For oropharyngeal tumors, Shah [2] did not observe any skip nodal metastasis. In our retrospective study, we removed only levels II and III in 54 patients presenting an oropharyngal tumor with N0 neck. We observed two neck failures (3.7%) respectively in level IV and level V.

For hypopharyngeal tumors, Shah [2] did not report any neck failure. We preferred to perform MND in this primary site except for T1 tumors because of the high rate of node metastasis. For this reason, only 29 patients underwent an SND in levels II and III. We reported one node failure in contralateral level II (3.4%).

Results of Selective Node Dissection

Out of 464 patients with negative neck who underwent an SND at our Institute, we observed 29 neck failures (6.3%) without local recurrence. Thirteen nodal recurrences were outside treated neck out of six didn't have the right protocol: bilateral SND for midline involvement or MND for positive nodes at frozen sections examination. Finally seven patients (1.5%) really had a skip nodal metastasis. Four of these seven recurrences were controlled. We can conclude that SND is a reliable procedure.

Sentinel Node Biopsy

SNB is used in cutaneous melanomas [13] to access patient's nodal status. It could be an alternative diagnostic method of SND. We could perform a preoperative radionuclide lymphoscintigraphy and then an intraoperative localization of sentinel nodes with the use of the gamma probe and isosulfan blue dye technique.

At the present time, not much information has been reported about this technique in HNSCC.

Pitman [14] has reported on 16 patients that no isosulfan blue-stained cervical lymph nodes were identified after injection of the mucosa surrounding the primary site.

Koch [15] has shown in 5 patients with oral or oropharyngeal primaries some limitations of this technique due to:
- the inaccessibility of many primary sites to local injection of Tc99m colloid or blue dye without general anesthesia
- the primary tumor site can be close to the first nodal basin obscuring the dynamic lymphoscintigram and the independent detection of the radioactive node with the gamma probe
- intra mucosal injection of radiolabeled colloid is technically more difficult to achieve than in intradermal injection.

To our mind, indications of SNB are limited to the patients with N0 neck, presenting tumors that are easily accessible to injections without general anesthesia: tumors of the oral cavity and upper part of the oropharynx. The tumor must be superficial to make it easy to map all the lymphatic drainage with mucosal injection of Tc99m colloid. If the surgeon determines that adequate resection of primary site requires an approach through the neck, then SND would certainly be more logical.

Finally, only those patients whose primary cancer can be resected intraorally are the subject of the SNB.

Patients presenting a small tumor (T1N0) of the oral cavity with a depth of the tumor less than 4 mm at CT Scan or MR imaging have a low risk of metastatic disease. At the present time, those patients could have a supraomohyoid neck dissection or a wait-and-see policy with the same results [16]. On one hand, SND is an overtreatment, on the other hand the wait-and-see policy is an undertreatment. SNB should be the right approach.

For these reasons, we have decided to begin an SNB protocol for these patients. They have a preoperative lymphoscintigraphy. After induction of general anesthesia, an injection of isosulfan blue dye is performed into the mucosa surrounding the primary tumor. After the neck incision for the supra-omohyoid neck dissection, we use the gamma probe and blue dye coloration of the lymph nodes to locate the SN. SND is completed after removing the SN. All the lymph nodes are checked at frozen sections examination. Patients with positive node undergo an MND.

In our limited experience on two patients presenting a T1 N0 of the oral cavity, we found SN at lymphoscintigram the day before the operation. We could isolate these nodes with the gamma probe during the operation in level I, but we did not obtain any blue dye coloration of the lymph nodes. One patient had negative nodes and the other had metastatic disease only in the SN, other nodes of MND being free of disease. These encouraging results have led us to continue this protocol to confirm the usefulness of this method.

Conclusion

The SN concept is now well established for HNSCC and gives us a strong basis to treat patients with N0 neck where the rate of occult node metastasis is high. At the present time, the most accurate method for staging N0 neck is pathologic examination of the neck content. In that way, SND and SNB are complementary surgical procedures. SNB has limited indications in HNSCC because of the inaccessibility of most of the primary sites to local injection of Tc99m colloid. However, it seems to be an encouraging approach for small tumors of the oral cavity. In other primary sites except for small glottic tumors, patients must undergo an SND.

References

1. Mamelle G., Pampurik J, Luboinski B, Lancar R, Lusinchi A, Bosq J: Lymph Node Prognostic Factors in Head and Neck Squamous Cell Carcinomas. Am J Surg 1994; 168: 494–498
2. Shah JP: Patterns of cervical lymph node metastasis from squamous carcinomas of the upper aerodigestive tract. - Am J Surg 1990 Oct;160(4): 405–499
3. Li XM, Wei WI, Guo XF, Yuen PW, Lam LK: - Cervical lymph node metastatic patterns of squamous carcinomas in the upper aerodigestive tract. J Laryngol Otol 1996 Oct;110(10): 937–411
4. Jones AS, Phillips DE, Helliwell TR, Roland NJ: Occult node metastases in head and neck squamous carcinoma. Eur Arch Otorhinolaryngol 1993;250(8): 446–499
5. van den Brekel M, Castelijns J, Snow G: Diagnostic evaluation of the neck. Otolaryngol Clin North Am 1999; 31: 601–619
6. Rouviere H: - Anatomy of the human lymphatic system. 1938

7. Lindberg R: Distribution of cervical lymph node metastases from squamous cell carcinomas of the upper respiratory and digestive tracts. Cancer 1972; 29: 1446–1449
8. Robbins T: Classification of neck dissections. Current Concepts and Future Considerations. Otolaryngol Clin North Am 1998; 31: 639–654
9. Shah JP, Candela FC, Poddar AK: The patterns of cervical lymph node metastases from squamous carcinoma of the oral cavity. Cancer 1990 Jul 1;66(1): 109–133
10. Byers RM, Weber RS, Andrews T, McGill D, Kare R, Wolf P: Frequency and therapeutic implications of "skip metastases" in the neck from squamous carcinoma of the oral tongue [see comments]. Head Neck 1997 Jan; 19(1): 14–99
11. Manni JJ, van den Hoogen FJ: Supraomohyoid neck dissection with frozen section biopsy as a staging procedure in the clinically node-negative neck in carcinoma of the oral cavity. Am J Surg 1991 Oct; 162(4): 373–366
12. Henick DH, Silver CE, Heller KS, Shaha AR, El GH, Wolk DP: Supraomohyoid neck dissection as a staging procedure for squamous cell carcinomas of the oral cavity and oropharynx. Head Neck 1995 Mar–Apr; 17(2): 119–233
13. Morton D, Wenn DR, Foshag L, Cochran A: Intraoperative lymphatic mapping and selective cervical lymphadenectomy for early-stage melanomas of the head and neck. - J Clin Oncol. 1993; 11: 1751–1756
14. Pitman KT, Johnson JT, Edington H, et al: Lymphatic mapping with isosulfan blue dye in squamous cell carcinoma of the head and neck. Arch Otolaryngol Head Neck Surg 1998 Jul; 124(7): 790–733
15. Koch WM, Choti MA, Civelek AC, Eisele DW, Saunders JR: Gamma probe-directed biopsy of the sentinel node in oral squamous cell carcinoma. Arch Otolaryngol Head Neck Surg 1998 Apr; 124(4): 455–499
16. Vandenbrouck C., Sancho-Garnier H., Chassagne D., Saravane D., Cachin Y., and Micheau C. Elective Versus Therapeutic Radical Neck Dissection in Epidermoid Carcinoma of the Oral Cavity. Cancer 1980; 46: 386–390

Sentinel Lymph Node Dissection for Thyroid Malignancy

P. I. Haigh[1] and A. E. Giuliano[2]

[1] Surgical Oncology, John Wayne Cancer Institute, 2200 Santa Monica Boulevard, Santa Monica, CA 90404, USA
[2] Chief of Surgical Oncology, John Wayne Cancer Institute, 2200 Santa Monica Boulevard, Santa Monica, CA 90404, USA

Abstract

Sentinel lymph node dissection (SLND) for melanoma and breast cancer has been validated as an accurate technique to assess the status of the lymph nodes in the regional drainage basin. The sentinel node concept has also been investigated in other solid tumors, and more recently, in thyroid carcinoma. SLND using a vital blue dye during thyroidectomy for suspected thyroid malignancy successfully identifies sentinel nodes, with minimal morbidity. Excised sentinel nodes can be examined for micrometastases, and if negative, then the rest of the cervical nodes are likely to be negative. The false negative rate of SLND for thyroid malignancy is unknown, however, because modified neck dissections have not accompanied all cases. The impact that lymph node metastasis in thyroid carcinoma has on prognosis is debatable, unlike breast cancer and melanoma, which therefore makes the utility of thyroid SLND less clear. The technique, results, and morbidity of SLND during thyroidectomy is presented, and its possible utility in well-differentiated and medullary thyroid carcinoma is discussed.

Introduction

Intraoperative lymphatic mapping and sentinel lymph node dissection (SLND) was first described by Morton et al. in 1992 for patients with melanoma [1]. This technique has since been validated by other independent investigators [2, 3]. It is based on the concept that the sentinel node, the first lymph node in the regional nodal basin that drains a primary tumor, reflects the tumor status of the remaining lymph nodes of that basin. At the John Wayne Cancer Institute (JWCI), our group adapted Morton's dye-directed SLND technique for use in patients with primary breast cancer, and we have validated the sentinel node concept for this disease [4, 5]. Our hypothesis was that the sentinel node

Recent Results in Cancer Research, Vol. 157
© Springer-Verlag Berlin · Heidelberg 2000

concept would also prove valid in patients with thyroid malignancy, and therefore proceeded with testing the hypothesis using SLND.

Thyroid SLND at JWCI

In 1998, we reported a feasibility study of thyroidectomy combined with SLND performed on 17 patients who underwent the procedure for the diagnosis of a thyroid nodule suspicious for malignancy [6]. No patient had palpable cervical lymphadenopathy. Pathologic review of the 17 nodules revealed 5 benign and 12 malignant lesions: 11 were papillary carcinomas, and 1 was follicular carcinoma. At least one blue-stained sentinel node, with a median number of 2 sentinel nodes, were identified and removed in 15 patients. Sentinel nodes were not identified in two patients who had blue lymphatics coursing beneath the clavicle. All patients had paratracheal sentinel nodes, while only 2 patients had additional jugular sentinel nodes, which is similar to the metastatic pattern in patients who underwent elective neck dissection for thyroid carcinoma [7].

In 5 of the 12 thyroid malignancies in our study, lymphatic metastases were present in the sentinel node [6]. Three of 4 patients who had sentinel node metastases identified by frozen section underwent central neck lymph node dissection, and in 2 of these the sentinel node was the only positive node. In the other patient, non-sentinel nodes and a jugular node had metastases, and subsequent modified lateral neck dissection revealed additional nodal metastases. In one case, the sentinel node was falsely negative, as metastases were found by immunohistochemistry in a perithyroidal node removed with the thyroidectomy specimen. There were no complications of permanent recurrent laryngeal nerve injury or hypoparathyroidism.

Since this study, we have performed SLND in an ongoing trial on 38 additional patients with thyroid nodules suspicious for malignancy. Sentinel nodes were detected in 33 patients, for an overall successful identification rate of 87%. The 5 failed procedures were due to fat misidentified as lymph nodes (2), a parathyroid gland within fat misidentified as a sentinel node, a lymphatic tract coursing retrosternally, and dye that failed to migrate from a nodule. Thyroidectomy specimens revealed 21 benign lesions, and 17 malignant lesions. Of these 17 malignant lesions, 1 SLND failed. In the remaining 16 malignant cases, metastases were identified in at least one sentinel node in 9 (56%) patients (Table 1) Not all patients had central neck dissections after SLND and therefore the false negative rate is unknown.

Technique of Thyroid SLND

After the thyroid gland is exposed through a standard transverse collar incision, 0.5–1.0 ml of isosulfan blue (Lymphazurin) is injected into the thyroid nodule using a tuberculin syringe. The thyroid gland is not extensively mobilized before dye injection so that lymphatic drainage remains intact. Usually within seconds,

Table 1. Recent series of SLND during thyroidectomy for suspected thyroid malignancy

Pathology	N	SN identified	SN metastases
Benign	21	17/21 (81%)	–
Follicular adenoma	7	6	–
Hurthle cell adenoma	3	2	–
Colloid nodule/multinodular goiter	7	5	–
Hashimoto thyroiditis	4	4	–
Malignant	17	16/17 (94%)	9/16 (56%)
Papillary	16	15	9
Follicular	1	1	0

but sometimes up to 1–2 min, which is much quicker than with breast SLND, blue lymphatic channels can be traced to a blue sentinel node which is removed. Unfortunately in our recent series, the blue lymphatic channel that drained from a benign colloid nodule tracked directly into or beside a parathyroid gland surrounded by fat, which was mistaken for the sentinel node and removed. A thyroid lobectomy was performed on this patient who remains eucalcemic. Extreme caution must be exercised, especially during a total thyroidectomy, so that parathyroid glands are not removed with SLND. When in doubt, a small incisional biopsy of the blue stained structure can be done to confirm it is a lymph node.

As in melanoma and breast cancer, after removal of sentinel nodes, nodes are submitted for frozen section; after the node is bivalved on its long axis, it is examined with Diff-Quik stain. Permanent sections are examined with hematoxylin and eosin staining, and if negative at two levels, immunohistochemistry using anti-cytokeratin antibodies on an additional two sections are performed.

Utility of Thyroid SLND

Whether thyroid SLND and the identification of sentinel lymph node micrometastases will influence patient outcome centers around the debate on whether lymph node metastases have an impact on prognosis in well-differentiated thyroid malignancy. Although lymph nodes are involved in up to 80% of patients with papillary thyroid carcinoma who have clinically negative neck nodes, the effect of lymph node involvement on recurrence and survival is uncertain [8, 9]. Several studies suggest that survival is unaffected in patients with nodal metastases [10–13], or at least is only minimally decreased [14] compared to risk factors of age, distant metastases, extent of invasion, and size of primary tumor (AMES) [15]. However, the contrary view is supported in other studies, which suggest that positive lymph nodes portend a worse outcome for both recurrence [16, 17] and survival [9, 18]. Therefore, SLND, a procedure that only refines the diagnosis of occult nodal involvement and does not change the biology of the disease, will likely not help to clarify the controversy. However, it may identify those patients more likely to develop a difficult central neck recurrence.

The question of prophylactic or elective modified radical neck dissection for patients with occult nodal metastases from well-differentiated carcinoma is also controversial. Although many patients have occult metastases diagnosed after elective lymph node dissection, if similar patients do not have a lymph node dissection, the recurrence rate is low [7]. Nevertheless, recurrences are usually first found in the regional lymph nodes [17]. It may be possible that SLND could refine the stage of patients with both low and high risk lesions, and possibly change the operative approach. For young patients with a small carcinoma confined to the thyroid gland who might otherwise be treated with subtotal thyroidectomy alone, micrometastases identified in the sentinel node by SLND could change the operative approach to total thyroidectomy plus postoperative radioiodine for ablation of residual disease. Although the total number of patients who would benefit from such an approach may be small, it is a more logical approach than routine prophylactic node dissection, which is associated with a significant risk of hypoparathyroidism and recurrent laryngeal nerve injury [18, 19]. SLND in patients with high risk lesions undergoing total thyroidectomy with planned radioiodine ablation might also identify occult metastases, such that resection may decrease recurrence rates of close to 35% [20].

The greatest benefit from SLND may be the identification of a sentinel node outside the central neck that contains occult metastases from medullary thyroid carcinoma (MTC). This would identify disease that would have been left unresected with only a central neck dissection, and provide for a more logical approach to lateral neck dissection. With rates of persistent MTC indicated by hypercalcitoninemia after thyroidectomy and central neck dissection as high as 83% for hereditary disease [21], we hypothesize that SLND may be superior to jugular node sampling [22] in detecting residual nodal metastatic disease.

A final theoretical benefit of SLND is that it may assist in the diagnosis of carcinoma for an atypical follicular or Hurthle cell neoplasm that does not reveal or has questionable capsular or vessel invasion on frozen section: if metastases are identified in the sentinel node, then invasion can be assumed and total thyroidectomy performed without a second operation.

Conclusion

SLND can be performed successfully in thyroid carcinoma. The sentinel nodes can be easily identified using blue dye, and removed with minimal morbidity. The role of SLND in the surgical management of patients with differentiated thyroid carcinoma remains to be fully defined. The use of SLND is less defined in this disease because of the questionable influence that lymph node metastases have on survival. The procedure may be most useful for patients with MTC so that micrometastases in nodes other than the central neck can be identified. SLND is successful for melanoma, breast cancer and now thyroid carcinoma, and will likely become applicable in many other solid tumors.

References

1. Morton DL, Wen DR, Wong JH, et al (1992) Technical details of intraoperative lymphatic mapping for early stage melanoma. Arch Surg 127:392–399
2. Reintgen D, Cruse CW, Wells K, et al (1994) The orderly progression of melanoma nodal metastases. Ann Surg 220:759–767
3. Thompson JF, McCarthy WH, Bosch CM, et al (1995) Sentinel lymph node status as an indicator of the presence of metastatic melanoma in regional lymph nodes. Melanoma Res 5:255–260
4. Giuliano AE, Kirgan DM, Guenther JM, et al (1994) Lymphatic mapping and sentinel lymphadenectomy for breast cancer. Ann Surg 220:391–401
5. Giuliano AE, Jones RC, Brennan M, et al (1997) Sentinel lymphadenectomy in breast cancer. J Clin Oncol 15:2345–2350
6. Keleman PR, Van Herle AJ, Giuliano AE (1998) Sentinel lymphadenectomy in thyroid malignant neoplasms. Arch Surg 133:288–292
7. Noguchi S, Muranaki N (1987) The value of lymph-node dissection in patients with differentiated thyroid cancer. Surg Clin North Am 67:251–61
8. Frazell EL, Foote FW (1955) Papillary thyroid carcinoma: Pathologic findings in cases with and without clinical evidence of cervical node involvement. Cancer 8:1164
9. Scheumann GFW, Gimm O, Wegener G, et al (1994) Prognostic significance and surgical management of locoregional lymph node metastases in papillary thyroid cancer. World J Surg 18:559–568
10. Sato N, Oyamatsu M, Koyama Y, et al (1998) Do the level of nodal disease according to the TNM classification and the number of involved cervical nodes reflect prognosis in patients with differentiated carcinoma of the thyroid gland? J Surg Oncol 69:151–5
11. Carcangiu ML, Zampi G, Pupi A, et al (1985) Papillary carcinoma of the thyroid. A clinicopathologic study of 241 cases treated at the University of Florence, Italy. Cancer 55:805–28
12. Mazzaferri EL, Young RL (1981) Papillary thyroid carcinoma: a 10 year follow-up report of the impact of therapy in 576 patients. Am J Med 70:511–8
13. Cunningham MP, Duda RB, Recant W, et al (1990) Survival discriminants for differentiated thyroid cancer. Am J Surg 160:344–7
14. Hamming JF, Roukema JA (1997) Management of regional lymph nodes in papillary, follicular, and medullary thyroid carcinoma. In: Clark OH, Duh QY (eds) Textbook of Endocrine Surgery. Philadelphia, WB Saunders, p 155
15. Cady B, Rossi R (1988) An expanded view of risk-group definition in differentiated thyroid carcinoma. Surgery 104:947–53
16. Mazzaferri EL, Jhiang SM (1994) Long-term impact of initial surgical and medical therapy on papillary and follicular thyroid cancer. Am J Med 97:418–28
17. McHenry CR, Rosen IB, Walfish PG (1991) Prospective management of nodal metastases in differentiated thyroid cancer. Am J Surg 162:353–356
18. Hamming JF, Van de Velde CJH, Fleuren GJ et al (1988) Differentiated thyroid cancer: a stage-adapted approach to the treatment of regional lymph node metastasis. Eur J Cancer Clin Oncol 24:325–330
19. Henry JF, Gramatica L, Denizot A et al (1998) Morbidity of prophylactic lymph node dissection in the central neck area in patients with papillary thyroid carcinoma. Langenbecks Arch Surg 383:167–169
20. Cady B, Sedgewick CE, Meissner WA et al (1979) Risk factor analysis in differentiated thyroid cancer. Cancer 43:810–820
21. Harwood J, Clark OH, Dunphy JE (1978) Significance of lymph node metastases in differentiated thyroid cancer. Am J Surg 136:107–110
22. Block MA, Jackson CE, Tshjian AH Jr (1980) Clinical characteristics distinguishing hereditary from sporadic medullary thyroid carcinoma: Treatment implications. Arch Surg 115:142–148
23. Russell CF, van Heerden JA, Sizemore GW et al (1983) The surgical management of medullary thyroid carcinoma Ann Surg 197:42–48

Lymphoscintigraphy and Ultrasound-Guided Fine Needle Aspiration Cytology of Sentinel Lymph Nodes in Head and Neck Cancer Patients

E. J. C. Nieuwenhuis[1], D. R. Colnot[1], H. J. Pijpers[2], J. A. Castelijns[3], P. J. van Diest[4], R. H. Brakenhoff[1], G. B. Snow[1], and M. W. M. van den Brekel[1]

[1] Department of Otolaryngology/Head and Neck Surgery, University Hospital Vrije Universiteit, P.O. Box 7057, 1007 MB Amsterdam, The Netherlands
[2] Department of Radiology, University Hospital Vrije Universiteit, P.O. Box 7057, 1007 MB Amsterdam, The Netherlands
[3] Department of Nuclear Medicine, University Hospital Vrije Universiteit, P.O. Box 7057, 1007 MB Amsterdam, The Netherlands
[4] Department of Pathology, University Hospital Vrije Universiteit, P.O. Box 7057, 1007 MB Amsterdam, The Netherlands

Abstract

Accurate staging of the regional lymph nodes is crucial for the appropriate management of patients with squamous cell carcinoma of the head and neck (HNSCC). However, the current diagnostic modalities have low accuracy for N0 neck, and even the most optimal procedure, ultrasound-guided fine needle aspiration cytology (USgFNAC), still has a sensitivity of only 42%–73%. In this study we evaluated whether the identification of the sentinel node might improve the selection of lymph nodes for USgFNAC. Twelve HNSCC patients received 3–4 peritumoral injections of 10–30 MBq 99mTc-labeled colloidal albumin, and the sentinel node was identified by dynamic scintigraphy and marked on the skin using a handheld probe, and/or by scintillation counting of the aspirates. After sentinel node identification USgFNAC was performed. Correct aspiration of the identified sentinel node(s) was confirmed by scintillation counting. In 11 out of 12 cases the sentinel node(s) could be visualized by dynamic planar imaging. In one case the sentinel node(s) were identified by scintillation counting only. In a number of patients different or supplementary lymph nodes were aspirated on the basis of sentinel node identification. These initial data strongly suggest that sentinel node identification might improve the staging of the neck by USgFNAC.

Introduction

In head and neck squamous cell carcinoma (HNSCC) the lymph node status of the neck is the most important prognosticator. In case of cervical lymph node metastases, survival is reduced by a factor of 2. Moreover, if at histopathological examination lymph node metastases are absent (pN–), regional failure occurs in only 2.6%, whereas recurrence in the neck occurs in 9.7% of the pN+ cases (Leemans et al. 1990). Failure in the neck after neck dissection is almost invariably fatal. The failure rate at distant sites, with controlled locoregional disease, varies from 6.9% in pN0 cases to 46.8% for patients with more than 3 lymph node metastases (Leemans et al. 1993). In contrast to malignancies like breast cancer or melanomas, where staging of regional lymphatic spread is a more accepted prognosticater for development of distant metastases, HNSCC is often considered a locoregional disease. Furthermore, it should be realized that effective systemic treatment is not available for HNSCC.

In many institutions throughout the world the neck is mainly staged by palpation. In view of the high false negative rate of this approach, a neck without palpable metastases (N0) is at risk of harboring occult metastases. The management of N0 neck is a source of continuous controversy among clinicians. In contrast to elective axillary dissection in breast cancer, elective neck dissection has a low morbidity, especially when limited to the levels at high risk (selective neck dissection). Because of this low morbidity, the policy of elective neck dissection is widely accepted if the risk of occult metastases, based on characteristics of the primary tumor such as site and stage, is estimated to be higher than 20% (Weiss et al. 1994). Although current diagnostic imaging techniques like computed tomography (CT), magnetic resonance imaging (MRI) or ultrasonography (US) in general have increased diagnostic accuracy of the status of the lymph nodes in the neck, these modalities still have a relatively low accuracy for N0 neck (Table 1). Therefore there remains a great need for more accurate staging techniques.

Table 1. The sensitivity and specificity of different imaging modalities found by several authors for the palpatory N0 neck (electively operated)

Author	Modality	Sensitivity	Specificity	Number of patients
Stern et al. 1990	CT	40	92	53
Friedman et al. 1990	CT	68	90	68
	MRI	80	82	16
Van den Brekel et al. 1993	CT	49	78	86
	US	58	75	88
	MRI	55	88	83
	US-FNAC	73	100	43
John et al. 1993	US	50	82	28
Takes et al. 1996	US–FNAC	42	100	118
Righi et al. 1997	CT	60	100	25
	US-FNAC	50	100	25
Moreau et al. 1990	CT	50	86	32

Ultrasound-guided fine needle aspiration cytology (USgFNAC) has gained popularity because cytology is more reliable than radiological criteria. In experienced hands its sensitivity can reach 73% with a specificity of 100% for N0 neck (van den Brekel et al. 1991). However, others reported a sensitivity of 42%–50% (Takes et al. 1996; Righi et al. 1997). In a recent study with oral cancer patients treated with transoral tumor excision, using USgFNAC for initial work up as well as follow-up, almost 20% of patients with negative USgFNAC developed a neck node metastasis during follow-up (van den Brekel et al. 1999). Of these neck failures 71% could still be salvaged by neck dissection followed by radiotherapy. These data indicate that USgFNAC does not enable detection of all occult metastases, and even more important, that it is not an easy technique and may have a long learning curve with high interobserver variance. Possible causes of false negative results are aspiration of the wrong node, aspiration of the wrong part of a node containing a small metastasis, and false interpretation of the cytopathologist.

In recent years, the sentinel node (SN) concept, where a cancer metastasizes first to a specific lymph node from which it can further spread, has allowed selective targeting of early lymph node metastases in malignancies like breast cancer and melanoma (Borgstein et al. 1998; Pijpers et al. 1997a). Allowing that the SN concept holds for HNSCC as well, improvement of the sensitivity of USgFNAC may be possible with better selection of lymph nodes at risk, i.e., selective aspiration of the SN. Moreover, with improved analyses of aspirates using molecular techniques, as described in the chapter by van Houten et al., in this issue, the rate of false negative cytology results might even be further diminished.

This study describes our initial experiences with the combined use of lymphoscintigraphic SN detection and aspiration of this SN by ultrasound guidance. The final aim of the study is to investigate whether the SN procedure is able to improve the ultrasound detection and subsequent fine needle aspiration of the lymph nodes at risk of harboring metastases.

Materials and Methods

Patients

Twelve patients with a squamous cell carcinoma of the oral cavity and oropharynx were included in the study, 9 men and 3 women. All were treated between May 1998 and February 1999 at the Department of Otorhinolaryngology/Head and Neck Surgery, University Hospital Vrije Universiteit in Amsterdam. Ten patients had a carcinoma in the oral cavity (tongue, n=7; floor of mouth, n=2; retromolar trigone, n=1) and 2 patients in the oropharynx (Table 2). All patients had clinically N0 neck as assessed by palpation.

Table 2. Patient characteristics and summary of the results

Patient	Sex	Age (years)	Localization	TN	Visible SN	Level SN	USgFNAC SN	USgFNAC other nodes	Level	Histopathology SN	Histopathology other nodes	Follow-up
1	female	67	tonsil right	T3N0	1	II	neg	neg	II	neg	neg	1x USgFNAC pos[a]
2	male	59	tongue right	T3N0	1	II	neg	neg		neg	neg	3x USgFNAC neg
3	male	57	oropharynx left trigonum	T3N0	2	III	neg	neg	III	neg	neg	1x USgFNAC neg
4	male	72	retromolare right	T4N0	2	II, III	neg	neg	I, II, III	neg	neg	1x USgFNAC neg
5	male	46	tongue left	T2N0	1	I	pos	pos	I, II	pos	pos	no USgFNAC[b]
6	female	64	floor of mouth left	T4N0	0			1 pos?[1]	I	pos	4 pos?[3]	no USgFNAC[b]
7	male	59	tongue right	T1N0	1	II	neg	2 neg?[2]	-	neg	neg	
8	male	44	tongue right	T1N0	1	II	neg	neg	-			
9	male	73	tongue right	T2N0	2	II	no FNAC	neg	I			
10	male	52	tongue right	T2N0	2	II	neg	neg	-			
11	male	49	tongue left	T2N0	2	I, II	neg	neg	I			
12	female	59	floor of mouth left	T2N0	2	II, III	neg	neg	I, II			

Patient died after 6 months of liver metastases.

[a] within 3 months USgFNAC revealed positive and a subsequent neck dissection was performed, patient developed liver metastases and died within 5 months;

[b] these patients underwent transoral excision recently, therefore did not get follow-up USgFNAC until now.

[1] This lymph node contained radioactivity, therefore considered as SN, was tumor positive at cytological and histopathological examination.

[2] These 2 lymph nodes contained radioactivity as well, but were tumor negative at cytological and histopathological examination.

[3] Four other nodes were tumor positive but not radioactive.

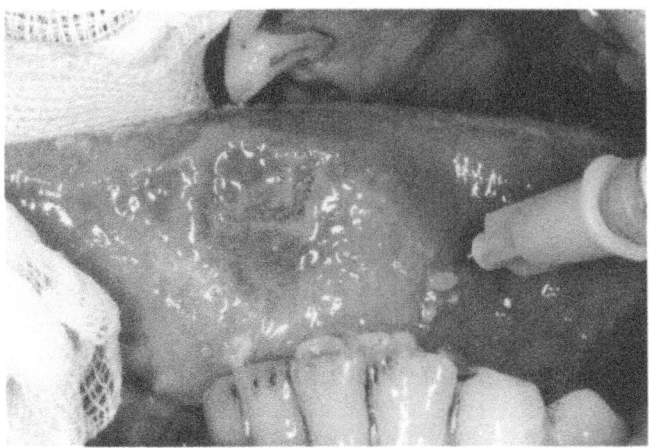

Fig. 1.

Injection of ⁹⁹ᵐTc Labeled Colloidal Albumin

The patients received 3 or 4 peritumoral injections of 30–40 MBq ⁹⁹ᵐTc-labeled colloidal albumin (CA) (particle size 3–80 nm; 77±12% < 30 nm) in 2 ml saline (Nanocoll, Sorin Biomedica, Saluggia, Italy;) injected submucosally 0.5 cm from the tumor (Fig. 1). The radiochemical purity of ⁹⁹ᵐTc labeled CA had to be at least 95%. These particles are known to be captured in lymph nodes and have shown selective targeting and prolonged intranodal retention in the SNs of 92% of breast cancer patients (Pijpers et al. 1997).

Imaging

Directly after administration of ⁹⁹ᵐTc-labeled colloidal albumin dynamic planar imaging (20 frames of 60 s, 64×64 matrix) of the neck was performed using a large field of view gamma camera (300 s acquisition in a 128×128 matrix) in order to determine the presence and localization of SNs. Images were made in antero-posterior and lateral projection in order to reduce over-projection of radioactive scatter from the injection site over the sentinel nodes in the neck. A handheld gamma probe (Navigator, Gamma Guidance System, RMD, Watertown, MA) was then used to detect the localization of the SN, after which its place was marked on the overlying skin.

Ultrasound-Guided Fine Needle Aspiration

Within 1 h after scintigraphy the SN was identified by ultrasound using a 7 MHz linear array transducer (Acuson 1,28 system, Acuson Company, Mountain View, CA) and subsequently aspirated. Prior to aspiration, the handheld gamma probe was used to confirm that the ultrasound-detected lymph node was indeed the SN. The aspirate was partially processed for cytologic examination, and residual material was cryopreserved for molecular diagnostics. As the aspirate was not radioactive as assessed with the handheld probe, the aspirate residue from the last 4 patients was counted for radioactivity in a liquid scintillation counter (1282 Compugamma, Wallac, Turku, Finland) in order to confirm that the aspirated lymph node was an SN, i.e., contained radiolabeled CA. Routine USgFNAC of the neck was continued and other suspicious lymph nodes based on ultrasound criteria were aspirated as well.

Surgery

Five out of twelve patients were scheduled for surgery with an elective unilateral neck dissection as to get adequate exposure for excision of the primary tumor or for reconstruction of the resulting defect. To distinguish the SNs from the remaining cervical lymphatics, the handheld gamma probe was used to confirm content of radioactive CA when the specimen was removed from the patient. All specimens were examined histopathologically by complete paraffin embedding after formalin fixation, taking 1 hematoxylin and eosin (H&E) slide per block. The sentinel lymph nodes were processed separately. Cytology of the aspirated SNs was correlated to the histopathological findings for each patient. Seven out of twelve patients underwent transoral excision of the primary tumor without elective treatment of the neck.

Follow-up

From the patients who underwent surgery without an elective neck dissection USgFNAC of the neck was performed every 8 weeks during follow-up. If lymph nodes larger than 4 mm were detected, aspiration was repeated.

Results

Detection of Sentinel Lymph Nodes with Scintigraphy

In 11 out of 12 patients at least 1 SN was visible with lymphoscintigraphy within 20 min after peritumoral injection of ^{99m}Tc-CA. In patient 6 with an anterior floor of mouth carcinoma, the SN could not be identified. In 5 patients 1 lymph node was visible and in 6 patients 2 lymph nodes were visible (Table 2, Fig. 2). In 10 cases the SN was located in level II, and in 2 cases another SN was depicted in level III, whereas in 1 case another SN was located in level I. In case 5, a patient with a T2 tongue carcinoma the SN was located in the lower part of level I. Also with use of the handheld probe, it

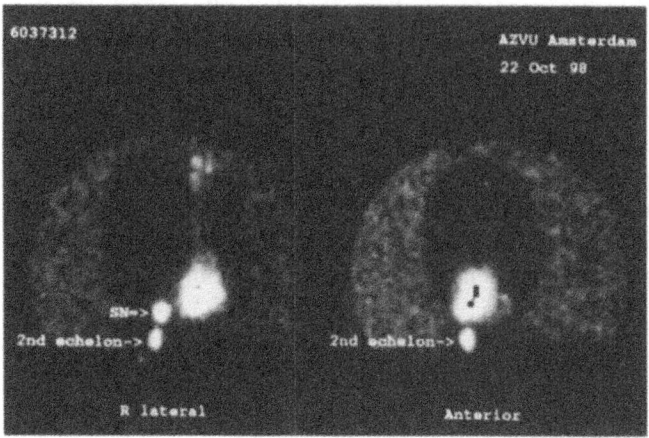

Fig. 2.

proved to be difficult to reliably detect SNs in level I, because of the proximity to the primary tumor. Scintigraphy at later time points was not performed.

Ultrasound-Guided Aspiration

Ultrasound detection and aspiration of the depicted lymph nodes was possible in 10 patients. Patient 9 had 2 level II SNs measuring 3 mm, which were considered too small for aspiration. In 3 patients the SN-USgFNAC was performed some days after SN assessment using conventional USgFNAC. In all 3 patients different or supplementary lymph nodes were aspirated. Confirmation of SN aspiration by counting radioactivity content of the aspirate was feasible. Counts per minute (cpm) for SN aspirates ranged from 600 to 12500, whereas mean background activity was 30 cpm. From patient 6 in whom no SN was visible at scintigraphy, 3 level I lymph nodes were aspirated, of which 2 were considered SNs based on the presence of radioactivity.

Cytologic Examination of the Aspirates

In 9 cases cytology was reported to be tumor negative. One patient (case 5) with a T2 tongue carcinoma of which the SN measured 11 mm, had a positive SN cytology. Cytological examination of aspirates of case 6, a patient with a floor of mouth carcinoma in whom no SN was visible at scintigraphy, revealed SCC in 1 submental lymph node and the aspirate proved to be radioactive. A second aspirated submandibular lymph node which appeared to contain reactivity did not show SCC.

Histopathological Examination

After excision of the primary tumor and removal of the neck dissection specimen the SN could be identified with the gamma probe. Routine histopathological examination of the separately processed SNs, as well as the other lymph nodes in the neck dissection specimen, did not show lymph node metastases in 4 out of 6 patients who underwent a neck dissection.

The 2 remaining patients had nodal metastases. Patient 5 had not been planned for elective neck dissection but based on a positive USgFNAC examination of the SN just before transoral excision, a therapeutic neck dissection was performed 12 days after transoral tumor excision. Histopathological examination of the neck dissection specimen revealed 6 lymph node metastases. The neck dissection specimen of patient 6, in whom no SN was identified at scintigraphy, showed metastatic disease in 1 radioactive lymph node, as identified with the handheld probe, in level I on the left. The lymph node aspirate was positive at cytological examination as well. Two other radioactive lymph nodes, in level II on the left and level IV on the right, did not contain metastases. However, 2 non-radioactive lymph nodes in level II on the left were infiltrated by metastatic disease as well, both for 10%. Furthermore, in level I on the right 2 lymph nodes showed metastases, of which 1 lymph node was replaced by tumor for 20% and the other for 80%.

Follow-up

All patients were regularly followed with USgFNAC after transoral excision. In patient 7, USgFNAC three months after transoral excision showed lymph node metastases and subsequently a unilateral neck dissection was performed. Histopathological examination demonstrated a large tumor mass containing multiple lymph node metastases through levels II–IV. The other 5 patients have not developed a lymph node metastasis during follow-up with UsgFNAC so far. The follow-up ranged from 1 to 10 months (mean 5 months).

Discussion

The SN concept is based on the principle that lymphatic tumor spread follows a route specific for the site of the primary tumor. The first echelon lymph node or SN can be visualized using peritumoral injection of radiolabeled particles and subsequent lymphoscintigraphy. The histopathological examination of the SN should be predictive for the N-stage of the neck, i.e., if the SN is tumor negative, all other nodes should be negative, whereas if other nodes are tumor positive, the SN should be tumor positive as well. The concept and predictive value of the SN in patients with breast carcinoma and melanoma has been confirmed in large studies (Giuliano et al. 1994; Veronesi et al. 1997; Borgstein et al. 1998; Pijpers et al. 1997a,b; Krag et al. 1998). Based on these studies, it has convincingly been demonstrated that sentinel node biopsy is an accurate and workable technique and can be exploited as a selection procedure for nodal dissection in patients with breast carcinoma or melanoma.

The sentinel node procedure has not yet gained popularity or acceptance in head and neck cancer. Even in patients with a relatively low risk of occult metastases, elective neck dissection is a widely accepted procedure due to its relatively low morbidity. A selective neck dissection takes only 1 or 2 h and is considered a curative treatment in case of limited neck disease. Furthermore, dissection of the neck can render histopathologic arguments like multiple metastases or extranodal tumor spread for postoperative radiotherapy. However, in spite of these arguments, it has never been proven unequivocally that elective treatment of the neck is beneficial in terms of prognosis as compared to observing the neck (van den Brekel 1999). Furthermore, elective treatment means overtreatment for the majority of patients and therefore might disturb the lymphatic spread, possibly resulting in unpredictable patterns of metastasis and early distant metastases.

Until now, few research groups have investigated the possibility of lymphatic mapping of HNSCC. Pitman used peritumoral injections of isosulfan blue dye in 16 HNSCC patients in an attempt to identify the sentinel node during surgery (Pitman et al. 1998). However, in none of her patients, both N0 and N+, were any stained lymphatic channels or cervical lymph nodes identified intraoperatively. Double tracer lymphoscintigraphy was performed by Klutmann in 78 HNSCC patients to examine the correlation of cervical lymph nodes and the anatomic structures of the head and neck region (Klutmann et al. 1997). Images were obtained at 30 min and 4–6 h after injection. In 64% of the patients sentinel lymph nodes were detected of which 28% showed bilateral lymphatic drainage. However, no histopathological or surgical correlation was made. In another trial performed by Koch et al. (1998), 5 patients with a T1 or T2 SCC and a clinically N0 neck received peritumoral injections of ^{99m}Tc sulfur colloid. SNs were identified in 3 patients. In 2 of these 3 cases the SN did accurately predict cervical node involvement. In the third patient the SN, located in level IV, was false negative since 3 nodes in level II–III were extensively infiltrated by metastatic disease. One of the 2 patients in whom no SN was identified had received prior radiation therapy for a T2N0 SCC of the right retromolar trigone. Biopsy performed 4 months later showed persistent tumor in the primary site. Subsequent lymphoscintigraphy showed no SN, neither could radioactivity be detected in nodes found on dissection. At histopathological examination, several nodes in levels I and III contained metastatic disease. The other patient in whom no SN was visible had a SCC of the anterior oral cavity. Three lymph nodes in level I, in close proximity to the primary tumor, and 1 in level III contained radioactivity as assessed with the handheld gamma probe at surgical exploration. All nodes were tumor negative.

In our study we found that lymphoscintigraphy, gamma probe guided detection and USgFNAC of the sentinel node is feasible in N0-staged HNSCC patients with primary tumor sites accessible for injection. In the 6 patients who underwent a neck dissection, the earlier cytopathological findings in the sentinel node(s) aspirate(s) correctly reflected the lymph nodes status in the neck (2 positive, 4 negative). Although in one of these 6 patients the SN could not be detected by lymphoscintigraphy, two aspirate residues of lymph nodes located in level I contained radioactivity, and were therefore considered as SNs. Their location in close proximity to the primary tumor therefore might have led to overprojection by radioactive scatter from the injection site.

One of these SNs showed metastases both at cytological and histopathological examination. However, in this patient two other lymph nodes were radioactive but tumor negative at histopathological examination whereas 4 other nodes were tumor positive but not radioactive. Although only one of four SNs was found tumor-positive, it still correctly predicted lymphatic spread in the neck.

In 5 of the 6 patients who were managed with neck observation because of a negative USgFNAC of the SN, lymph node metastasis did not develop so far, although it should be noted that the follow-up period is still limited. In one of these patients (case 9) the SN measured only 3 mm and was thus not aspirated and considered tumor negative. In patient 7 the USgFNAC of the depicted SN was tumor negative whereas he developed a lymph node metastasis in the neck 4 months later. This false negative USgFNAC can be due either to aspiration from a wrong part of the sentinel node, a false negative cytology or aspiration from the wrong lymph node in the same level. This patient had very aggressive disease, as he developed distant metastases and died within 5 months after his neck dissection.

Molecular detection of small tumor deposits may improve the sensitivity of sentinel node-USgFNAC. In melanoma cells it was found that tyrosinase RT-PCR improved the detection of micrometastases compared to routine histopathological examination and immunohistochemistry (Wang et al. 1994; van de Velde-Zimmerman et al. 1997). Furthermore, the application of PCR and differential hybridization detection of mutated p53 can identify submicroscopic levels of HNSCC tumor cells in lymph nodes (Brennan et al. 1995). In our department, the RT-PCR method based on the E48 cDNA was found to be feasible for detection of squamous tumor cells in blood and bone marrow (Brakenhoff et al. 1998). At this moment optimalization of this assay is performed to allow its use in lymph node aspirates.

This study shows that identification of the SN is possible in the majority of oral and oropharyngeal cancer patients. Confirmation of aspirating the SN by radioactivity counting is possible as well. Identification of sentinel nodes in level I is still difficult because of the close proximity to the primary tumor. In this respect, digital subtraction techniques and dynamic scintigraphy might be helpful. Of course, a longer follow-up and a larger series of patients is necessary to determine the accuracy of this concept. We believe that enhanced sensitivity in nodal assessment may be possible using a combination of the SN procedure and molecular tumor cell detection in aspirates from these sentinel nodes. A reliable and accurate technique may have far-reaching consequences for the staging and treatment of head and neck cancer patients.

References

1. Borgstein PJ, Pijpers R, Comans EF, van Diest PJ, Boom RP, Meijer S (1998) Sentinel lymph node biopsy in breast cancer: guidelines and pitfalls of lymphoscintigraphy and gamma probe detection. J Am Coll Surg 186:275–283
2. Brennan JA, Mao L, Hruban RH, Boyle JO, Eby YJ, Koch WM, Goodman SN, Sidransky D (1995) Molecular assessment of histopathological staging in squamous-cell carcinoma of the head and neck. N Engl J Med 332:429–435
3. Brakenhoff RH, Stroomer JGW, Ten Brink CBM, De Bree R, Weima SM, Snow GB, Van Dongen GAMS (1999) Sensitive detection of squamous cells in bone marrow and blood of head and neck cancer patients by E48 reverse transcriptase polymerase chain reaction. Clin Cancer Res, in press
4. Friedman M, Mafee MF, Pacella BL, JR., Strorigl TL, Dew LL, Toriumi DM (1990) Rationale for elective neck dissection in 1990. Laryngoscope 100:54–59
5. Giuliano AE, Kirgan DM, Guenther JM (1994) Lymphatic mapping and sentinel lymphadenectomy for breast cancer. Ann Surg 220:391–401
6. John DG, Anaes FC, Williams SR, Ahuja A, Evans R, To KF, King WW, van Hasselt CA (1993) Palpation compared with ultrasound in the assessment of malignant cervical lymph nodes. J Laryngol Otol 107:821–823
7. Klutmann S, Bohuslavizki KH, Höft S, Kröger S, Brenner W, Tinnemeyer S, Werner JA, Henze E (1997) Lymphoscintigraphy in double tracer technique in patients with head and neck carcinomas. Laryngo-Rhino-Otologie 76:740–744
8. Koch WM, Choti MA, Civelek C, Eisele DW, Saunders JR (1998) Gamma probe-directed biopsy of the sentinel node in oral squamous cell carcinoma. Arch Otolaryngol Head Neck Surg 124:455–459
9. Krag DN, Weaver DL, Ashikaga T, Moffat F, Klimberg VS, Shriver C, Feldman S, Kusminsky R, Gadd M, Kuhn J, Harlow S, Beitsch P (1998) The sentinel node in breast cancer. N Engl J Med 339:941–946
10. Leemans CR, Tiwari R, van der Waal I, Karim ABMF, Nauta JJP, Snow GB (1990) The efficacy of comprehensive neck dissection with or without postoperative radiotherapy in nodal metastases of squamous cell carcinoma of the upper respiratory and digestive tracts. Laryngoscope 100:1194–1198
11. Leemans CR, Tiwari R, Nauta JJP, Van der Waal I, Snow GB (1993) Regional lymph node involvement and its significance in the development of distant metastases in head and neck cancer patients. Cancer 71(2):452–456
12. Moreau P, Goffart Y, Collignon J (1990) Computed tomography of metastatic cervical lymph nodes. Arch Otolaryngol Head Neck Surg 116:1190–1193
13. Pijpers R, Borgstein PJ, Meijer S, Hoekstra OS, van Hattum LH, Teule GJ (1997a) Sentinel node biopsy in melanoma patients: dynamic lymphoscintigraphy followed by intraoperative gamma probe and vital dye guidance. World J Surg 21:788–792
14. Pijpers R, Meijer S, Hoekstra OS, Collet GJ, Comans EFI, Boom RPA, Van Diest PJ, Teule GJJ (1997b) Impact of lymphoscintigraphy and tracer kinetics on sentinel node identification with Technetium-99m-colloidal albumin in breast cancer. J Nucl Med 38:366–368
15. Pitman KT, Johnson JT, Edington H, Barnes EL, Day R, Wagner RL, Myers EN (1998) Lymphatic mapping with isosulfan blue dye in squamous cell carcinoma of the head and neck. Arch Otolaryngol Head Neck Surg 124:790–793
16. Righi PD, Kopecky KK, Caldemeyers KS, Ball VA, Weisberger EC, Radpour S (1997) Comparison of ultrasound fine needle aspiration and computed tomography in patients undergoing elective veck dissection. Head and Neck 19:604–610
17. Stern WBR, Silver CE, Zeifer BA, Persky MS, Heller KS (1990) Computed tomography of the clinically negative neck. Head Neck 12:109–113
18. Takes RP, Knegt P, Manni JJ, Meeuwis CA, Marres HAM, Spoelstra HAA, De Boer MF, Bruaset I, Van Oostayen JA, Lameris JS, Kruyt RH (1996) Regional metastases in head

and neck squamous cell carcinoma: revised value of US with US-guided FNAB. Radiology 198:819–823

19. Van den Brekel MWM, Castelijns JA, Stel HV, Luth WJ, Valk J, Van der Waal I, Snow GB (1991) Occult metastatic neck disease: detection with US and US-guidedfine-needle aspiration cytology. Radiology 180:457–461

20. Van den Brekel MWM, Castelijns JA, Stel HV, Golding RP, Meyer CJ, Snow GB (1993) Modern imaging techniques and ultrasound-guided aspiration cytology for the assessment of neck node metastases: a prospective comparative study. Eur Arch Otorhinolaryngol 250:11–17

21. Van den Brekel MWM, Castelijns JA, Reitsma LC, Leemans CR, Van der Waal I, Snow GB (1999) Outcome of observing the N0 neck using ultrasonographic-guided cytology for follow-up. Arch Otolaryngol Head Neck Surg 125:153–156

22. Van de Velde-Zimmermann D, Roijers JF, Bouwens-Rombouts A, de Weger RA, de Graaf PW, Tilanus MG, van den Tweel JG (1996) Molecular test for the detection of tumor cells in blood and sentinel nodes of melanoma patients. Am J Path 149:759–764

23. Veronesi U, Paganelli G, Galimberti V, Viale G, Zurrida S, Bedoni M, Costa A, De Cicco C, Geraghty JG, Luini A, Sacchini V, Veronesi P (1997) Sentinel-node biopsy to avoid axillary dissection in breast cancer with clinically negative lymph-nodes. Lancet 349: 1864–1867

24. Wang X, Heller R, Van Virhis N, Cruse CW, Glass F, Fenske N, Berman C, Leo-Messina J, Rappaport D, Wells K (1994) Detection of submicroscopic lymph node metastases with polymerase chain reaction in patients with malignant melanoma. Ann Surg 220:768–774

25. Weiss MH, Harrison LB, Isaacs RS (1994) Use of decision analysis in planning a management strategy for the stage N0 neck. Arch Otolaryngol Head Neck Surg 120:699–702

VII. Sentinel Node Detection
in Breast Cancer

Present and Future of Sentinel Node Lymphadenectomy in Breast Cancer

U. Veronesi and S. Zurrida

Istituto Europeo di Oncologia, Via Ripamonti 435, 20141 Milan, Italy

Introduction

Up to about 1960, it was generally thought that breast cancer was mainly a local-regional disease. This concept, inherited from Halsted, led to increasingly aggressive treatments of the primary lesion and the regional lymph nodes. Total mastectomy, which in the form developed by Halsted was already an extensive operation, became enlarged to include extensive removal of skin and use of skin transplants, sacrifice of important vessels and nerves such as the thoracodorsals, and meticulous dissection of the regional nodes, sometimes including those of the internal mammary chain via thoracotomy. Radiotherapy was given to the axillary, supraclavicular and retrosternal lymph node areas, as well as to the mastectomy scar.

This highly aggressive approach, which often left the patients in poor condition, was supposed to improve survival, but by the 1960s it became clear that it did not. On the contrary, it slowly became apparent that mortality was almost always related to the development of distant metastases, and that prognosis depended on whether occult metastases, carried in the blood, had spread to distant organs. These new concepts pushed the therapeutic trend in the opposite direction. The extent of surgery was reduced and randomized clinical studies on the safety of breast conserving procedures were carried out, although initially against considerable opposition.

That it was possible to avoid mastectomy was demonstrated in a careful randomized trial [1], while other important studies [2, 3] showed that removal of the axillary nodes and the internal mammary nodes did not improve the survival of breast cancer patients. From these latter findings the concept developed that regional lymph node dissection was useful more as a staging procedure than as a treatment, and metastases in the axillary nodes were more indicators of distant spread than a source of it. More attention was therefore directed to occult metastases in distant organs and many attempts were made to control the disease through systemic treatments, first by administering hormones, then by hormone deprivation (oophorectomy, adrenalectomy, hypophysectomy) and more recently by chemotherapy and anti-estrogens.

Thus, enlarged understanding of the biology of breast cancer gave rise to the trend to breast conservation and to greater attention to quality of life in breast cancer patients. There has been a tendency also to limit axillary dissection in breast cancer, for example by random biopsy of nodes, lymph node sampling, or removal of the first level only. Unfortunately, all these approaches have serious drawbacks as staging procedures. Furthermore, the currently available non-surgical methods for evaluating the axilla are inadequate. Neither ultrasonography (including colour Doppler), nor lymphangiography, nor lymphoscintigraphy are able to determine the presence or extent of axillary lymph node involvement, while positron emission tomography (PET) and magnetic resonance imaging (MRI) are still experimental modalities as far as the diagnosis of metastatic axillary lymph nodes is concerned.

It is in this context that sentinel node lymphadenectomy appears interesting as a method of disease staging in breast cancer: it is minimally invasive, does not compromise quality of life and as discussed below, under defined circumstances, can reliably diagnose the real state of the axilla.

The Sentinel Node

The term "sentinel node" was first used in 1977 by Cabanas [4] to refer to the first involved inguinal node in penile cancer. Before that, in 1954, Gallico [5] described the results of node mapping, using blue dye in 23 patients 12 of whom had breast cancer. In 1963 Cope [6] referred to the "Delphian node" as the lymph node that will "foretell the nature of a disease process" affecting a nearby organ.

Specifically, therefore, the idea of sentinel node lymphadenectomy is to identify, remove and pathologically examine the first node to receive lymph from the area of the breast harbouring the tumour. The assumption is that if this node is free of metastases, all other axillary lymph nodes will be negative. The result of the examination can therefore be used to select patients for total axillary lymphadenectomy versus no further axillary treatment.

The validity of the sentinel node concept was first demonstrated for melanoma by Morton and colleagues [7]. Patent blue V dye was injected close to the primary lesion and the blue-stained sentinel node was later found by dissection. Various dyes have been tested to optimize the kinetics, both in terms of take-up and transport by lymph and retention by the first node to receive that lymph. Blue dyes are also used to identify the sentinel node in breast cancer, either alone or in conjunction with other methods. Giuliano and colleagues [8] have clearly shown the utility of the blue dye technique in detecting the sentinel node in breast cancer. Its disadvantages are that a considerable training period is necessary to learn the dissection technique and, above all, the incision to the armpit must be wide since the exact location of the sentinel node cannot be known in advance and a long search is often necessary to isolate the blue node after the identification of the lymphatic channels.

The Italian Experience

Our group at the European Institute of Oncology in Milan started clinical research on sentinel nodes in breast cancer a few years ago, employing radiolabelled particles, lymphoscintigraphy and a hand-held gamma probe to locate
the sentinel node and facilitate its removal during surgery. The gamma probe
allows dissection of the hot node that is detectable a few hours after the injection of tracer around the primary carcinoma. The shortest access path
from the skin to the hot node is used, and only a small incision is necessary.
   The inoculation method depends on tumour site. When the tumour is
superficial its lymphatic drainage is in close relation to that of the skin, and
subdermal injection identifies the sentinel node with ease. When the tumour
is deep, peritumoral inoculation is better.
   The method used to investigate the removed sentinel node is of the utmost importance, as the decision to forego axillary dissection or to remove
the axillary nodes will be taken while the patient is under general anaesthesia for removal of the primary tumour. In our early experience 17% of sentinel nodes found to be negative by intraoperative frozen section analysis
proved to be metastatic on definitive histological analysis. We therefore developed a new more extensive intraoperative frozen section method. This has
now been perfected and involves bisecting the removed node along its major
axis and embedding and freezing both halves. Fifteen pairs of adjacent sections, 4 μm thick, are then cut at 50 μm intervals in each half node, amount-
ing to 60 sections per node. Whenever residual tissue is left, additional pairs
of sections are cut at 100 μm intervals, until the node is completely sampled.
One section of each pair is routinely stained with hematoxylin and eosin and
examined. As soon as malignant cells are found the examination stops as the
result is positive. If there is any doubt as to the presence of malignant cells
in a given section, the other section is immunostained for cytokeratins,
using a rapid method with monoclonal antibodies.
   Thus, for sentinel node biopsy, the intraoperative frozen section examination has become the definitive histological examination at our institute, and
in this way the surgeon receives adequate information for deciding whether
or not to perform complete axillary lymphadenectomy during the operation
on the primary. Some centres now use a polymerase chain reaction for detecting micrometastases. The sensitivity and specificity of methods for detecting micrometastatic disease in sentinel nodes are likely to improve
further in the near future.
   In the initial Milan experience [9] the sentinel lymph node was identified
in 371 of 376 patients (98.7%). The method correctly predicted the state of
the axilla in a high percentage of cases (96.8%), as determined by complete
axillary dissection, although there were 12 patients in whom the sentinel
lymph node was negative but other axillary lymph nodes were positive (3.2%
of all patients) (Table 1). The finding of 73 patients (43.5% of positive sentinel lymph nodes) in whom the sentinel lymph node was the only positive
one confirms the rational basis of the sentinel lymph node technique.

Table 1. Concordance between sentinel node evaluation and definitive status of all axillary nodes in 371 patients with breast cancer

Sentinel node	Axillary nodes	Number	% of total
Positive	Positive*	168	45.3
Negative	Negative	191	51.5
Negative	Positive	12	3.2
Total		371	100

Concordance 359/371 (96.8%).
* In 70 patients the sentinel node was the only positive node.

$$\text{Sensitivity} = \frac{\text{Number of patients with a positive sentinel node biopsy}}{\text{Number of patients with axillary lymph node metastases}} = \frac{168}{198} = 93.3\%$$

$$\text{Specificity} = \frac{\text{Number of patients with a negative sentinel node biopsy}}{\text{Number of patients with no axillary lymph metastase}} = \frac{191}{191} = 100\%$$

$$\text{Positive Predictive Value} = \frac{\text{Number of patients with axillary lymph node metastases}}{\text{Number of patients with a positive sentinel node biopsy}} \frac{168}{168} = 100\%$$

$$\text{Negative Predictive Value} = \frac{\text{Number of patients without axillary lymph node metastases}}{\text{Number of patiens with a negative sentinel node biopsy}} = \frac{191}{203} = 94.1\%$$

$$\text{Overall Accuracy} = \frac{\text{Number of patients with true positive and true neagive sentinel node biopsies}}{\text{Number of patients in whom sentinel lymph nodes were identified}} = \frac{359}{371} = 96.8\%$$

$$\text{False Negative Rate} = \frac{\text{Number of patients with a negative sentinel node biopsy}}{\text{Number of patients with axillary lymph node metastases}} = \frac{12}{180} = 6.7\%$$

(From Veronesi U, Paganelli G, Viale G, et al. J Natl Cancer Inst 91 (4):368–373, 1999)

World Wide Experience

More than 3500 cases of sentinel node biopsy for breast cancer have been described in the literature. Sentinel node identification rates vary from 71% to 99% and appear higher when radioactive tracer techniques are used [10]. The false negative rates range from 1% to 11% [11]. The results show in particular that radio-guided biopsy of the sentinel node in breast cancer is an effective procedure, characterized by a high rate of identification, no risk of radioactivity exposure to staff, and low rate of false negatives (particularly in relation to the non-negligible rate of false negatives in complete axillary dissection). Furthermore radio-guided sentinel node dissection is quick and easy for surgeons who are experienced in axillary lymph node dissection, and requires no special training. This contrasts to the blue-dye method for which it is suggested that 30–50 dissections are required to reach full competence.

The Future

Two decades ago, the treatment of breast cancer was transformed by the demonstration that conservative surgery is as effective as mastectomy. Today we are on the threshold of extending conservative treatment to the axilla by means of sentinel node biopsy, which promises to make it possible to safely forego axillary dissection in a considerable percentage of patients with small size breast cancer. This is important since removal of the axillary lymph nodes deprives the patient of immunocompetent tissue, which if healthy is best retained. Furthermore axillary dissection may be accompanied by other sequelae, such as reduced arm motility, reduced skin sensitivity, pain, lymphoedema and increased susceptibility to infections.

A pivotal aspect of surgical research in breast cancer will be to assess the precise prognostic significance of the various types of micrometastatic involvement of the sentinel node. Perhaps the finding of few positive cells confined to the subcapsular sinus may not justify total axillary dissection and may also indicate that systemic treatments are not necessary. At present our data suggest that sentinel lymph nodes involved by microfoci of cancer cells are associated with a non-negligible rate of metastatic involvement in the remaining axillary lymph nodes. We therefore believe that the presence of microfoci in the sentinel lymph node represents an indication for total axillary lymphadenectomy.

A future clinical application of the sentinel node technique might be to stage the axilla before neoadjuvant chemotherapy, since this treatment can alter axillary status.

Another aspect of the sentinel node technique is that it may allow direct reduction of treatment costs by reducing the duration of surgery and length of hospital stay. Indirect cost reduction may arise from the complete absence of motor sequelae in patients who have sentinel node biopsy but no axillary clearance and improvement of the patients' quality of life.

This new development is particularly important considering the changing presentation of primary breast cancer. Small tumours are found with greater frequency, and the percentage of patients with axillary metastatic involvement has declined. Furthermore, sufficient prognostic information can be obtained by investigation of the biologic properties of the primary, so that the information derived from histological examination of all the axillary nodes is becoming less important.

Another advantage of sentinel node biopsy is that it can enlarge surgical staging possibilities. Our experience is that in some cases lymphoscintigraphy reveals that lymph flow from the tumour area is to the internal mammary chain. This occurs more often if the tumour is located in the internal quadrants.

The internal mammary chain consists of a few lymph nodes alongside the retrosternal internal mammary vessels. To access them requires cutting the intercostal muscles and for this reason they have been largely ignored in breast cancer surgery. However, in the 1950s and 1960s some surgeons devoted considerable effort to removing the internal mammary nodes, together with the axillary nodes, in order to determine their prognostic significance and perhaps improve the cure rate. In these studies the internal mammary node was involved in around 20% of cases. And while their radical removal did not improve survival, their pathological status was found to be a significant prognostic variable.

We have recently started removing sentinel nodes from the internal mammary chain. The approach is to separate the longitudinal fibres of the pectoralis major to expose the rib cage. The intercostal muscle is severed above the hot spot, and the internal mammary vessels are easily identified. The sentinel node is located and removed without difficulty with the aid of the probe, taking care not to damage the underlying pleura. Examination of this node adds significant prognostic information, and in particular the finding of metastatic involvement may indicate the need for radiotherapy to the internal mammary chain.

In conclusion, sentinel node lymphadenectomy with selective lymphadenectomy appears a very attractive approach in breast-cancer patients since it is based on logical anatomical and physiological principles and promises to reduce the number of axillary node dissections. Regional control and survival will certainly remain unaffected and it is possible that the sparing of normal immunological tissue (the axillary lymph nodes) may even be beneficial. However, it is still unclear to which extent the benefits of this technique will outweigh the risks and, if so, in which patient groups. It is currently impossible to propose absolute indications for sentinel node lymphadenectomy because evidence from randomized trials on the efficacy of this approach is not yet available. The technique is therefore still in the developmental stage and standardization has not yet been achieved. Randomized clinical studies are in progress in the United States and Europe and preliminary results will hopefully be available in a short time.

References

1. Veronesi U, Saccozzi R, Del Vecchio M, et al. Comparing radical mastectomy with quadrantectomy, axillary dissection, and radiotherapy in patients with small cancers of the breast. N Engl J Med 1981; 305: 6–11
2. Veronesi U, Cascinelli N, Bufalino R, et al. Risk of internal mammary lymph node metastases and its relevance on prognosis of breast cancer patients. Ann Surg 1983; 198: 681–684
3. Veronesi U, Marubini E, Mariani L, et al. The dissection mammary nodes does not improve the survival of breast cancer patients. 30 years of a randomized trial. Eur J Cancer, 1999; 35:1320–1325
4. Cabanas RM. An approach for the treatment of penile carcinoma. Cancer 1977; 39:456–466
5. Gallico E, Giacomelli V, Pricolo V. La colorazione vitale dei linfatici nella chirurgia dei tumori. Chirurgia 1954; 9(3):1–8
6. Cope O. Surgery of the thyroid. In: The thyroid and its diseases. By JH Means, LJ De Groot, JB Stanbury. McGraw-Hill, New York 1963:561–598
7. Morton D, Wen D, Wong JH, et al. Technical details of intraoperative lymphatic mapping for early stage melanoma. Arch Surg 1992; 127:392–399

8. Giuliano AE. Sentinel lymphadenectomy in primary breast carcinoma: an alternative to routine axillary dissection. J Surg Oncol 1996; 62 (2):75–77
9. Veronesi U, Paganelli G, Viale G, et al. Sentinel lymph node biopsy and axillary dissection in breast cancer: results in a large series. J Natl Cancer Inst 1999; 91(4):368–373
10. Borgstein PJ, Pijpers, Comans EF, et al. Sentinel lymph node biopsy in breast cancer: guidelines and pitfalls of lymphoscintigraphy and gamma probe detection. J Am Coll Surg 1998; 186:275–283
11. Krag D, Weaver D, Ashikana T, et al. The sentinel node in breast cancer – a multicenter validation study. New Engl J Med 1998; 339(14):941–946

Specification of Potential Indications and Contraindications of Sentinel Lymph Node Biopsy in Breast Cancer

P. M. Schlag and A. Bembenek

Department of Surgery and Surgical Oncology, Robert-Rössle-Clinic, Charité, Campus Buch, Humboldt University, Berlin, Germany

Abstract

The promising results of various studies applying different methods of SN biopsy in heterogeneous patient subpopulations, show that sentinel lymph node biopsy is a reliable and minimally invasive method for the determination of the nodal status in breast cancer patients. While multicenter studies for the evaluation of the method's accuracy are still ongoing, future indications and contraindications are discussed. Based on our own experience, we try to give an actual overview of the potentials and problems of sentinel node biopsy in breast cancer.

Sentinel node detection was performed in 146 patients with breast cancer stages I–III, consisting of 127pT1/2 tumors and 19pT3/4. All of them underwent standard axillary dissection after SN biopsy. Using the radionuclide method including preoperative lymphoscintigraphy and intraoperative γ. Probe detection, the detection rate varied in relation to the tumor size between 94% for tumors with a diameter <1 cm, 85% (1–3 cm), 70% (3–5 cm) and 63% (>5 cm). The accuracy of the SN-biopsy in the prediction of the nodal status varied also with tumor diameter ranging from 100% for very small tumors (<1 cm), over 97% (1–3 cm) and 88% (3–5 cm), to 67% (>5 cm). In the subgroup of patients with pT1–2 tumors (n = 106), 57 patients (53%) showed true negative sentinel nodes, 38 (36%) revealed tumor cells in the H&E staining and an additional 7 patients (7%) solely in the immunohistochemical staining. 4 (4%) of these patients, all of them from the first half of the study period, underwent false-negative SN-biopsy, all of them showing lymphangiosis carcinomatosa and/or extensive infiltration of the metastatic lymph node(s).

The results presented show, that in about 50% of early breast cancer patients surgical intervention could potentially be avoided after a negative SN-biopsy, and an additional 5–10% of conventionally nodal negative patients can be found by immunohistochemical examination of the sentinel node. The SN concept is not recommended in clinically nodal positive patients or advanced disease. Potential applications include the evaluation of parasternal lymph nodes and patients with recurrent tumor. Before clinical application, quality control of the medical center and the performing surgeon have to be established potentially including the performance of about 20 procedures under supervision for each surgeon, an individual accuracy of at least 93%, and the possibility of immunohistochemical staining as well as a regular follow-up.

Introduction

The promising results of Veronesi et al. (preceding chapter) and various studies of the sentinel node biopsy using different methods in heterogeneous patient subpopulations, show that sentinel lymph node biopsy is a reliable and minimally invasive method for the determination of nodal status in breast cancer patients [6, 7, 8, 15]. Taking these results into consideration, it is now important to specify exactly the subgroup of patients who benefit from this procedure and to determine exactly the indications and contraindications of the method. Before broad application, however, the requirements of general quality control have to be defined, as well as the standardization of the method(s). Based on our own experience, we try to specify the indications and give an overview of the potentials of the method.

Patients and Methods

Using the radionuclide method, as previously described by Veronesi et al. [15], we performed SN biopsy in 146 patients with invasive breast cancer (142 female and 4 male, aged between 35 and 84 years). Two of them had undergone neoadjuvant radiochemotherapy for histopathologically proven advanced breast cancer, and nine of them had recurrent tumors after breast conserving surgery.

After informed consent 0.5–1 ml of a Tc^{99m}-colloid-solution (Nanocoll) was injected in the parenchyma surrounding the tumor 17 h before surgery. In the case of a non-palpable tumor, the injection was performed under ultrasound-guidance. Just before surgery, a scintigraphic picture was taken with a y-camera. The demonstrated radionuclide accumulation(s) was (were) localized intraoperatively with a hand-held y-probe and the corresponding lymph node was selectively excised. If there was more than one node detected we excised all of them, up to 4 nodes depending on the count rate. After sentinel node biopsy all patients underwent standard axillary dissection, including level I and II.

The histopathologic examination of the sentinel node included 2–6 serial sections with H&E staining and, if no tumor cells were found, immunohistochemistry with anti-CK-19-ab (Biogenex) was performed.

Results

The postoperative histopathologic tumor classifications revealed 127 pT1–2 and 19 pT3/4. The detection rate varied in relation to the tumor size between 94% in tumors with a diameter <1 cm, 85% (1–3 cm), 70% (3–5 cm) and 63% in tumors greater than 5 cm (Fig. 1).

The accuracy of the sentinel node biopsy was examined by comparing the sentinel node and non-sentinel node specimens. As for the detection rate, the consensus varied in relation to the tumor diameter between 100% (tumor diameter up to 1 cm), 97% (1–3 cm), 88% (3–5 cm) and 67% (>5 cm/T4) of the cases (Fig. 2).

In the subgroup of patients with a tumor-diameter up to 5 cm (106 patients) 57 patients (53%) showed true negative SN biopsies. 38 patients (36%) showed primarily tumor cells in the H&E staining, 7 patients (7%) were negative in the H&E, but positive in immunohistochemical staining (Fig. 3).

4 patients (4%), all of them belonging to the first half-period of the study, revealed a false negative SN biopsy meaning, that the SN examination (H&E and immunohistochemistry) showed no tumor cells, whereas other lymph nodes in the axilla-specimen revealed metastasis (Table 1).

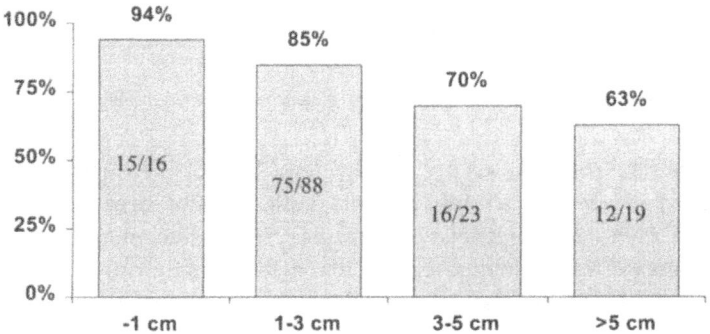

Fig. 1. Detection rate (%), depending on the tumor size (n = 146 patients)

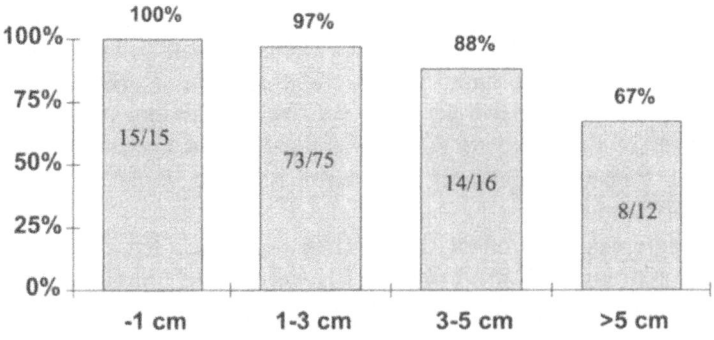

Fig. 2. Accuracy in the prediction of the nodal status of the SN biopsy, depending on the tumor-size

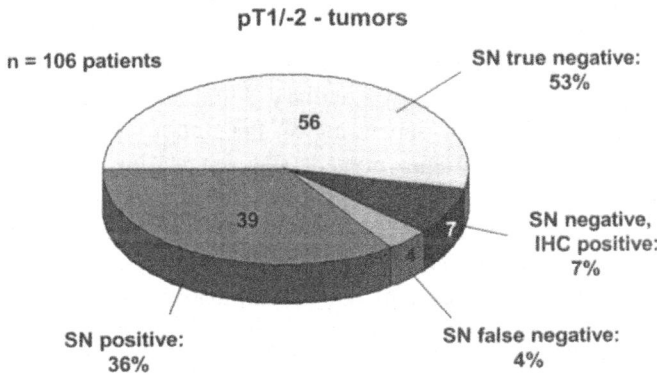

Fig. 3. Histopathologic results in patients with pT1/pT2 tumors. *IHC,* Immunohistochemistry

Table 1. Histologic tumor characteristics of patients with false-negative SN biopsies and pT1/T2 tumors

Pat.	pT	Tumor size	Type of invasive carcinoma	pN	Metastatic lymph nodes	Lymphangiosis carcinomatosa
1	pT1b	0.9 cm	tubular	pN2	4/29	no information
2	pT2	2.9 cm	ductal	pN1biii	1/16	yes
3	pT2	2.1 cm	ductal	pN1biii	1/26	yes
4	pT2	2.3 cm	ductal	pN1bi	1/20	yes

Table 2. Potential applications of sentinel lymph node biopsy

	Patients	Detection rate	Positive nodes
Local tumor recurrence	13	4/13 (31%)	2
Post neoadjuvant therapy	3	3/3	3

Two patients showed a parasternal SN, both of whom had undergone prior breast-conserving surgery with axillary dissection. In one of the two cases, the nodal status was formerly N0, now switching to rpN+. In total, 13 patients with recurrent cancer underwent sentinel lymph node biopsy: in 4 of the patients (31%) a sentinel node was excised, containing tumor cells in 2 cases. In all 3 patients with SN biopsy after neoadjuvant therapy a sentinel lymph node could be excised and all of the three nodes revealed tumor metastasis (Table 2).

Discussion

The results presented showed a highly predictive accuracy (97–100%) of the SN biopsy in regard to the axillary nodal status for patients with tumors up to 3 cm in diameter, depending on the tumor size. The detection rates in the same group of patients ranged, also in relation to the tumor size between 86% and 94%. According to the results presented, which are comparable to) the results of other studies [1, 8, 11, 15], the method is expected to identify a negative nodal status in about 50% of the patients with pT1/2 tumors. This means that, in the case of clinical application, about 50% of the early breast cancer patients could be spared from axillary dissection.

On the other hand, 39 out of 106 patients (36%) would have been selected for standard axillary dissection for proven axillary lymph node metastases and may be dissected with maximal thoroughness because of the proven malignancy in the axilla.

The patients with false-negative SN biopsies in 4/106 pT1/2-patients (3.8%), [respectively 4/46 nodal positive pT1/2-patients (8.7%)] stand in contrast to 7/106 (7%) patients with micrometastases being solely positive in immunohistochemical examination. Very probably, these metastases would not have been detected in an axillary specimen after standard dissection. Beside this, an additional percentage of lymph nodes with micrometastases in the H&E staining is exclusively detected by the SN-method, because of the higher number of serial sections, which can be performed in one sentinel lymph node compared to a whole axillary specimen that is routinely examined. In total, most of the recent studies expect a percentage of at least 10% additional metastases detected by microstaging of the SN biopsy, overriding the percentage of false negative SN biopsies [2, 6, 10, 12].

While most of the former studies did not provide data concerning the relationship between tumor-size and the results of SN biopsy [4, 8, 11, 15], the data presented showed that for patients with tumors bigger than 5 cm the detection rate as well as the accuracy declined to 63% (detection rate) and 67% (accuracy) respectively. In contrast, Hill et al., could not confirm any dependence of the detection rate or accuracy on the tumor size, but did not differentiate between pT2 and pT3 tumors [7]. Extensive infiltration of lymph nodes by metastatic tumor was found to cause negative lymphoscintigraphies and false-negative SN biopsies [2] too, probably also reflecting a generally negative influence of advanced disease on SN biopsy. One explanation for these findings could be that infiltration and obstruction of lymphatic channels or lymph nodes may cause a deviation of the lymph flow, leading to the detection/biopsy of a lymph node which is not or not yet infiltrated. This mechanism, however, may not be reserved only for advanced disease, but could be responsible for false-negative results in patients with smaller tumors, too. As was shown in the 4 cases presented with false-negative results (Table 1), all of these patients had lymphangiosis carcinomatosa and/or extensive infiltration of the lymph node beyond the capsule. Beside this, false-negative results may also be caused by multifocal tumors, as described by

Veronesi et al. [15] or by major changes of the immunologic interactions between lymph nodes and tumor cells, which has not been sufficiently evaluated up to now.

As mentioned by Veronesi et al. (preceding chapter), the detection of internal mammary lymph nodes is another interesting aspect of the SN biopsy.
About 6–16% of all axillary negative breast cancer patients show parasternal
metastases [3], which have the same prognostic significance as metastatic axillary lymph nodes [3, 9]. Thus, the nodal status of the parasternal node
seems to be of major importance, even if it was largely neglected in recent
decades, because parasternal dissection failed to reveal any survival benefit
[14]. It has yet to be proven that the SN concept could resolve this problem:
as published earlier [10], we performed SN biopsy in two formerly axillary
dissected patients with locally recurrent tumors (0.28% of the detected sentinel nodes) and found two metastatic sentinel nodes. In one of them, formerly classified as nodal negative, the nodal status switched. Borgstein et al.,
found in 21 out of 122 patients with pT1/T2-breast cancer parasternal hot
spots, but only in 2 patients (0.8%) the axilla was free of accumulation at the
same time. Parasternal SN biopsy in these two patients revealed that one was
tumor-infiltrated, whereas the other was tumor-free, but had an axilla with
many tumor-infiltrated nodes [2].

In total, in the present study, 13 patients with local recurrence after tumor
resection and axillary dissection underwent SN biopsy and showed detection
of a sentinel node in 4 cases (31%). Two of them, both parasternal, contained tumor cells, one of them therefore switching from formerly nodal negative to nodal positive disease. Such results may play a major role for the indication to systemic therapy, mainly in premenopausal patients, and may
support the continuing evaluation of sentinel node biopsy even after previous surgery with axillary dissection. In an additional 3 patients the method
was used after neoadjuvant induction therapy for advanced cancer and in
every case a positive sentinel node was found, confirming the indication for
axillary dissection. However, SN biopsy may play a role in patients where no
tumor cells are found at the primary tumor site after induction therapy. In
these cases SN biopsy may add in the decision of axillary dissection, if there
are no clinically suspicious nodes.

In this study's patients we exclusively performed preoperative lymphoscintigraphy in combination with a hand-held gamma-probe for intraoperative
SN detection without injection of blue dye. This form of radionuclide method is exact, easy to learn, and requires minimal surgical trauma. It is favored
by Veronesi et al., and other centers in Europe [11, 15]. A special problem
with the radionuclide method is the signal of the primary injection site overlapping the axilla, if the tumor is located in the upper outer quadrant near
the axilla while the SN biopsy is performed. Guiliano et al., still perform the
blue dye technique, which seems to be technically more difficult and requires
a somewhat more extended surgical trauma. They also report high detection
rates and a reliable predictive value, both close to 100% [6]. However, this
study group certainly has by far the greatest experience with this method

and had to go through a several-year learning phase also, with much worse results at the beginning [5]. In contrast, it seems much easier to become experienced with the radionuclide technique. Several study groups have begun to evaluate the combination of both methods [1, 4]. But, in contrast to melanoma patients, where the blue dye method helps to distinguish between first and second-tier nodes [13], this "pass-through", effect of the draining lymph nodes is obviously not as pronounced in breast cancer. Beside this, the blue dye method can lead to an accumulation of blue dye in the breast as result of a lymphatic block after axillary dissection [6]. A slight increase of the detection rate up to 8% by the addition of the blue dye technique is reported by Barnwell et al., and Hill et al. [2, 7]. But both study groups used the radionuclide technique without preoperative lymphoscintigraphy and, thus, probably reduced the potential of the radionuclide method significantly. In conclusion, up to now we see no striking argument for the addition of a second, more difficult method with the danger of a potentially cosmetic derangement to an already very accurate procedure.

While awaiting the results of the ongoing multicenter studies that are expected to prove the predictive value of SN biopsy for the axillary status, it becomes important to define who will or will not be elective to undergo the procedure and who will be allowed to perform it. This means, first of all, quality control for the medical center offering SN biopsy as a diagnostic tool and for the surgeon performing the procedure. Based on the recommendations of Cox et al., from the Lee Moffit Cancer Center in Tampa, FL [4], the following criteria may be useful as guidelines for quality control for medical institutes and surgeons performing SN biopsy:
- At least 20 self-conducted SN biopsies under supervision, followed by axillary dissection
- Individual accuracy for prediction of the nodal status of more than 92% of the personally performed procedures of each surgeon
- Possibility of immunohistochemical staining
- Regular follow-up controls in an ambulant care setting
- Performance of routine axillary dissection in the case of no detectable sentinel node

Even if it is not yet the time to define exactly the indications for SN biopsy in the clinical management of breast cancer, some contraindications seem to be preliminarily reasonable:
- Clinically positive axilla
- Tumor size >5 cm, tumor infiltration of the skin
- Multifocal tumors

Further studies should evaluate, if the following additional applications reach clinical importance:
- Detection of internal mammary lymph nodes
- SN biopsy before and/or after neoadjuvant therapy
- SN biopsy in patients with recurrent tumors

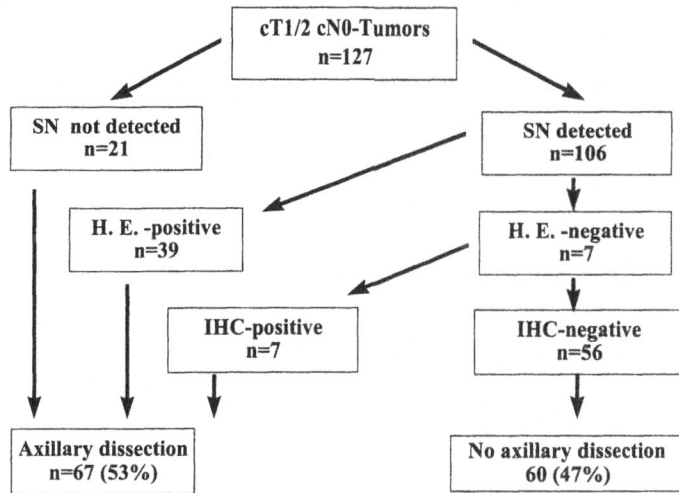

Fig. 4. Algorithm for the application of SN biopsy *IHC*, Immunohistochemistry

Figure 4 shows a possible algorithm for the clinical application of SN lymphonodectomy.

In conclusion, besides the demonstration of its reliability and clinical applicability in multicenter studies, future efforts must focus on the determination of clear indications and contraindications of SN lymphonodectomy. Additionally, standard detection methods and quality standards will have to be defined and training programs with individual quality controls will have to be established before a general routine use can be recommended.

References

1. Barnwell JM, Arredondo MA, Kollmorgen D, Gibbs JF, Lamonica D, Carson W, Zhang P, Winston J, Edge SB (1998) Sentinel node biopsy in breast cancer. 5(2) 126–130
2. Borgstein PJ, Pijpers R, Comans EF, van Diest PJ, Boom RP, Meijer S (1998) Sentinel lymph node biopsy in breast cancer: guidelines and pitfalls of lymphscintigraphy and gamma probe detection. J Am Coll Surg 186:275–283
3. Cody III HS, Urban JA (1995) Internal mammary lymph node status: A major prognostic factor in axillary node negative breast cancer. Ann Surg Oncol 2:32–37
4. Cox CE, Pendas S, Cox JM, Joseph E, Shons A, Yeatman T, Ku NN, Lyman GH, Berman C, Haddad F, Reintgen DS (1998) Guidelines for sentinel node biopsy and lymphatic mapping of patients with breast cancer. Ann Surg 227:645–653
5. Giuliano AE, Kirgan DM, Guenther JM, Morton DL (1994) Lymphatic mapping and sentinel lymphadenectomy for breast cancer. Ann Surg 220:391–401
6. Giuliano AE, Jones RC, Brennan MF, Statman R (1997) Sentinel lymphadenectomy in breast cancer. J Clin Oncol 15:2345–2350
7. Hill ADK, Tran KN, Akhurst T, Yeung H, Yeh SDJ, Rosen PP, Borgen PI, Cody III HS (1999) Lessons learned from 500 cases of lymphatic mapping for breast cancer. Ann Surg 229:528–535
8. Krag D, Weaver D, Ashikaga T, Moffat F, Klimberg VS, Shriver C, Feldman S, Kusminsky R, Gadd M, Kuhn J, Harlow S, Beitsch P (1998) The Sentinel Node in breast cancer. N Engl J Med 339 (14):941–946

9. Lacour JL, Monique LE, Caceres E, Koszarowski T, Veronesi U (1983) Radical mastectomy versus radical mastectomy plus internal mammary dissection. Cancer 51:1941–1943
10. Reuhl T, Kaisers H, Markwardt J, Haensch W, Hohenberger P, Schlag PM (1998) Axillaausräumung bei klinisch nodal-negativem Mammakarzinom. Dtsch Med Wochenschr 123:583–587
11. Roumen RMH, Valkenburg JGM, Geuskens LM (1997) Lymphoscintigraphy and feasibility of sentinel node biopsy in 83 patients with primary breast cancer. Eur J Surg Oncol 23:495–502
12. Schreiber RH, Pendas S, Ku NN, Reintgen DS, Shons AR, Berman C, Boulware D, Cox CE (1999) Microstaging of breast cancer patients using cytokeratin staining of the sentinel lymph node. Ann Surg Oncol 6:95–101
13. Uren RF, Howman-Giles RB, Thompson JF (1998) Demonstration of second-tier lymph nodes during preoperative lymphscintigraphy for melanoma: Incidence varies with primary tumor site. Ann Surg Oncol 5:517–521
14. Veronesi U, Valagussa P (1981) Inefficacy of internal mammary nodes dissection in breast cancer surgery. Cancer 47:170–175
15. Veronesi U, Paganelli G, Galimberti V, Viale G, Zurrida S, Bedoni M, Costa A, De Cicco C, Geraghty JG, Luini A, Sachini V, Veronesi P (1997) Sentinel-node biopsy to avoid axillary dissection in breast cancer with clinically negative lymph-nodes. Lancet 349: 1864–1867

Potential and Pitfalls of Sentinel Node Detection in Breast Cancer

K. U. Chu and A. E. Giuliano

John Wayne Cancer Institute, 2200 Santa Monica Boulevard, Santa Monica, CA 90404, USA

Abstract

The last decade has seen the development of a minimally invasive technique to identify representative nodes – sentinel nodes – that reflect the tumor status of nodes in the axillary lymphatic basin draining a primary breast carcinoma. Sentinel lymph node dissection (SLND), originally developed as an alternative to elective complete lymph node dissection in patients with primary cutaneous melanoma, has been applied successfully to the management of patients with breast cancer. SLND holds promise as a staging technique to replace formal level I and II axillary lymph node dissection in selected patients with breast carcinoma, thus avoiding an unnecessary procedure that has no role in many patients with tumor-free axillae. Under way are two large randomized trials examining the role of SLND for the management of patients with invasive breast carcinoma. Even when tumor is detected in the sentinel node, a focused examination of this node may indicate whether or not completion axillary lymph node dissection is necessary. However, although SLND has great potential, its successful widespread use requires more stringent definition of the sentinel node and standardized guidelines for lymphatic mapping. Each institution must carefully assess the accuracy and consistency of results obtained by its multidisciplinary SLND team.

Introduction

Intraoperative lymphatic mapping and sentinel lymph node dissection (SLND) is a highly accurate means for identifying axillary nodal metastasis in patients with invasive breast carcinoma. SLND is a promising technique that could potentially replace routine level I and II axillary lymph node dissection (ALND). The utility of SLND in breast cancer patients is being examined in two large randomized trials conducted by the National Surgical Adjuvant Breast and Bowel Project (NSABP) and the American College of Sur-

Recent Results in Cancer Research, Vol. 157
© Springer-Verlag Berlin · Heidelberg 2000

geons Oncology Group (ACSOG). This chapter briefly describes the development and current status of SLND, outlines the technique of SLND, and discusses its potential and pitfalls in patients with breast cancer.

Development of SLND in Breast Cancer

Lymphatic mapping in patients with breast cancer actually dates back to 1972 when Haagensen [1] first illustrated the axillary nodal uptake of a vital blue dye during mastectomy. Five years later, Cabanas [2] used the term 'sentinel node' to describe a fixed-location node receiving lymphatic drainage from penile cancer. However, the concept of operative lymphatic mapping to identify the first lymph node draining a primary tumor was not popularized until 1990 when Morton et al. [3] from the John Wayne Cancer Institute (JWCI) described the technique of SLND in patients with malignant cutaneous melanoma. SLND was developed as a practical means of identifying patients with regional nodal metastases and thereby eliminating routine lymph node dissection in patients with no clinical evidence of nodal involvement [4]. Because the sentinel node (SN) is the first regional lymph node to receive tumor cells that metastasize along the lymphatic pathway from a primary tumor, its tumor status should reflect the tumor status of the entire regional lymphatic drainage basin.

In October of 1991, we first applied this technique in patients with breast carcinoma, and began to test its feasibility. Our initial goal was to eliminate routine ALND without losing its staging advantage. Three years later, we reported our cumulative experience in 174 patients with primary breast tumors (176 cases) [5]. Intraoperative lymphatic mapping was performed with 1% isosulfan blue dye, and SLND was always followed by completion ALND (levels I and II) to verify the procedure's accuracy. An SN was identified in 114 (66%) procedures and accurately predicted axillary status in 109/114 (96%) cases. Three of the 5 false-negative results were dye-stained axillary fat misidentified as an SN early in the series; this prompted the routine use of frozen section to confirm lymph node recovery and prepare our pathologists for frozen sections that, if tumor-free, would eventually obviate completion ALND. A fourth false-negative was identified as a true-positive when a "tumor-free" SN was reexamined using immunohistochemistry (IHC), a highly sensitive technique that has since become routine for nodal specimens that do not contain metastases detectable with hematoxylin and eosin (H&E). To determine if the SN could predict axillary status by chance alone, we examined the ALND specimens of patients with histologically involved nodes. Of the 751 lymph nodes removed from 34 patients, 63 (8%) were SNs and 688 (92%) were nonsentinel nodes (NSNs) [5]. Tumor was found in 39 SNs compared with 93 NSNs (62% vs. 14%; $p < 0.0001$). This suggests that a primary breast tumor spreads to the axilla along a specific pathway of lymph nodes that cannot be identified by random axillary sampling.

In 1995, we evaluated the first 162 patients undergoing successful SLND followed by completion ALND (SLND group), and compared them with 134 patients undergoing ALND alone (ALND group) [6]. Each SN was evaluated by H&E and anti-cytokeratin IHC staining; NSNs were evaluated by H&E alone. We detected a significantly higher incidence of axillary metastasis in the SLND group than the ALND group (42% vs. 28%; $p < 0.05$), which was primarily due to detection of more micrometastases (≤ 2 mm) in SNs than NSNs (16% vs. 3%; $p < 0.05$), particularly with IHC staining. We used these results to define our standard of focused histopathologic examination with IHC staining. This time-consuming and expensive technique is not practical for routine examination of the much larger ALND specimen; however, a focused examination of the lymph node most likely to contain cancer cells (the SN) may be more accurate than routine examination of all axillary lymph nodes and may enhance the staging accuracy of axillary surgery by detecting metastases that would be missed by routine tissue processing. Our IHC study of 1087 NSNs confirmed that the SN is always the first node to harbor tumor cells metastasizing from a primary breast lesion [7]; this study showed that when the SN is tumor-free by both routine H&E and IHC, the probability of tumor in an NSN is 1/1087, or 0.09%.

Over the last few years, investigators at several other institutions have verified the SN concept in breast cancer. Krag and associates [8] were the first to report lymphatic mapping of breast cancer using a gamma probe to follow the path of a radiolabeled isotope. In their 1993 pilot study of probe-directed mapping, 22 patients received an injection of unfiltered technetium sulfur colloid 1–4 h before SLND. No dye was used. The SN was identified in 18 (82%) patients, and predicted the histopathologic status of the axilla in each case. A study by Albertini and colleagues [9] combined isosulfan blue dye and filtered technetium sulfur colloid for lymphatic mapping. An SN was identified in 57 of 62 patients (92%). Forty-five SNs were identified by both blue dye and radiolabeled colloid, and 12 were identified by colloid alone. Metastases were found in 18 SNs, all of which had been identified by both dye and colloid. No patient had a tumor-positive NSN if the SN was free of tumor. Albertini's group concluded that the combination of dye and colloid increases identification of the SN, and in their hands this method was superior to colloid or dye alone. Veronesi and colleagues [10] reported the results of probe-directed lymphatic mapping using technetium-labeled human serum albumin injected subdermally and superficial to the tumor. The SN was identified in 160 of 163 patients and was predictive of axillary status in 156 of the 160 (97%) patients.

Table 1 summarizes the results of numerous studies on the SN as a predictor of axillary status in patients with primary breast cancer [5–22]. Taken as a group, these studies confirm that the lymphatic drainage of a breast cancer can be identified and traced to the SN intraoperatively, and that the histologic status of the SN accurately predicts the tumor status of the entire axilla.

Table 1. Studies examining the success rate and accuracy of SLND in breast cancer

Study	N	Mapping technique	Histo-pathologic technique	Rate of SN identifi-cation	Accuracy of SN as indicator of axillary status	Average number of SN examined	Rate of metastasis only to SN
Krag [8]	22	Probe	H&E	18/22 (82%)	18/18 (100%)	–	43%
Giuliano [5]	174	Dye	H&E	114/174 (66%)	109/114 (96%)	1.8	38%
Albertini [9]	62	Dye +Probe	H&E	57/62 (92%)	57/57 (100%)	2.2	67%
Pijpers [11]	37	Probe	H&E	34/37 (92%)	32/32 (100%)[a]	2.2	64%
Veronesi [10]	163	Probe	H&E	160/163 (98%)	156/160 (98%)	1.4	38%
Giuliano [12]	107	Dye	H&E +IHC	100/107 (94%)	100/100 (100%)	1.8	67%
Guenther [13]	145	Dye	H&E	103/145 (71%)	100/103 (97%)	–	43%
Dale [14]	21	Dye	H&E	14/21 (66%)	14/14 (100%)	1.2	60%
Borgstein [15]	130	Probe	H&E +IHC	122/130 (94%)	103/104 (99%)[b]	1.2	59%
Barnwell [16]	42	Dye +Probe	H&E	38/42 (90%)	38/38 (100%)	1	33%
O'Hea [17]	59	Dye +Probe	H&E	55/59 (93%)	52/55 (95%)	2.2	41%
Miner [18]	42	Probe	H&E	41/42 (98%)	40/41 (98%)	2.9	57%
Offodile [19]	41	Probe	H&E IHC	40/41 (98%)	40/40 (100%)	3	–
Cox [20]	466	Dye +Probe	H&E +IHC	440/466 (94%)[c]	–	1.9	–
Koller [21]	98	Dye	–	96/98 (98%)	93/96 (97%)	2.7	27%
Crossin [22]	50	Probe	–	42/50 (84%)	41/42 (98%)	2	–

[a] Two patients refused completion ALND and were censored from this analysis
[b] Eighteen patients refused completion ALND and were censored from this analysis
[c] The majority of patients with tumor-negative SNs did not undergo completion ALND

Current Status of SLND

During the developmental phase of SLND and subsequently for approximately 100 cases using the fully modified technique, we did not consider
abandoning routine ALND because we were still proving the accuracy of
SLND. In 1997 we reported a series of 107 consecutive patients undergoing
SLND followed by completion ALND [12]: the rate of SN identification was
94%, and there were no false-negative results – a sensitivity and specificity of

100%. Based on these results and the results of IHC on NSNs [7], in 1995 we abandoned routine ALND for SN-negative patients and began a trial to study outcome and clinical recurrence rate in patients undergoing SLND followed by completion ALND *only* if the SN has tumor cells. Candidates for this trial are patients with clinically negative axillary lymph nodes and primary breast tumors no greater than 4 cm (T1 and T2). Patients with primary tumors in the inner hemisphere undergo preoperative lymphoscintigraphy to document axillary drainage. SLND is performed using dye-directed mapping, except for inner hemisphere tumors, where we use both dye and probe. The excised SN is intraoperatively examined by frozen section with H&E or DiffQuik (Dade International, Miami, FL); if it contains tumor, then completion ALND is performed before the patient leaves the operating room. IHC staining, which is a 2-day process at our institution, is performed postoperatively on multiple levels of all SNs that are tumor-free by H&E.

Our trial has now accrued over 500 cases. In those patients with at least 2 years of follow-up, 40% had SN metastases and underwent completion ALND; the remaining 60% had no evidence of SN metastases and therefore did not undergo ALND. No patient in either group has developed an axillary recurrence, and no patient in the SLND group has experienced lymphedema or numbness. Based on our data and that reported by other investigators, we have started a prospective randomized trial through ACSOG to examine the efficacy of SLND, and the clinical significance of ALND in patients who have micrometastatic disease in the axilla.

Sentinel Lymph Node Dissection at JWCI

The SN to be excised during SLND is identified intraoperatively by lymphatic mapping using a vital blue dye and/or a radioactive tracer. In either case, the technique can be done with local anesthesia and heavy sedation, or with light general anesthesia. If the primary tumor is in the medial hemisphere, dye-directed lymphatic mapping should be preceded by preoperative lymphoscintigraphy to determine whether the tumor drains to axillary nodes.

At the time of surgery, 3–5 ml of isosulfan blue dye (Lymphazurin®) is injected into the breast parenchyma immediately adjacent to the breast mass laterally and below the subcutaneous fat, to avoid tattooing the overlying skin. If the primary tumor was excised previously, dye is injected into the wall of the biopsy cavity. If the primary tumor is not palpable, a needle inserted under mammographic guidance for tumor localization is used to inject the dye. Approximately 5 min after dye injection, a transverse incision is made just below the hair-bearing area in the axilla. Blunt dissection is performed to identify the dye-filled lymphatic tract. This tract is then followed proximally and distally until a blue-stained sentinel node is identified. If more than one dye-filled lymphatic tract is identified, each is followed. These tracts usually drain to the same SN.

Probe-directed mapping using a radioactive tracer is performed by inject-ing technetium-99m (Tc-99m) labeled sulfur colloid or Tc-99m albumin col-loid 2–24 h prior to operation. A lymphoscintigram is obtained preoperative-ly to determine the axillary drainage pattern from the primary tumor. At the time of surgery, a hand-held gamma-ray counter (Neoprobe® or C-Trak®) is held over the axilla to identify the area of greatest radioactivity in counts per second. A background count is established by measuring radioactivity over a neutral site. The skin is incised over the area of greatest radioactivity, and the probe is held over the incision to measure the in vivo radioactivity of axillary lymph nodes. The SN is usually the node with the highest abso-lute count. After this node is excised, in vivo radioactivity of the axillary basin is reassessed. Some SLND investigators will continue to search for ad-ditional SNs if the absolute count of the basin still exceeds background. Despite lack of clear definition of an SN by radioactive count, probe-directed mapping has the advantage of detecting any "hidden" SNs with a count high-er than background. In contrast, dye-directed mapping allows surgeons to visualize the SN before its excision. The blue dye technique is especially helpful when the primary tumor is close to the lymph node basin, because the radioactivity of the primary can obscure counts in the lymph node basin (shine-through effect).

Because the SLND specimen contains only one or two lymph nodes, it can be routinely examined in multiple sections with IHC staining for cytokeratin. Each SN removed during SLND is bisected and a frozen section is obtained to look for metastatic cells. The SN is then processed routinely for perma-nent section with H&E. Each node is blocked individually, with preparation of two permanent-section levels per paraffin block. If H&E staining is nega-tive for tumor cells, the SN is examined with IHC using an antibody cocktail (MAK-6: Ciba-Corning, Alameda, CA) directed against low and intermediate molecular weight cytokeratin. Approximately six to eight histologic sections (including the frozen section) of each SN are examined. The ALND speci-mens are examined using standard pathologic techniques. Lymph nodes are identified visually or with manual palpation; no lymph node clearing solu-tion is employed. Lymph nodes greater than 3–4 mm are grossly sectioned and all nodal tissue is embedded in paraffin; one or two histologic sections, H&E stained, are prepared for diagnostic evaluation. Cytokeratin IHC stains are not routinely used.

Potentials of SLND

As better screening for breast cancer increases the number of patients who have small primary lesions, the incidence of axillary involvement will con-tinue to decline. Only about one-third of patients with clinically negative ax-illae have nodal metastases after histopathological examination of the ALND specimen [23–26], and this rate is even lower for patients with small lesions [27–30]. The use of SLND can avoid unnecessary surgery with its potential

for significant morbidity. Furthermore, axillary status does not affect the selection of adjuvant therapy in approximately 40% of patients [31, 32],
although the tumor status of axillary lymph nodes remains the single most
significant indicator of prognosis [33, 34]. With minimal risk of morbidity,
SLND can accurately distinguish patients who would not benefit from ALND
from those who would benefit from complete axillary staging.

Permanent lymphedema has been documented in 7%–37% of patients who
undergo ALND [35–38], and the frequency and severity of lymphedema increase with the extent of axillary dissection [39, 40]. Other complications
such as wound infection, seroma, arm weakness, decreased shoulder range of
motion, and neurologic changes also occur after ALND [41]. These complications, which are considered minor and often ignored in the literature, can
lead to significant emotional stress and functional impairment [38, 42]; they
also significantly increase the costs of treatment. Removing only a few SNs is
minimally invasive and has few complications. We have yet to see lymphedema in a patient undergoing SLND without ALND, although we suspect it is
possible.

SLND is a staging procedure that has therapeutic potential. The therapeutic role of ALND is controversial; several studies have suggested that ALND
is without therapeutic benefit, even in patients with tumor-involved axillary
lymph nodes [43], whereas others believe that routine use of ALND can improve survival by ensuring regional control [44]. If there is any real survival
advantage to ALND, SLND can identify patients who may benefit (those with
SN metastases) and those who are unlikely to benefit (patients with tumor-
free SNs). The SN is frequently the only lymph node containing tumor cells.
In our previous study of 107 consecutive patients [12], 67% (28/42) of those
with SN involvement had no other tumor-positive nodes in the axillary basin. Corresponding rates of 40% (32/81), 59% (26/44), 67% (12/18), and 33%
(5/15) have been reported by Veronesi et al. [10], Borgstein et al. [15], Albertini et al. [9], and Barnwell et al. [16], respectively.

We have found that the size of SN metastases and the size of the primary
tumor accurately predict the likelihood of metastases in NSNs [45]. In our
studies, the rate of NSN involvement in patients with SN micrometastases
(<2 mm in maximum diameter) was <10% when the primary tumor was
<5 cm in maximum diameter. Furthermore, patients with IHC-detected me-
tastases in an SN were unlikely to have H&E-positive NSNs. Thus a focused
examination of the SN removed during SLND could indicate not only the tumor status of the SN but also the probable tumor status of NSNs in the same
basin. Our data indicate that patients with small tumors and micrometastatic
involvement of the SN are unlikely to benefit from ALND.

Historically, the axillary specimens from standard level I and II ALND
were evaluated by bivalving the nodes and performing routine H&E examination. However, the more focused examination possible with the much smaller
SLND specimen can identify metastases that might be missed by standard
H&E examination. In our study, the 42% rate of axillary metastasis in 162
patients undergoing SLND followed by ALND was significantly (p < 0.03)

higher than the 29.1% rate in 134 patients undergoing ALND alone [6]. The corresponding rates of axillary micrometastasis (≤2 mm) were 38.2% (26/68) and 10.3% (4/39). Eleven of the 26 micrometastases in the SLND group were identified by IHC staining after H&E stains were negative. Thus, the detailed examination of the SN "upstaged" an additional 16% (11/68) of axillary lymph node basins. In general, more sections and IHC examination of the nodes increased the detection of metastases from 25% to 40%–50%. However, most of these additional tumor foci were micrometastases, the importance of which remains controversial.

Although the clinical significance of axillary micrometastases has not been examined in a prospective fashion, several retrospective studies suggest that micrometastases are associated with poor outcome [46–54]. The International (Ludwig) Breast Cancer Study Group used serial sectioning of axillary lymph nodes to identify micrometastases in 9% (83/921) of breast cancer patients whose nodes were tumor-free by routine histopathological examination [50]. Patients with micrometastases had lower rates of 5-year disease-free survival (p = 0.0003) and overall survival (p = 0.002) than those whose nodes remained negative: 58% and 79%, respectively, versus 74% and 88%, respectively. Two subsequent large (n > 100) retrospective analyses also demonstrated the prognostic importance of identifying occult micrometastases when H&E stains were negative. De Mascarel et al. [52] used IHC to identify micrometastases in 50 of 218 patients (23%) whose ALND specimens stained negative for tumor cells with H&E. In patients with invasive ductal carcinoma, IHC-detected micrometastases were the most significant factor associated with recurrence (multivariate p-value = 0.011). Although IHC-detected micrometastases were not significant for survival in this subset of patients on univariate analysis (p = 0.07), they were significant on multivariate analysis (p = 0.027). Hainsworth et al. [53] identified occult metastases in 41 of 343 "node-negative" patients (12%) whose nodal specimens were reexamined with IHC. The presence of occult metastases increased the 5-year recurrence rate from 16% to 32%. If micrometastases have clinical significance, SLND could be used to identify those patients at risk for recurrence or distant disease. Accurate staging of these patients might eliminate or at least decrease the incidence of early recurrence that we observe in many patients with small primary tumors. In addition, SLND offers an opportunity to identify candidates for clinical trials of adjuvant therapies.

Pitfalls of SLND

The tremendous degree of variation in the SLND technique and its results was clearly demonstrated in the first prospective multicenter feasibility trial [55]. Although the overall staging accuracy was 97%, the false-negative rate ranged from zero to 29% (mean 11%) and the rate of SN identification ranged from 79% to 98%. These findings underline the need for quality control; consistently accurate results with SLND require substantial training and total commitment from the surgeon.

How many cases of SLND followed by completion ALND must be performed before the surgeon can undertake SLND alone? Recently, Morton [56] recommended approximately 60–80 cases to develop an "acceptable level of technical skill (90% accuracy in identifying sentinel node)." ACSOG requires 30 cases with ≥85% accuracy and a false-negative rate ≤5% before participating in the trial. The exact number of cases to reach a high degree of accuracy with a low rate of false-negatives varies from surgeon to surgeon. Quick-learning surgeons who have performed many axillary operations will master SLND after fewer cases, whereas others may never develop the skills necessary to accurately identify an SN.

The SN can be identified by radiocolloid and/or blue dye. At present, there is no standardization of the SLND technique. The "best" technique depends on the experience and training of the individual surgeon and his or her team. Many surgeons believe that blue dye alone is too difficult for the beginner, and many prefer a combination of dye and colloid. However, adding a radiocolloid does not necessarily increase mapping accuracy and may introduce additional technical problems such as "shine-through" when the tumor is near the axillary nodal basin. In this case, an SN cannot be detected by the probe without special techniques such as removing the primary site or shielding the tumor from even the most collimated probe.

Probe-directed mapping is complicated by numerous variables, all of which have been interpreted differently. An example is the site of injection: some groups use peritumoral injection, whereas others use intratumoral or even subcutaneous or cutaneous injection. A second variable is the radiocolloid, which may be filtered sulfur colloid, unfiltered colloid, or radiolabeled albumin. This difference in the radioactive tracers used to map lymphatic drainage has prohibited the development of uniform criteria for identifying an SN by its radioactive count. Krag et al. [8] used unfiltered sulfur colloid and defined an SN as any node with radioactivity 3 times over the background and at least 15 counts per 10 seconds. Veronesi et al. [10] used albumin colloid and defined an SN as the node with the highest radioactive count. Albertini et al. [9] used sulfur colloid and defined the SN as the node with more than 10 times the radioactivity of neighboring NSNs; these authors also searched for additional SNs if the basin count remained 150% higher than background. Yet another variable is the time from injection to operation. These subtle technical variations – type of gamma counter, type of colloid, injection site, timing – make probe-directed mapping very subjective.

Our initial experience with probe-directed lymphatic mapping was extremely unsatisfying and we were unable to reproduce the results of others after many modifications. We have found that the detection of an SN with blue dye is much more predictable and consistent. Surgical fellows training at JWCI generally learn dye-directed SLND after about 10–15 cases, and visiting surgeons who observe our technique usually find it easy to master when they return to their practice. Surgeons learning the technique of SLND in breast cancer might feel more secure with a "back-up" mapping agent that allows a "second chance" to identify an SN not stained by the blue dye. However, the surgeon must understand the drawbacks of probe-directed mapping. We strongly advise surgeons learning SLND to perform this technique without variation or modification. Results must be consistent and reproducible before any "improvements" are considered in the technical details of SLND.

As SLND becomes more widely publicized, more surgeons are confronted by patient requests for SLND instead of ALND. However, surgeons who are not yet proficient at SLND must not abandon routine ALND. Any surgeon interested in providing SLND must establish an institutional protocol to accurately perform SLND, organize a committed team of pathologists, nuclear medicine physicians, nurses and surgeons, and apply rigorous controls to assure proficiency at every stage of the technique. During the learning phase, SLND should be followed immediately by ALND; comparing the tumor status of SNs and NSNs removed during SLND and ALND, respectively, will allow the surgeon and other members of the team to determine when they can reproduce the excellent results reported in the literature. Without vigorous quality control and a well-organized team, SLND may yield a high false-negative rate that increases the potential for significant locoregional recurrence and poor outcome.

Conclusion

Although the issues regarding consensual definition of an SN by the radioactive tracer technique, kinetics of the different radioactive tracers, and quality control in the community setting must be resolved, SLND is a promising procedure that may play a major role in the management of patients with invasive breast cancer. There is no doubt that SLND can accurately stage patients with breast cancer, and the literature shows that when the SN can be identified with accuracy it can predict axillary status. The question is whether its potential can be fully translated into general practice. Quality control is paramount for successful application of this technique, and each surgeon must learn how to do the procedure and must ensure that members of the multidisciplinary SLND team are equally committed and skilled in their roles. Those surgeons who have performed a sufficient number of mapping procedures will be convinced of their own accuracy in identifying the SN and can comfortably abandon ALND. Underway are two large prospective randomized trials that will indicate the role of SLND in the management of patients with invasive breast cancer.

References

1. Haagensen CD. Lymphatics of the breast. In: Haagensen CD, Feind CR, Herter FP, Stanetz CA, Weinberg JA. The Lymphatics in Cancer. Philadelphia, Pa: WB Saunders Co; 1972:300–398
2. Cabanas RM. An approach for the treatment of penile carcinoma. Cancer 1977; 39:456–466
3. Morton DL, Cagle LA, Wong JH, Economou JS, Foshag LJ, Wen DR, et al. Intraoperative lymphatic mapping and selective lymphadenectomy: technical details of a new procedure for clinical stage I melanoma. Presented at the Society of Surgical Oncology, March 1990, Washington, DC
4. Morton DL, Wen DR, Wong JH, et al. Technical details of intraoperative lymphatic mapping for early stage melanoma. Arch Surg 1992; 127:392–399
5. Giuliano AE, Kirgan DM, Guenther JM, Morton DL. Lymphatic mapping and sentinel lymphadenectomy for breast cancer. Ann Surg 1994; 220:391–401
6. Giuliano AE, Dale PS, Turner RR, Morton DL, Evans SW, Krasne DL. Improved axillary staging of breast cancer with sentinel lymphadenectomy. Ann Surg 1995; 222:394–401
7. Turner RR, Ollila DW, Krasne DL, Giuliano AE. Histopathologic validation of the sentinel lymph node hypothesis for breast carcinoma. Ann Surg 1997; 226:271–278
8. Krag DN, Weaver DL, Alex JC, Fairbank JT. Surgical resection and radiolocalization of the sentinel node in breast cancer using gamma probe. Surg Oncol 1993; 2:335–340
9. Albertini JJ, Lyman GH, Cox C, et al. Lymphatic mapping and sentinel node biopsy in the patient with breast cancer. JAMA 1996; 276:1818–1822
10. Veronesi U, Paganelli G, Galimberti V, et al. Sentinel-node biopsy to avoid axillary dissection in breast cancer with clinically negative lymph-nodes. Lancet 1997; 349:1864–1867
11. Pijpers R, Meijer S, Hoekstra OS, et al. Impact of lymphoscintigraphy on sentinel node identification with technetium-99m-colloidal albumin in breast cancer. J Nucl Med 1997; 38:366–368
12. Giuliano AE, Jones RC, Brennan M, Statman R. Sentinel lymphadenectomy in breast cancer. J Clin Oncol 1997; 15:2345–2350
13. Guenther JM, Krishnamoorthy M, Tan LR. Sentinel lymphadenectomy for breast cancer in a community managed care setting. Cancer J Sci Am 1997; 3:336–340
14. Dale PS, Williams JT. Axillary staging utilizing selective sentinel lymphadenectomy for patients with invasive breast carcinoma. Am Surg 1998; 64:28–32
15. Borgstein PJ, Pijpers R, Comans EF, et al. Sentinel lymph node biopsy in breast cancer: guidelines and pitfalls of lymphoscintigraphy and gamma probe detection. J Am Coll Surg 1998; 186:275–283
16. Barnwell JM, Arredondo MA, Kollmorgen D, et al. Sentinel node biopsy in breast cancer. Ann Surg Oncol 1998; 5:126–130
17. O'Hea BJ, Hill ADK, El-Shirbiny AM, et al. Sentinel lymph node biopsy in breast cancer: initial experience at Memorial Sloan-Kettering Cancer Center. J Am Coll Surg 1998; 186:423–427
18. Miner TJ, Shriver CD, Jaques DP, et al. Ultrasonographically guided injection improves localization of the radiolabeled sentinel lymph node in breast cancer. Ann Surg Oncol 1998; 5:315–321
19. Offodile R, Hoh C, Barsky SH, et al. Minimally invasive breast carcinoma staging using lymphatic mapping with radiolabeled dextran. Cancer 1998; 82:1704–1708
20. Cox CE, Pendas S, Cox JM, et al. Guidelines for sentinel node biopsy and lymphatic mapping of patients with breast cancer. Ann Surg 1998; 227:645–653
21. Koller M, Barsuk D, Zippel D, et al. Sentinel lymph node involvement – a predictor for axillary node status with breast cancer – has the time come? Eur J Surg Oncol 1998; 24:166–168
22. Crossin JA, Johnson AC, Stewart PB, et al. Gamma-probe-guided resection of the sentinel lymph node in breast cancer. Am Surg 1998; 64:666–669

23. Fisher B, Wolmark W, Bauer M et al. The accuracy of clinical nodal staging and of limited axillary dissection as a determinant of histologic nodal status in carcinoma of the breast. Surg Gynecol Obstet 1981; 152:765–772

24. Pamilo M, Soiva M, Lavast EM. Real-time ultrasound, axillary mammography, and clinical examination in the detection of axillary lymph node metastases in breast cancer patients. J Ultrasound Med 1989; 8:115–120

25. Sacre RA. Clinical evaluation of axillary lymph nodes compared to surgical and pathological findings. Eur J Surg Oncol 1986; 12:169–173

26. De Freitas R, Jr, Costa MV, Schneider SV. Accuracy of ultrasound and clinical examination in the diagnosis of axillary lymph node metastases in breast cancer. Eur J Surg Oncol 1991; 17:240–244

27. Osteen RT, Karnell LH. The National Cancer Data Base report on breast cancer. Cancer 1994; 73:1994–2000

28. Silverstein MJ, Gierson ED, Waisman JR, et al. Axillary lymph node dissection for T1a breast carcinoma. Is it indicated? Cancer 1994; 73:664–667

29. Reger V, Beito G, Jolly PC. Factors affecting the incidence of lymph node metastases in small cancers of the breast. Am J Surg 1989; 157:501–502

30. Dowlatshahi K, Snider HC, Jr, Kim R. Axillary node status in nonpalpable breast cancer. Ann Surg Oncol 1995; 2:424–428

31. Menard S, Bufalino R, Rilke F, et al. Prognosis based on primary breast carcinoma instead of pathological nodal status. Br J Cancer 1994; 70:709–712

32. Reynolds JV, Mercer P, McDermott EW, et al. Audit of complete axillary dissection in early breast cancer. Eur J Cancer 1994; 30 A:148–149

33. Fisher ER, Sass R, Fisher B. Pathologic findings from the National Surgical Adjuvant Project for Breast Cancers (protocol no. 4). X. Discriminants for tenth year treatment failure. Cancer 1984; 53:712–723

34. Carter CL, Allen C, Henson DE. Relation of tumor size, lymph node status, and survival in 24,740 breast cancer cases. Cancer 1989; 63:181–187

35. Kissin MW, Querci della Rovere G, Easton D, et al. Risk of lymphoedema following the treatment of breast cancer. Br J Surg 1986; 73:580–584

36. Keramopoulos A, Tsionou C, Minaretzis D et al. Arm morbidity following treatment of breast cancer with total axillary dissection: A multivariated approach. Oncology 1993; 50:445–449

37. Cabanes PA, Salmon RJ, Vilcoq JR, et al. Value of axillary dissection in addition to lumpectomy and radiotherapy in early breast cancer. The Breast Carcinoma Collaborative Group of the Institut Curie. Lancet 1992; 74:126–129

38. Velanovich V, Szymanski W. Quality of life of breast cancer patients with lymphedema. Am J Surg 1999; 177:184–187

39. Penzer RD, Patterson MP, Hill LR. Arm edema in patients treated conservatively for breast cancer: Relationship to patient age and axillary node dissection technique. Int J Radiat Oncol Biol Phys 1986; 12:2079–2083

40. Larson D, Weinstein M, Goldberg I, et al. Edema of the arm as a function of the extent of axillary surgery in patients with stage I-II carcinoma of the breast treated with primary radiotherapy. Int J Radiat Oncol Biol Phys 1986; 12:1575–1582

41. Ivens D, Hoe AL, Podd TJ, et al. Assessment of morbidity from complete axillary dissection. Br J Cancer 1992; 66:136–138

42. Tobin MB, Lacey HJ, Meyer L, et al. The psychological morbidity of breast cancer-related arm swelling: Psychological morbidity of lymphedema. Cancer 1993; 72:3248–3252

43. Cady B. Case against axillary lymphadenectomy for most patients with infiltrating breast cancer. J Surg Oncol 1997; 66: 7–10

44. Moore MP, Kinne DW. Axillary lymphadenectomy: a diagnostic and therapeutic procedure. J Surg Oncol 1997; 66: 2–6

45. Chu KU, Turner RR, Hansen NM, Brennan M, Bilchik A, Giuliano AE. Do all patients with sentinel node metastasis from breast carcinoma need complete axillary node dissection? Ann Surg 1999; 229:536–541

46. Nasser IA, Lee AKC, Bosari S, et al. Occult axillary lymph node metastases in "node-negative" breast carcinoma. Hum Pathol 1993; 24:950–957
47. Bettelheim R. Price KN, Gelber RD, et al. Prognostic importance of occult axillary lymph node micrometastases from breast cancer. Lancet 1990; 335:1565–1568
48. Trojani M, de Mascarel I, Bonichon F, et al. Micrometastases to axillary lymph nodes from carcinoma of breast: detection by immunohistochemistry and prognostic significance. Br J Cancer 1987; 55:303–306
49. Sedmak DD, Meineke TA, Knechtges DS, et al. Prognostic significance of cytokeratin-positive breast cancer metastases. Mod Pathol 1989; 2:516–520
50. International (Ludwig) Breast Cancer Study Group. Prognostic importance of occult axillary lymph node micrometastases from breast cancer. Lancet 1990; 335:1565–1568
51. Chen ZL, Wen DR, Coulsen WF, et al. Occult metastases in the axillary lymph nodes of patients with breast cancer node negative by clinical and histologic examination and conventional histology. Dis Markers 1991; 9:239–248
52. De Mascarel I, Bonichon F, Coincre JM, Trojani M. Prognostic significance of breast cancer axillary lymph node micrometastases assessed by two special techniques: re-evaluation with longer follow-up. Br J Cancer 1992; 66:523–527
53. Hainsworth PJ, Tjandra, Stillwell RG, et al. Detection and significance of occult metastases in node-negative breast cancer. Br J Surg 1993; 80:459–463
54. Clare SE, Sener SF, Wilkens W et al. Prognostic significance of occult lymph node metastases in node-negative breast cancer. Ann Surg Oncol 1997; 4:447–451
55. Krag D, Weaver D, Ashikaga T, et al. The sentinel node in breast cancer: a multicenter validation study. N Engl J Med 1998; 339:941–995
56. Morton DL. Intraoperative lymphatic mapping and sentinel lymphadenectomy: community standard care or clinical investigation? Cancer J Sci Am 1997; 3:328–330.

VIII. Sentinel Node Detection in Gastric Cancer

Gastric Lymphography and Detection of Sentinel Nodes

T. Sano, H. Katai, M. Sasako, and K. Maruyama

Gastric Surgery Division, National Cancer Center Hospital, Tokyo, Japan

Abstract

The lymphatic drainage system of the stomach was studied using lymphography with various dyes, and several major routes have been shown. Gastric lymph channels are multidirectional and form complex networks. We conducted a retrospective study to know the first site of metastasis from small gastric cancers by examining 89 cases with only one lymph node metastasis. The perigastric nodal area close to the primary tumor was the first site of metastasis in only 62% of the cases. N2 metastasis without N1 involvement was seen in 13%. In order to identify sentinel nodes for local resection of gastric cancer, a novel method needs to be developed.

Lymphography of the Stomach

Lymphography of the stomach has a long history and the first report of its clinical study for gastric cancer was as early as in 1950. Weinberg et al. [1] utilized sky blue injection to visualize the lymphatic system around the stomach during gastrectomy. Japanese surgeons have shown particular interest in lymphatic mapping around the stomach and meticulously studied the possible pathways of lymph node metastasis [2]. Endoscopic or intraoperative injections of various kinds of dye or radioisotope were tested, and the solution of activated fine carbon particle CH40 was developed by Hagiwara et al. [3].

The solution of CH40 shows high affinity with lymphatic tissue and remains in nodes for a long time. A direct injection of CH40 to a perigastric node immediately visualizes the lymphatic channels and connected nodes (Fig. 1). This intraoperative lymphography has enabled surgeons to recognize the anatomical structure of the lymphatic system and to perform a precise lymphadenectomy. The dye in the nodes also makes the postoperative nodal retrieval by surgeons or pathologists easy.

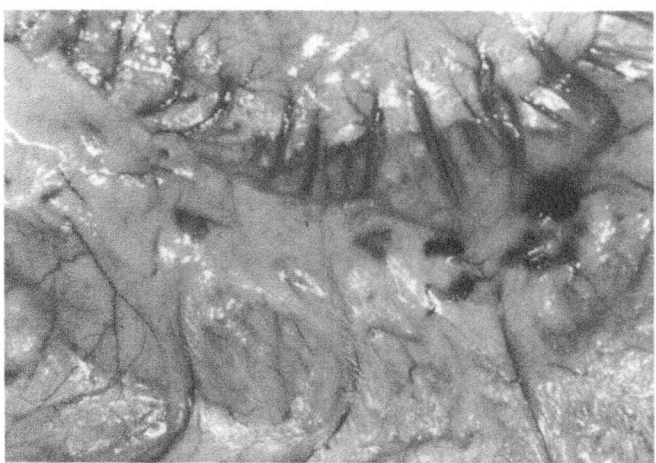

Fig. 1. Intraoperative lymphography using CH40 solution. The lymphatic channels and lymph nodes along the right gastroepiploic artery are stained black

Lymphatic Drainage of the Stomach

The lymphatic drainage system of the stomach has been studied by dye-assisted lymphography. Endoscopic or intraoperative injections of various dyes visualize the draining lymphatic network. One of the anatomical features of the stomach is the existence of two mesenteria, the lesser and greater omenta. The dye injected in the subserosa of the stomach, therefore, flow out to the two opposite directions through the lymphatic channels.

Outside the stomach, the lymphatic vessels form fine networks along the arterial arcades and make nodal chains. The following four major routes are known (Fig. 2): (1) Channels along the left gastric artery from the proximal two-thirds of the lesser curvature to the celiac nodes. (2) Channels along the right gastric artery from the distal third of the lesser curvature to the celiac nodes via the common hepatic nodes. (3) Channels along the right gastroepiploic artery from the distal half of the greater curvature to the infrapyloric nodes. They then flow either to the celiac nodes crossing the pancreatic surface or to the paraaortic nodes along the superior mesenteric artery. (4) Channels along the splenic artery from the proximal half of the greater curvature and the posterior wall of the cardia, via the left gastroepiploic artery, posterior gastric artery or the short gastric arteries, to the celiac nodes.

Besides these four, the route along the left subphrenic artery is important in cardia tumors. It drains the gastric fundus into the paraaortic nodes without passing through the celiac route.

It should be noted that most of lymphatic channels from the stomach gather around the celiac axis along its main branch arteries. The exceptions are the infrapyloric-superior mesenteric route and the fundus-paraaortic route.

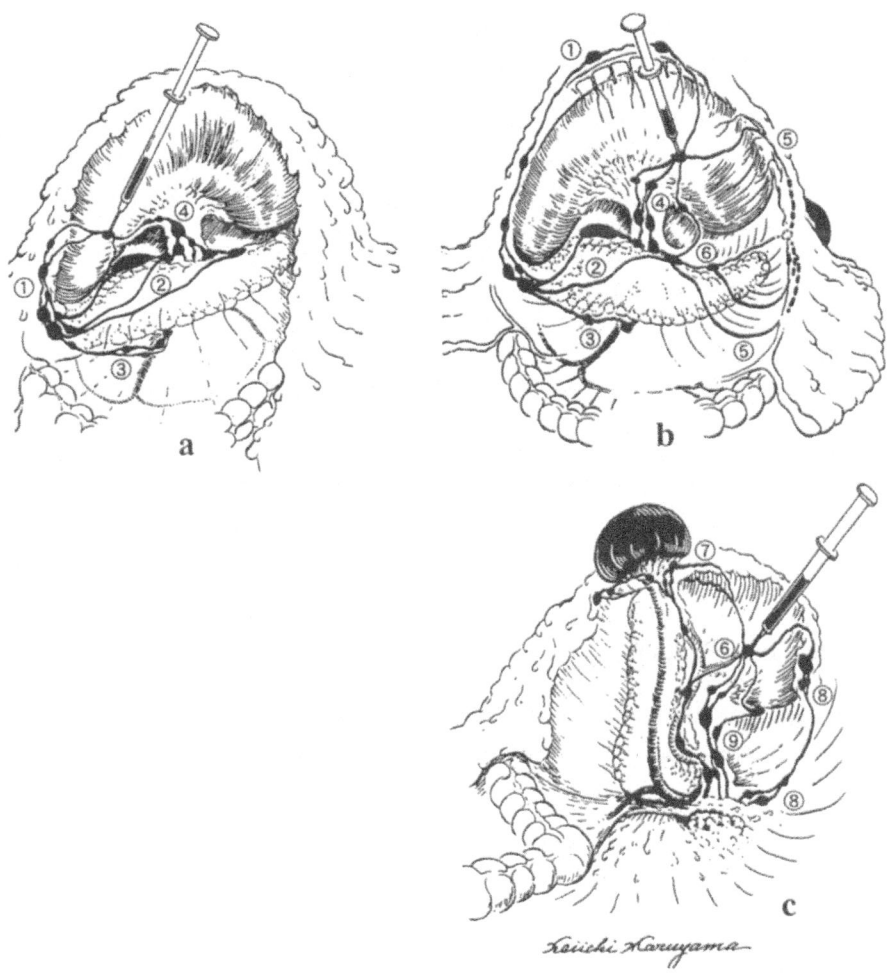

Fig. 2. Major lymphatic channels from the lower third (**a**), the middle third (**b**), and the upper third (**c**) of the stomach. (1) Channel along the right gastroepiploic artery. (2) Channel crossing the pancreas to the celiac nodes. (3) Channel along the superior mesenteric artery. (4) Channel along the left gastric artery. (5) Channel along the left gastroepiploic artery. (6) Channel along the posterior gastric artery. (7) Channel at the splenic hilum. (8) Channel along the left subphrenic artery. (9) Channel from the right cardia

The location of a gastric tumor can be precisely determined before operation by endoscopy with or without barium meal study. The possible lymphatic spread should, therefore, be preoperatively predicted on the basis of the lymphatic routes mentioned above. Preoperative endoscopic dye injections around the tumor help operative recognition of lymphatic channels.

The First Site of Nodal Metastasis from Small Gastric Cancer

If the site of lymph nodes to which gastric cancer first metastasizes were known, it could serve as a sentinel site for metastasis. The problem is that the gastric lymphatic channels are multidirectional and complex and that a tumor area is often drained by more than one lymphatic route listed above. Furthermore, each route consists of fine lymph channels that can be connected to, or independent from, each other. Under these anatomical conditions, it does not seem simple to identify the site of the first nodes at which metastatic tumor cells would arrive.

In Japan, resected lymph nodes have been grouped and given anatomical "station numbers" according to the Japanese Classification of Gastric Carcinoma [4] (Fig. 3). In this system, the location of primary tumor is recorded as upper, middle or lower-third of the stomach. These classifications are quite simple for surgeons to use and may serve to identify the "sentinel group" of nodes to each tumor location. We retrospectively studied whether it would be possible to identify the first nodal group of metastasis by the location of the primary tumor.

Materials and Methods

In our database of gastric cancer, we searched for cases of small tumor with only one lymph node metastasis. Among 3568 patients undergoing curative

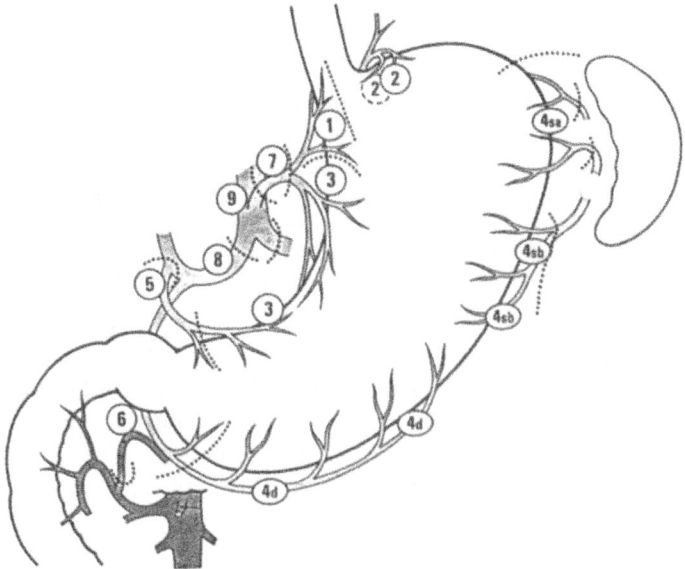

Fig. 3. Lymph node station numbers in Japanese Classification of Gastric Carcinoma

resection for gastric cancer in our institution between 1970 and 1990, 89 cases (2.5%) were selected by the following criteria: (1) The tumor was smaller than 3 cm and solitary. (2) The tumor was located at least 2 cm away from the cardia or the pylorus. (3) A curative gastrectomy with lymphadenectomy was performed. (4) The histological examination of all resected lymph nodes revealed only one positive node.

The conditions (1) and (2) were set in order to exclude tumors that would not be fit for local resection. The histological mapping of lymph nodes was based on the station numbers (1 to 16) and the group numbers (N1 to N3) defined by the Japanese Classification.

Results

The distribution of the single positive node is shown in Table 1 according to the location of the primary tumor. In 20 (54%) out of 37 tumors in the lower-third of the stomach, the single node metastasis was found in either the lesser (No. 3) or greater curvature (No. 4) perigastric area close to the tumor. In 16 cases (43%), the metastasis was found in either the suprapyloric (No. 5) or infrapyloric (No. 6) area, both of which were N1 but somewhat remote from the primary tumor. In one case, the metastasis was found in the left gastric area (No. 7, N2) without perigastric involvement.

In 31 (72%) out of 43 tumors in the middle-third, the single node metastasis was found in either the lesser (No. 3) or greater curvature (No. 4) perigastric area close to the primary tumor. In 6 cases (7%), the metastasis was found in the remote perigastric area (Nos. 1, 5, 6), and in another 6 cases in the N2 area (Nos. 7, 8).

In nine cases with an upper-third tumor, four (44%) had the single metastasis in the perigastric node close to the tumor (Nos. 1, 3, 4). In the other five patients, the metastasis was found in an N2 area (Nos. 7, 11).

In total, the single nodal metastasis was found in the nearest perigastric nodal area in 62% of cases, in a fairly remote perigastric area in 25% of them, and in the N2 area without N1 involvement in 13%.

Table 1. The site of single nodal metastasis from 89 small gastric cancers

	Primary tumor		
	Lower third n=37	Middle third n=43	Upper third n=9
1 Right cardiac nodes		2	1
3 Lesser curvature nodes	13	22	2
4 Greater curvature nodes	7	9	1
5 Suprapyloric nodes	3	2	
6 Infrapyloric nodes	13	2	
7 Left gastric artery nodes	1	5	3
8 Common hepatic artery nodes		1	
11 Splenic artery nodes			2

Discussion

The stomach is one of the organs in which the lymphatic drainage system is highly developed. Even in a simple distal gastrectomy, 20 or more lymph nodes are retrieved. The number of regional nodes sometimes reaches 100 after total gastrectomy with extended lymphadenectomy. These numbers are far greater than those in the surgery of breast cancer or colorectal cancer.

Gastrectomy with D2 lymphadenectomy (dissection of N1 and N2 nodes) is the standard surgery for gastric cancer in Japan. This procedure covers the celiac lymph nodes where most of the lymphatic drainage routes of the stomach gather. There can be plural pathways from any location of the stomach to the celiac nodes, and in each pathway, highly developed lymph channels cross each other. Metastatic nodes can be seen anywhere between the nearest perigastric area and the celiac area.

We studied the location of the first metastasis from small gastric cancers by retrospectively examining the cases with only one positive node. In 62%, the positive node was located in the perigastric area close to the primary tumor. In 13%, the node was in N2 area without involvement of N1 nodes. These results indicate that the blind examination of the nodal area close to the primary tumor cannot be a reliable method to detect the first metastasis.

Prospective studies should be conducted to establish the methodology to detect sentinel nodes in gastric cancer. Injections of a dye or isotope would be able to show the first nodal site, and the histological results of these possible sentinel nodes should be analyzed after gastrectomy with sufficient lymphadenectomy. Problems to be solved include what material should be injected in which part of the stomach wall at what timing. These have also been the problems in breast cancer surgery for which the technique of sentinel node biopsy has almost been established. However, considering the anatomical features of the complex lymphatic system in the stomach, breast cancer techniques or conventional lymphography methods seem unlikely to accurately hit the sentinel nodes. Novel techniques need to be developed. When a reliable method is established, many small gastric cancers will be treated by local wedge resection without lymphadenectomy.

References

1. Weinberg JA, Greaney EM (1950) Identification of regional lymph nodes by means of avital staining dye during surgery of gastric cancer. Surg Gyn Obst 90:561
2. Aikou T, Natugoe S, Tenabe G, Baba M, Shimazu H (1987) Lymph drainage originating from the lower esophagus and gastric cardia as measured by radioisotope uptake in the regional lymph nodes following lymphoscintigraphy. Lymphology 20(3):145–151
3. Hagiwara A, Takahashi T, Sawai K, et al (1992) Lymph nodal vital staining with newer carbon particle suspensions compared with India ink: experimental and clinical observations. Lymphology 25:84–90
4. Japanese Gastric Cancer Association (1998) Japanese Classification of Gastric Carcinoma – 2nd English Edition. Gastric Cancer 1:10–24

Potential and Futility of Sentinel Node Detection for Gastric Cancer

J. R. Siewert and A. Sendler

Chirurgische Klinik und Poliklinik der Technischen Universität München, Klinikum rechts der Isar, Ismaningerstrasse 22, 81675 Munich, Germany

Abstract

The technique and scientific background of sentinel node dissection has spread extremely rapidly over the surgical community. Following the addition of this technique to the tools of oncologic surgery for treatment of malignant melanoma and breast cancer, questions arise regarding the use of this method in gastric cancer also. While the lymphatic flow on the surface of the body can be defined easily, the lymphatic drainage of the stomach is much more complicated. Following rotation of the stomach during embryonic development, the lymphatic flow is not directed in a simple fashion. It is questionable whether a specific area of the stomach will drain into one lymph node echelon only. This is one of the essential obstacles for SLND in gastric cancer. Furthermore, skip metastasis seems to be quite common in cancer of the stomach. In gastric cancer, the value and the extent of classical lymph node dissection itself is still under scientific discussion. The rationale, aims, and extent of LA in gastric cancer are addressed. The scientific discussion on whether D1 or an extended lymphadenectomy are appropriate is not finally closed as yet. The possibilities and problems concerning an individualised indication for a selective lymphadenectomy in gastric cancer are discussed.

Introduction

Since the studies of Morton, who invented the strategy of sentinel lymph node dissection (SLND) in patients with malignant melanoma, this method spread extreme rapidly over the surgical oncologic community (Morton et al. 1992). However, even for melanoma and for breast cancer, the method is still under scientific evaluation. The aim of the SLND concept is a meticulous pathohistological staging of the N-category, the so-called „ultra-staging". This is done with the help of a minor and uncomplicated operation. Following this, an adjuvant therapy regimen could be applied on a new basis.

Up to now, SLND is done for malignomas on the surface of the body. This is a region with a well-defined lymphatic flow, which can be made visible using lymphoscintigraphy. For gastric cancer, the route of tumour spread and the question of skip metastasis is rather more complicated.

Furthermore, the therapeutical value and the extent of lymphadenectomy (LA) in gastric cancer is still under discussion. Following the work of the „Japanese Research Group for Gastric Cancer" between 1970 and 1980, extended lymphadenectomy (D2-resection) in gastric cancer came more and more into the focus of interest for surgeons in the Western world. In retrospective analyses and in non-randomised large studies in the Western world, D2 dissection proved its benefit. However, in two prospective, randomised Western studies (the British [MRC] and the Netherlands trail), the method of radical LA in gastric cancer failed to demonstrate any survival advantage in the entire study population (Bonenkamp et al. 1999; Cuschieri et al. 1996). In the German, non-randomized study, a survival advantage was demonstrated for stage II tumours at least (Siewert et al. 1998).

In this chapter, we will consider the reasons, aims and problems of lymphadenectomy in gastric cancer first. This is followed by a discussion of possibilities and the possible futility of SLND in this tumour entity.

Rationale of Lymphadenectomy

The aim of every operation for gastric cancer has to be the complete resection of the tumour. This means not only the complete resection of the primary, but also the resection of the adjacent lymphatic tissue. This situation corresponds to the „R0-category" of the UICC. Only if an operation is performed following this principle, can the prognosis of the patient be ameliorated.

Complete tumour resection in this respect refers to:

- the primary tumour, i.e., no residual tumour at the oral and aboral resection margins and the tumour bed (the so-called third dimension) and
- the lymphatic drainage, i.e., as a minimal requirement no residual tumour in the peripheral or border lymph nodes.

In order to improve the prognosis of a patient not only does the primary have to be removed with an adequate safety margin, but this margin should also be respected in the area of the lymphatic drainage. During the first period of tumour growth, lymph node metastasis follows the anatomic lymphatic vessels. Only in the late stage of the disease may extra-anatomic lymphatic spread occur.

Safety margins of the primary can be measured simply by the distance of affected to non affected tissue. For lymph nodes, this margin can defined by the so-called „lymph node ratio". The number of removed lymph nodes has

Table 1. Ranking of independent prognostic factors on multivariate analysis in all patients with resected gastric cancer

Prognostic factor	Relative risk (95% Confidence interval)	p value
1. Lymph node ratio		
0	1	
< 20%	1.8 (1.5–2.2)	
> 20%	2.8 (2.2–3.4)	< 0.0001
2. R category		
R0	1	
R1	1.6 (1.3–1.9)	< 0.0001
R2	2.0 (1.6–2.4)	
3. pT category		
T1	1	
T2	3.0 (2.1–4.2)	
T3	4.5 (3.2–6.4)	< 0.0001
T4	6.2 (4.2–9.1)	
4. Postoperative complications		
No complications	1	
Multiple complications	2.1 (1.7–2.6)	
Anastomotic leak Cardiopulmonary	1.7 (1.3–2.1)	< 0.0001
5. M category		
M0	1	
M1	1.4 (1.2–1.6)	< 0.003

to exceed the number of obviously invaded nodes by a factor of five. In recent studies, the number of involved lymph nodes and the ratio of involved to examined lymph nodes correlates significantly with survival. Therefore, a lymph node ratio <0.2, i.e., less than 20% of the removed nodes are invaded by tumour, is required to improve prognosis (Siewert et al. 1993). If there are more than 20% of the lymph nodes affected by tumour cells, the reason for lymphadenectomy is merely the prevention of loco-regional recurrences (Table 1).

Furthermore, the necessity of extended lymph node dissection can be explained by the high prevalence of micrometastases in lymph nodes of tumours staged as N0 on histological routine examination (HE). In recent studies, the prognostic value of so-called „micro-involvement" of lymph nodes which were negative by routine histology was demonstrated. The presence of three or more tumour cells in more than 10% of the lymph nodes in pN0 cases was revealed by multivariate analysis to be an independent prognostic factor (Siewert et al. 1996). The independent prognostic influence of lymph node-ratio and microinvolvement stresses the importance of lymph node dissection in gastric cancer. These arguments are proven by multivariate analyses in the German Gastric Cancer Study (GGCS). The R0 resection and the lymph node ratio are strong and decisive independent prognostic factors (Roder et al. 1993; Siewert et al. 1996).

Only extended lymphadenectomy is able to influence the number of resected lymph nodes, which in turn directly influences the lymph node ratio.

However, in this respect it has to be stated that lymphadenectomy is not a principle on its own, but is a part of the whole strategy in treating gastric cancer.

Aims of Lymphadenectomy

There are three aims for radical LA in gastric cancer:
1. Accurate staging
2. Reduction of local recurrences (unproven)
3. Amelioration of the prognosis (unproven)

Reliable tumour staging is a prerequisite for any scientific approach to the problem of lymphadenectomy and the comparison of treatment results. This means not only the pretherapeutic staging of tumour spread, but also the pathohistological staging following resection. According to the rules of the UICC, a minimum of 15 dissected lymph nodes is necessary to define the N-category correctly. This is supported by the authors' and others' experience. It was shown that staging is only reliable when at least more than 15 nodes are removed and assessed by the pathologist (Roder et al. 1998; Siewert et al. 1996). Following this, the new N-category, applied since 1997, is based only on the number of affected lymph nodes (UICC 1997).

Since a more radical lymph node dissection will also allow a more accurate staging, extended lymphadenectomy may result in a higher prevalence of patients with lymph node metastases thus biasing the results of any comparison between various extents of lymph node dissection. This problem, termed 'stage migration', has become an important argument in the discussions around the benefits of extended lymphadenectomy (Bonenkamp and van de Velde 1995).

This is particularly in contrast to the observation of the GGCS (Fig. 1) that stage distribution was not significantly different between patients with standard and extended lymphadenectomy if patients with less than 15 removed lymph nodes were excluded from the analysis (Siewert et al. 1998). Furthermore, in patients with stage II tumours, the beneficial effect of extended lymph node dissection persisted when only those with more than 15 removed nodes were included in the analysis. Consequently the data of the present study strongly indicate that the observed survival differences in patients with stage II tumours are not due to 'stage migration' but rather reflect a real benefit of extended lymphadenectomy.

The value of staging for the patient lies in the future in a more precise indication for an adjuvant treatment. Up to now, the benefit of adjuvant therapy is still unproven (Hermans et al. 1993b), but there might be indications in the future if subgroups, which might profit from the treatment, are more properly evaluated (Hermans and Bonenkamp 1993a).

For some patients, knowledge about their own statistical prognosis could be useful. The reduction of local recurrences by extended LA is still un-

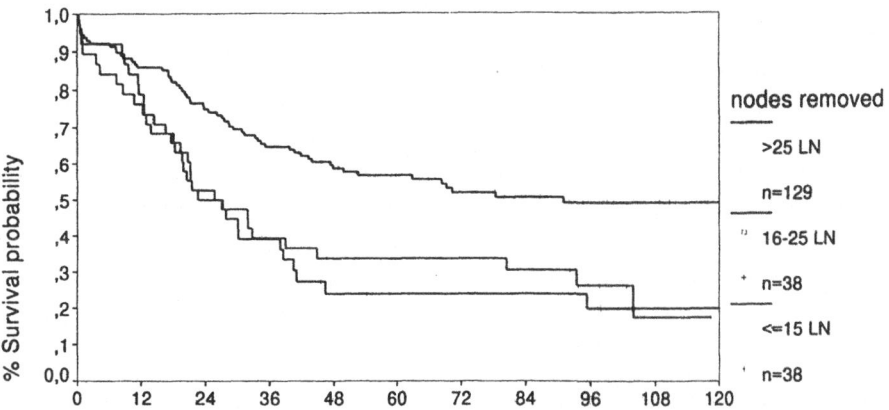

Fig. 1. 10-year survival data of 205 patients with UICC stage II gastric cancer; 10-year results of the German gastric cancer study. A significant survival advantage is achieved in patients in which more than 25 lymph nodes were removed (*upper line*); own data

proven. However, from retrospective analyses of populations operated on at different time intervals, a reduction of local recurrences seems to be possible (Nishi et al. 1993; Siewert et al. 1995).

The influence of extended (D2) lymphadenectomy on survival is still controversial. Multivariate analysis which compared non-randomised patients after extended lymphadenectomy with a historical control group with "classical" surgery found a significant survival benefit for the D2 operation. The fact that extended lymph node dissection can be performed without increased surgical morbidity and mortality was demonstrated by comparison with historical controls in Japan as well as in non-randomised studies in Europe. On the other hand, both large prospective and randomised trials have failed to demonstrate a survival advantage for the entire study population so far.

However, these studies pose serious problems, which may account for the high morbidity and mortality. In both studies, significantly more splenectomies and left pancreatic resections were performed in the D2 group than in the D1 group (Dutch trial: 32% vs. 3%, British trial 56.5% vs. 4%). Following this, a lot of pancreatic fistulas led to a high morbidity and mortality. Furthermore, the training of the surgeons for performing D2 LA was low in both studies. In the Dutch trial, 331 D2 lymphadenectomies were done by 82 surgeons at 51 centres, that is, 4 operations per surgeon in 4 years. In the British trail, 200 D2 LA were done at 31 centres, accounting for 6 D2 lymphadenectomies per centre in 7 years. The training of the individual surgeon and the experience of his or her hospital are main factors regarding the outcome following this operation.

A major problem in performing D2 resection is quality control. In the Dutch study, an attempt was made to assure quality in D2 resection. All operations were attended by one of eight specially trained regional supervising surgeons. Unfortunately, this good approach failed. In 51% of the patients who underwent D2 dissection, no lymph nodes were obtained from at least two of the lymph node stations that were supposed to have been dissected (Brennan 1999).

Similar to several randomised trials, the long-term results of the GGSC did not show a survival benefit of extended lymphadenectomy when the entire patient population was analysed. However, the analysis of the ten-year results indicated an improved survival rate after extended lymphadenectomy in patient subgroups (Siewert et al. 1998). Extended lymph node dissection significantly increased the 10-year survival rate and median survival time in patients with UICC stage II tumours. In this patient subgroup, extended lymphadenectomy resulted in a marked improvement of the 10-year survival rate from 19.9% with standard lymphadenectomy to 49.2%.

Since patients with UICC stage II tumours constitute only 15%–20% of the patients resected for gastric cancer in the Western world, even a marked improvement of the prognosis in this small subgroup will not significantly affect the overall prognosis of patients with resected gastric cancer. An improvement of the long-term survival rate from 20% to 50% in patients with stage II tumours translates into an increase of the overall long term survival rate of patients with resected gastric cancer of less than 5%. Well above 1000 patients would have to be randomised in order to detect such a marginal change of the overall prognosis with a power of 90% at a significance level 0.05. None of the randomised studies contains a large enough number of patients to detect this effect. Consequently, a beneficial effect of extended lymphadenectomy has so far only been demonstrated following subgroup analyses.

If patients with UICC stage II tumours were analysed according to the individual pTN subgroups, a survival benefit after extended lymphadenectomy could be demonstrated in patients of pN0 and pN1 categories (pT2N1 and pT3N0). This indicates that lymphadenectomy is beneficial not only in patients with frank lymph node metastases but also in patients in whom no lymph node metastases can be detected by standard histopathologic assessment (see above). This benefit of radical removal of apparently non involved lymph nodes can be explained by the phenomenon of 'lymph node microinvolvement' or 'micrometastases', i.e., minute tumour islands with stromal reaction, which are usually not detected by standard histopathologic assessment. These observations suggest that radical lymph node removal could be associated with an improvement of long-term survival particularly in patients with incipient lymph node metastases.

The recent published long term results of the Dutch Gastric Cancer trial indicate no survival advantage in any UICC stage (Stadium II D1: 38%, D2: 42% five-year survival, p=0.29, Stadium IIIA: 11% vs. 28%, p=0.07) (Bonenkamp et al. 1999). However, if complications following splenectomy and left-sided pancreatectomy are excluded, a survival advantage is demonstrable for both groups (van der Velde 1998, personal communication).

In conclusion, both in retrospective studies and in the Dutch trial, there are subgroups of patients, (Stadium II and IIIA) which will benefit from extended LA. In this patients, extended LA is indicated.

Side Effects of Lymphadenectomy

It is not possible to perform lymphadenectomy without any side effects. However, overall they are rare. In our own experience and reflecting the results of the German Gastric Cancer Study (GGCS), extended lymphadenectomy has no more complications than a D1 lymphadenectomy (Table 2). The precondition is that D2 lymphadenectomy is performed according to the rules of the JRSGC: a left-sided pancreas resection and splenectomy are avoided. In the Dutch and the British trial, in which a higher complication rate following D2 lymphadenectomy was seen, these rules were not followed. Nearly all the septic complications seen were observed following splenectomy and/or left-sided pancreatectomy.

After correction of the published data of the Dutch trial (exclusion of patient with left-sided pancreatectomy and splenectomy), no differences in complications between D1 and D2 lymphadenectomy can be demonstrated. In 1997 Sasako and co-workers published an analysis of the main risk factors in the Dutch gastric cancer trial (Sasako 1997). This investigation revealed splenectomy as the most important risk factor (relative risk 2.13) for overall complications. Whole pancreatectomy and type of gastrectomy were the only factors significantly influencing the occurrence of major surgical complications. In this analysis, where lymphadenectomy was also performed in centres with only limited numbers of the procedure, the extent of nodal dissection (D1 vs. D2) was a significant risk factor for death (relative risk 2.13).

These arguments stress two prerequisites:
- gastrectomy and D2 lymphadenectomy in gastric cancer should be performed only in well-trained and experienced centres (high volume hospitals)
- as a potential dangerous procedure, D2 LA needs an individual indication.

Table 2. Morbidity and mortality rates of standard versus radical lymph node dissection, results of the German Gastric Cancer Study

Type of complication	Standard (n = 558)	Radical (n = 1096)
Suture insufficiency	8.2	8.0
Bleeding	1.8	1.9
Wound healing	3.9	3.8
Abscess	3.2	4.7
Cardiopulmonary	9.5	9.3
Other	2.3	2.7
Total rate	29.0	30.6
Mortality rate		
30-day	5.2	5.0
90-day	10.0	10.9

Values are percentages.

Towards an Individual Indication for Lymphadenectomy in Gastric Cancer: The Potential of SLND

Individual indication for lymphadenectomy in gastric cancer, although highly warranted, at times poses several problems.

While the overall accuracy in pretherapeutic staging is about 80%–85%, problems still remain staging the N-category. The nodal staging is still a "black hole" in the entire staging process. Endoluminal ultrasound, worthwhile in staging the T-category, can only identify enlarged, but not infiltrated lymph nodes in close vicinity of the primary. The accuracy of this method in N-staging, even according to the old TNM classification, is about 60% (Rösch 1995). It is still better to calculate affected lymph nodes according to the T-category: T3 tumours have positive lymph nodes in about 80%. But even then, the localisation of these affected nodes is unclear.

In modern staging, surgical laparoscopy should be mandatory in advanced gastric cancer (Niederhuber 1999). When evaluating positive lymph nodes, a biopsy has to be taken during the procedure. However, this may lead to artificial tumour spread in the abdomen, transforming a localised disease to a disease with distant metastases, i.e., peritoneal spread. Also, laparoscopic ultrasound can detect only enlarged lymph nodes, the infiltration being unclear.

The intraoperative assessment of affected lymph nodes in open surgery poses similar problems. Dissection and consecutive frozen section of every lymph node found may harm the patient rather more than a well-performed lymphadenectomy. Furthermore, the sensitivity of detecting tumour cells in frozen sections is much lower than after conventional H&E staining.

The whole problem of sentinel node dissection in gastric cancer is not properly funded in scientific surgery at this time. As mentioned above, lymphatic flow in the upper abdomen is much more complicated than on the surface of the body, where lymph flow is directed to the cervical, axillary and inguinal regions and can be properly defined following lymphoscintigraphy.

The lymphatic drainage of the stomach follows the anatomy of the larger vessels (veins). The stomach of the embryo is initially located strictly in the centre of the yolk sac and rotates during embryogenesis. Blood vessels and the lymphatic vessels originating from the centrally located celiac axis follow this rotation. Therefore, the lymphatic drainage of the stomach is directed towards the celiac trunk. Extraperitoneal gastric tumours located at the cardia, the posterior wall of the proximal fundus, and tumours that grow beyond the pylorus are exempt from these rules of lymph node metastasis. These tumours have a direct extraperitoneal lymphatic drainage towards the left and right para-aortic nodes.

In Japan, the lymphatic flow is made visible by the use of the so-called Indian-ink staining. However, Sasako reported skip metastasis for carcinoma of the corpus between 18%–20% (Sasako, personal communication, 1998). In contrast, Veronesi et al. (1997) reported that in breast cancer, skip metastasis does not occur as was reported previously. He found that different axillary levels were fed by various lymphatic vessels, originating from the primary tumour.

Studies are warranted to elucidate this problem in upper GI cancer, using Indian-ink or, maybe even better, Technetium labelled colloids intraoperatively on the basis of a well-conducted study. The method of SLND is a truly anatomic method. The sentinel node is the first anatomic node, not the first infiltrated node. Therefore, anatomy of lymphatic spread of the stomach has to be studied under these new auspices.

A possibility for detecting affected nodes in gastric cancer could be the radio-immuno-guided surgery (RIGS) method. For this, specific antibodies to tumour specific cytokeratin are labelled with radioactive technetium. They will bind to tumour cells specifically. Although the idea is brilliant, this method is only functioning well up to now in cell culture or animal models. There is still a lack of high specific antibodies, although this problem might be overcome in the near future. If these specific antibodies become available, this method would be very promising for an individual lymphadenectomy.

Up to now, the best method for the predetermination of affected lymph nodes in gastric cancer is a computer program, developed by K. Maruyama, based on the lymph node metastases of about 4200 well-documented patients of the National Cancer Centre, Tokyo (Maruyama et al. 1989) (Fig. 2). Using this program, individual indication could be possible. But this program does have a problem in that microinvolvement of lymph nodes has not been taken into account so far. The program is based on affected lymph nodes which are diagnosed in routine histology. Therefore, the group of patients which will profit best from LA (patients with microinvolvement) is not taken into account.

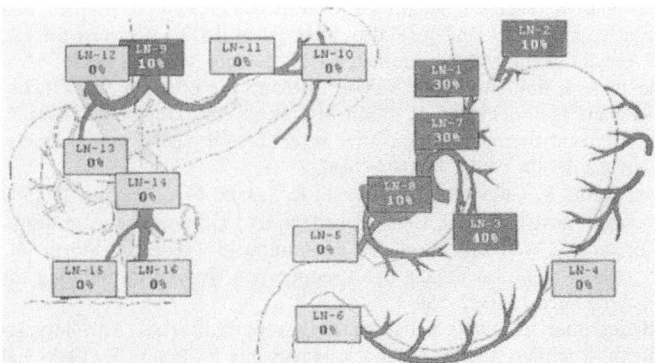

Fig. 2. The so-called Maruyama computer program for preoperative evaluation of lymphatic spread in gastric cancer. In this picture, LN metastases of a cT3 tumour are demonstrated. Adaptation of the program for the Department of Surgery, Technische Universität München

Conclusion

Nowadays, there is neither indication nor possibility for SLND in gastric cancer, nor the possibility for an individual indication for classical lymphadenectomy. However, both are highly warranted.

For the patient fit for surgery, extended lymphadenectomy (Compartment D1 and D2, as described by the Japanese Gastric Cancer Association) is the method of choice.

One possibility of a restricted operation could be the intraoperative frozen section analysis of lymph nodes of compartment 3. If these nodes are already infiltrated, the prognosis of the patient cannot be ameliorated by extended LA. However, this is a proven fact in UICC stage II and possible stage IIIA gastric cancer.

Currently, the lymphatic spread of the primary can be assessed only after a meticulous pathohistological work up of the resected specimen. Before the establishment of new and better technologies for LA in gastric cancer, no patient, fit for surgery, should be excluded from the chance for cure, which is given in the localised stages of the disease. There is an urgent need for studies addressing the anatomic lymphatic spread in gastric cancer, depending on the various primary sites.

References

Bonenkamp JJ, Hermans J, Sasako M, van de Velde CJ (1999) Extended lymph-node dissection for gastric cancer. Dutch Gastric Cancer Group. N Engl J Med 340:908–914

Bonenkamp JJ, van de Velde CJ (1995) Lymph node dissection in gastric cancer. Br J Surg 82:867–869

Brennan MF (1999) Lymph-node dissection for gastric cancer (editorial). N Engl J Med 340:956–958

Cuschieri A, Fayers P, Fielding J, Craven J, Bancewicz J, Joypaul V, Cook P (1996) Postoperative morbidity and mortality after D1 and D2 resections for gastric cancer: preliminary results of the MRC randomized trial. Lancet 347:995–999

Hermans J, Bonenkamp JJ (1993a) Letter to the Editor. J Clin Oncol 12:879–880

Hermans J, Bonenkamp JJ, Boon MC, Bunt AM, Ohyama S, Sasako M, van-de VC (1993b) Adjuvant therapy after curative resection for gastric cancer: meta-analysis of randomized trials. J Clin Oncol 11:1441–1447

Maruyama K, Gunven P, Okabayashi K, Sasako M, Kinoshita T (1989) Lymph node metastases of gastric cancer. General pattern in 1931 patients. Ann Surg 210:596–602

Morton DL, Wen DR, Wong JH, Economou JS, Cagle LA, Storm FK, Foshag LJ, Cochran AJ (1992) Technical details of intraoperative lymphatic mapping for early stage melanoma. Arch Surg 127:392–399

Niederhuber JE (1999) Neoadjuvant therapy [editorial]. Ann Surg 229:309–312

Nishi M, Ichikawa H, Nakajima T, Maruyama K, Tahara E (1993) Gastric cancer. 1, Springer, Tokyo, Berlin, Heidelberg, New York

Roder JD, Böttcher K, Busch R, Wittekind Ch, Hermanek P, Siewert JR (1998) Classification of regional lymph node metastasis from gastric carcinoma. Cancer 82:621–631

Roder JD, Böttcher K, Siewert JR, Busch R, Hermanek P, Meyer H-J, the German Gastric carcinoma study 1992 (1993) Prognostic factors in gastric carcinoma. Cancer 72:2089–2097

Rösch Th (1995) Endosonographic staging of gastric cancer: a review of literature results. Gastrointest Clin North Am 3:549–557

Sasako M (1997) Risk factors for surgical treatment in the Dutch Gastric Cancer Trial. Br J Surg 84:1567–1571

Siewert JR, Böttcher K, Roder JD, Busch R, Hermanek P, Meyer H-J (1993) Prognostic relevance of systematic lymph node dissection: results of the German Gastric Carcinoma Study 1992. Br J Surg 80:1015–1018

Siewert JR, Böttcher K, Stein H, Roder JD, and the German Gastric Carcinoma Study Group (1998) Relevant prognostic factors in gastric cancer. Ann Surg 228:449–461

Siewert JR, Huber FT, Sendler A, Fink U (1995) Abdominelle Rezidive nach Eingriffen am Intestinum. Chirurg 66:941–948

Siewert JR, Kestlmeier R, Busch R, Bottcher K, Roder JD, Muller J, Fellbaum C, Höfler H (1996) Benefits of D2 lymph node dissection for patients with gastric cancer and pN0 and pN1 lymph node metastases. Br J Surg 83:1144–1147

UICC (1997) TNM classification of malignant tumors. Springer, Berlin, Heidelberg, New York, Berlin, Heidelberg, New York

Veronesi U, Paganelli G, Galimberti V, Viale G, Zurrida S, Bedoni M, Costa A, de CC, Geraghty JG, Luini A, Sacchini V, Veronesi P (1997) Sentinel-node biopsy to avoid axillary dissection in breast cancer with clinically negative lymph-nodes. Lancet 349:1864–1867

IX. Sentinel Node Detection in Colorectal Cancer

Probe-Guided Surgery for Colorectal Cancer

P. Lechner[1], P. Lind[2], M. Snyder[3], and H. Haushofer[4]

[1,4] Community Hospital of Klosterneuburg, Department of Surgery,
Kreutzergasse 12–14, 3400 Klosterneuburg, Austria
[2] Public Hospital of Klagenfurt, Institute of Nuclear Medicine,
St. Veiter-Str. 12, 9020 Klagenfurt, Austria
[3] Immunomedics, Inc. World Headquarters, 300 American Road, Morris Plains,
New Jersey 07950, USA

Abstract

Anti-CEA-scintigraphy turned out to be very reliable in detecting primary and recurrent colorectal cancer, its overall accuracy being more than 90%. The intraoperative application of this technology should provide similar results when focussing at extrahepatic tumor deposits, for example in lymph nodes, thus allowing accurate staging of the underlying disease. To test this hypothesis we launched the following feasibility study the results of which are compared to those reported in the recent literature.

We investigated 20 patients, six with rectum and 14 with colon cancer. 24 hours before surgery they were intravenously given 1 ml of a fab'-fragment-antibody to CEA, labeled with 25 mCi of 99mTc (CEA-Scan™). During surgery the radioactivity in lymph glands regional to the tumors was measured and compared to the much lower activity in healthy nodes.

For this we used a scintillation probe (C-Trak™, Care Wise, Inc., Morgan Hill, CA). All lymph nodes of interest were then excised and submitted to frozen section pathology. In 7 out of 20 cases scintimetry led to an up-staging of the disease. In addition we found metastatic spread to lymph nodes that were basically not regional to the primary tumor (retroperitoneum, renal hilum etc.).

Scintimetry can precisely identify even very small tumor deposits. So it leads to accurate staging while surgery is still ongoing. In a further step the concept of sentinel node diagnosis, which is right now being clinically evaluated, may some day be applied in colorectal surgical oncology.

Introduction

Surgeons treating patients with breast cancer routinely perform stage-adjusted procedures. Modified radical mastectomies, gold standard until few years ago, are performed only in a very small percentage of cases today. By contrast, in colorectal cancer, surgeons are resistant – mostly for good reasons – to abandoning their standardized procedures, because it took a great deal of time and effort to establish these standards, and to get them broadly accepted. We are afraid that, if we make any changes, we might get worse results than we get right now.

That is why we apply our standardized protocols [1] to every primary colectomy. We open, look around for potential metastases, perform the colectomy, remove the regional lymph nodes, and close. Between a few months and a few years later, up to 40% [2, 3] of patients deemed surgical cures develop "recurrence" – widely attributed to "micrometastases" that weren't observable during the primary procedure [4]. Many oncologists believe that such "recurrent" tumors are probably there at the time of the primary [5]. That is why we suggest looking for them more aggressively, both with every available preoperative diagnostic modality and intraoperatively, and finding them, if only for staging purposes!

One of these new modalities is CEA-Scan^{TM} (arcitumomab). This nuclear imaging agent is a murine monoclonal antibody fragment (fab') specific to carcinoembryonic antigen (CEA). This antigen is, as we learned from previous investigations [6, 7], expressed by virtually every colorectal cancer cell. The antibody fragment is labeled with technetium-99-m, the most common nuclear imaging isotope, with a radiological half-life of 6 hours. Originally conceived as an external imaging agent [8, 9], CEA-Scan^{TM} has meanwhile undergone evaluation as an intraoperative target for "gamma probes" in the treatment of various types of cancer [10–12]. These probes are hand-held scintillation detectors. The centerpiece is an Iodine-Cesium-crystal. At between 24 and 48 hours postinjection, most of the labeled antibody fragments not attached to tumor cells are eliminated from the bloodstream via the kidneys. The probes are now capable of picking up the residual radiation emitted by tumors thus providing acceptable target-to-background ratios of over 1.5:1 [13].

CT and MRI have proved of minor value in staging patients with primary or recurrent colorectal cancer. Because both have an unacceptably low accuracy for identifying the early stages of primary colorectal cancers, their routine use for preoperative staging is not recommended [14].

On the other hand, CEA-Scan has been proven to contribute significantly to the preoperative evaluation of patients undergoing surgery for primary colorectal cancer. In our own series overall accuracy was over 93%. External SPECT-immunoscintigraphy turned out to have a decisive influence on treatment planning in every third primary colorectal cancer patient and was by far superior to CT scan [6].

Current pathological evaluations are not really satisfying either: they usually can tell the surgeon what he has *removed* from the patient, after having closed. But they do not afford the surgeon the opportunity to learn what has been left *in* the patient. This is our major problem. At the end of our procedures, we – and our patients even more – suffer from misstaging, especially our Dukes' B patients, all of whom we *should* be able to cure.

Nevertheless, up to 50% of patients who undergo potentially curative resections develop local, regional, or widespread recurrence [2, 3].

These statistics have remained relatively constant over several decades despite improved methods of early diagnosis and surgical treatment [14]. Other studies demonstrate that approximately 30% of Dukes' B patients will suffer recurrent disease [1, 15], and many will be dead within five years of their primary surgery. If this was truly Stage B cancer, it should have been curable at the time of the primary procedure by adequate resection.

The only logical explanation is that a certain percentage of those patients we believe to be Dukes' B are really Dukes' C, and we don't know it [16].

Pathologists can't know, because they can evaluate only the tissue that is sent to them. The most accurate examining, slicing and staining doesn't tell them anything about the lymph nodes that were not resected. This is where much of what we call 'recurrence' may arise, months or years later [16].

Patients

This prospective feasibility trial comprises 20 patients, all with endoscopically and histologically proven colorectal tumors in UICC-stages 1 A through 3 B (Table 1). Patients with known distant metastases were excluded, as no intraoperative staging modalities would have been able to provide additional information of clinical relevance.

The patients, 14 females and 6 males, were on average 69 (range 47–84) years old. In 6 of them the primary tumor was located in the rectum (i.e., less than 16 cm above the anal verge), in another 6 in the sigmoid colon. Four primaries had been found in the descending colon including the splenic flexure, 3 were in the transverse, and one was in the ascending colon.

Table 1. Patients included in prospective trial

Clinical/UICC stage	Rectum	Colon
I A T-1, N0, M0	1	1
I B T-2, N0, M0	2	2
II A T-3, N0, M0	1	5
II B T-4, N0, M0	0	0
III A T-X, N1, M0	2	2
III B T-X, N2, M0	0	4
Total no. of patients 20	6	14

Method

Various investigators from around the world used very different radioimmunotargeting agents with gamma probes in various types of cancer. Each patient had external planar and SPECT imaging with CEA-Scan^{TM} and was taken to probe-guided surgery 24 hours later, using a C-Trak^{TM} probe (Care Wise, Inc., Morgan Hill, CA).

Intraoperative use of CEA-Scan^{TM} doesn't require significant modification of the typical colorectal procedure. Once a clinician performs surgery guided by preoperative images and intraoperative probes, the operation will be extended by no more than 15 or 20 minutes.

Typically, after opening, the surgeon performs a thorough examination to confirm local resectability. Part of this examination is palpation of the liver, and we, like many others today, depend upon intraoperative ultrasound to obtain more accurate information.

The next step is to evaluate the extent of the primary tumor and of regional lymph node involvement.

The first use of the intraoperative probe must be to explore tissue stepwise, away from the tumor towards healthy tissue. Because of variations in vascularity and in residual blood pool activity, there are no absolutes for determining healthy tissue or tumor – one must "calibrate" each patient by taking a series of readings to determine what is "normal activity" for normal tissue, and "abnormal activity" for tumor in anatomically comparable areas.

For example, when the tumor is located in the descending colon, we take measurements in the ascending colon, recording the number of counts per 10 seconds. This figure appears on the display. We take three measurements from each spot, and calculate an average. Then, we squelch the sound indicator just to extinguish the sound over healthy tissue.

Then we turn to the mass. Taking measurements from the center of the mass is useful only for scientific purposes but it is not relevant to the performance of the procedure. The question is: where are the precise margins of the tumor? To find them, one has to move the probe in steps of 1 to 2 cm along the colon, away from the apparent center of the mass. We take 3 measurements from each spot, write them down, calculate the average, and compare that number to the average of the healthy tissue. As long as that average is at least 1.5 times higher than the average for healthy tissue, we have to consider the tissue involved [17].

In our 20-patient study, we found tumor-free margins as far as 7.8 cm from the visually apparent margins of the tumor.

The next step is to evaluate potentially involved lymph nodes. The most decisive lymph nodes for an individual patient's survival are often situated at the major blood vessels [1, 18, 19] – the mesenteric artery, or along the aorta, or the caval vein. We investigate the nodes in a fashion quite similar to the primary tumor: we identify lymph nodes that are regional to healthy colon, and we take three measurements at each of them. Then, we take similar measurements from lymph nodes that are regional to the tumor. Also, as in the case of determining the tumor margins, we define "probably involved" nodes as having average readings at least 1.5 times higher than healthy nodes.

The most precise way of calibrating one's procedure is to excise one of the probably-involved regional nodes and to measure it ex vivo. We have histopathologically determined that 25 counts per 10 seconds is a reliable threshold for calling a node positive for disease [13]. When we found 25 counts/10 seconds in an excised lymph nodes, it *always* turned out to be involved. When there were less than 25 counts/10 seconds, it was *always* non-involved. Thus, part of the staging can take place right in the operating room. This overcomes the obstacle of accurately evaluating lymph nodes along the great vessels, where blood pool activity at 24 hours may complicate in vivo measurements.

Whenever we find an involved node by this procedure, we follow the tract "downstream" and similarly check the next node. Once we find a noninvolved node, we check the next node or two and if they are clear too, we conclude we have excised all the involved nodes.

Then we proceed to resect the tumor and, with the probe, to check the tumor margins, both proximal and distal to the tumor. Residual tumor can easily be detected by probe evaluation of the tumor bed. This is especially valuable in the true pelvis: since the vascular supply is mirrored on both sides, it's useful to measure the activity of anatomically comparable regions at the left and right pelvic wall. The activity should be same on both sides. If we find a higher activity on one side, we must suspect tumor left behind here. We then excise several biopsy specimens, send them for frozen sectioning, and know for sure. If the probe reveals multiple areas of activity – particularly unresectable ones – then the surgeon must consider the procedure not to be sufficiently radical. At that point, many clinicians will decide to prepare their patient for adjuvant radiotherapy [20]. If, on the other hand, the presence of hepatic metastases can be documented at that point, one can, for example, use this opportunity to install a perfusion catheter into the hepatic artery for subsequent chemotherapy.

Clinical Results

Preoperative imaging detected 19 of the 20 known primary tumors, but the probe identified all 20. This was of little clinical significance, because all primary tumors had been identified by endoscopy, but the probe found one additional synchronous tumor in the ascending colon of a patient with known rectal tumor. Also of limited impact on care: involved N1 nodes were found in two patients by preoperative scan, 4 nodes by intraoperative probe – because all N1 nodes are routinely excised as part of most colectomies. However, the probe found unsuspected lesions and malignant distant nodes i.e.,
- Metastatic N2/3 nodes in four patients, vs. 1 by preoperative imaging
- Liver metastases missed by preoperative scan in one patient
- Peritoneal carcinomatosis missed in another (Table 2).

Table 2. Sensitivity of diagnostic imaging modalities, lesion-based analysis in 14 patients with colon cancer

Lesion	Preoperative		Intraoperative			Postoperative Histologie
	CT	US	Scan	Palpation	Probe	
Primary tumor	8	3	14	14	14	14
N1-nodes	3	0	9	12	19	31
N2/3-nodes	7	2	18	21	30	46
Peritoneal carcinoma	0	0	0	1	1	1
Liver metastases	0	0	0	2	4	4
Total no. of lesions	18	5	41	50	69	97

Table 3. Up-staging in rectal cancer (n = 6)

	Preop.	Intraop.
I A	1	1
I B	2	1
II A	1	0
II B	0	0
III A	2	3
III B	0	1

Table 4. Up-staging in colon cancer (n = 14)

Clin. stage	Preop.	Intraop.
I A	1	1
I B	2	2
II A	5	3
II B	0	0
III A	2	2
III B	4	4
IV	0	2

Thus, use of CEA-Scan^{TM} and an intraoperative probe led to upgrading in 7 of 20 patients in this small series (Tables 3, 4).

Conclusion

Intraoperative tumor targeting with CEA-Scan^{TM} offers surgeons the rationale for making minor but potentially lifesaving patient-specific modifications to standardized colectomies. Specifically, it enables us to:

- Determine the potential for a radical, curative procedure or, alternatively, a minimal procedure with only palliative intent.

- Confirm the thorough resection of the primary, providing a higher assurance of tumor-free margins than can be achieved under possible visual and tactile guidance only.
- Confirm the localization of metastases that are too small to be localized by an external imaging modality.
- Confirm the absence of tumor-bearing surgical debris in the peritoneum – debris that could form the nidus of a recurrence.
- More accurately and completely stage the patient, through intraoperative identification of lymph nodes that are normal in size and appearance, but contain metastatic disease [21].
- More accurately stratify the patients for postoperative adjuvant treatment modalities [22].

Prognosis for patients with the same stage of colorectal cancer can vary between 30% and 75% – even within the same institution – based on differences in surgical aggressiveness and technique of different clinicians [23].

Ultimately, the benefit of any new surgical procedure lies in the long-term statistics of its practitioners. The clinical contributions of CEA-Scan™ and gamma probes cannot yet be estimated, and further studies comprising greater numbers of patients are required.

However, this approach seems to be a reasonably objective and repeatable strategy for defining tumor margins, detecting involved lymph nodes, and assuring the radicality of resections, using the patient's own tissues as controls.

References

1. Gall FP, Hermanek P (1988) Die erweiterte Lymphknotendissektion beim Magen- und colorectalen Carcinom – Nutzen und Risken. Chirurg 59:202–210
2. Cesnik H, Lechner P (1989) Das Rezidiv des kolorektalen Karzinoms aus der Sicht des Chirurgen. Acta Med Austriaca 16(Suppl.):17–21
3. Jass JR (1990) Prognostic factors in colorectal cancer. Curr Top Pathol 81:295–322
4. Amato A, Scucchi L, Pescatori M (1994) Tumor budding and recurrence of colorectal cancer. Dis Colon Rectum 37(5):514–515
5. Quirke P, Dixon MF, Durdey P, Williams NS (1986) Local recurrence of rectal adenocarcinoma due to inadequate surgical resection. Histopathological study of lateral tumor spread and surgical excision. Lancet 2:996–999
6. Lechner P, Lind P, Binter G, Cesnik H (1993) Anticarcinoembryonic antigen immunoscintigraphy with a 99mTc-fab'-fragment (IMMU 4) in primary and recurrent colorectal cancer. Dis Colon Rectum 36(10):930–935
7. Lind P, Lechner P, Arian-Schad K, Klimpfinger M, Cesnik H, Kammerhuber F, Eber O (1991) Anti-carcinoembryonic antigen immunoscintigraphy (technetium-99m-monoclonal antibody BW431/26) and serum CEA levels in patients with suspected primary and recurrent colorectal carcinoma. J Nucl Med 32/7:1319–1325
8. Goldenberg DM, DeLand FH, Kim EE, Bennett SJ (1978) Use of radiolabeled antibodies to carcinoembryonic antigen in the detection and localization of diverse cancers by external photoscanning. N Engl J Med 298:1384–1388
9. Goldenberg DM, Goldenberg H, Ford EH (1989) Initial clinical imaging results with a new Tc-99-m-antibody method. J Nucl Med 30:809

10. Kuhn JA, Corbisiero RM, Buras RR, Carroll RG, Wagman LD, Wilson LA, Yamauchi D, Smith MM, Kondo R, Beatty JD (1991) Intraoperative gamma detection probe with presurgical antibody imaging in colon cancer. Arch Surg 126:1398–1404
11. Krag D, Weaver DL, Alex JC, Fairbank JT (1993) Surgical resection and radiolocalization of the sentinel lymph node in breast cancer using a gamma probe. Surg Oncol 2:335–340
12. Moffat FL, Vargas-Cuba RD, Serafini AN, Casillas VJ, Morillo G, Benedetto P, Robinson DS, Ardalan B, Manten HD, Clark KC (1994) Radioimmunodetection of colorectal carcinoma using technetium-99m-labeled fab'fragments of the IMMU-4 anticarcinoembryonic antigen monoclonal antibody. Cancer 73(Suppl.):836–845
13. Lechner P, Lind P, Binter G (1995) Tc-99m-labeled anti-CEA-antibodies in intraoperative diagnosis of colorectal cancer. Nucl Med 34(1):8–14
14. Thoeni RF (1997) Colorectal cancer radiologic staging. Radiol Clin North Am 35(2): 457–485
15. Eckhauser FE, Knol JA (1997) Surgery for primary and metastatic colorectal cancer. Gastroenterol Clin North Am 26(1):103–128
16. Adell G, Boeryd B, Franlund B, Sjodahl R, Hakansson L (1996) Occurrence and prognostic importance of micrometastases in regional lymph nodes in Dukes' B colorectal carcinoma: an immunohistochemical study. Eur J Surg 162(8):637–642
17. Hertel A, Baum RP, Auerbach B, Herrmann A, Hör G (1990) Klinische Relevanz humaner anti-Maus-Antikörper (HAMA) in der Immunszintigraphie. Nucl Med 29:46–47
18. Pezim ME, Nicholls RJ (1984) Survival after high or low ligation of the inferior mesenteric artery during curative surgery for rectal cancer. Ann Surg 200:729–733
19. Izbicki JR, Blochle C (1993) Colorectal carcinoma: impact of staging on surgical treatment. Endoscopy 25(1):117–124
20. Lechner P, Cesnik H (1992) Abdominopelvic omentopexy: preparatory procedure for radiotherapy in colorectal cancer. Dis Colon Rectum 35(12):1157–1160
21. Kronborg O (1993) Staging and surgery for colorectal cancer. Eur J Cancer 29A(4):575–583
22. Loh A, Jones D, Dickson GH (1994) Accuracy of intraoperative staging in colorectal cancer. J R Coll Surg Edinb 39(1):20–22
23. Averbach AM, Jacquet P, Sugarbaker PH (1995) Surgical technique and colorectal cancer: impaction on local recurrence and survival. Tumori 81(3 Suppl):65–71

Identification of Lymph Node Metastases in Recurrent Colorectal Cancer

S. Schneebaum, A. Troitsa, S. Avital, R. Haddad, H. Kashtan, G. Gitstein, M. Baratz, E. Brazovsky, J. Papo, and Y. Skornick

Radioguided Surgery Unit, Department of Surgery "A", Tel-Aviv Sourasky Medical Center, 6 Weizmann Street, Tel-Aviv 64239, Israel

Abstract

Lymph node metastases are an important prognostic prediction factor in patients with recurrent colorectal cancer, particularly those with liver metastasis.

Fifty-six patients with recurrent colorectal cancer were operated by us using the RIGS (radioimmunoguided surgery) technology. Patients were injected with 1 mg monoclonal antibody (MoAb) CC49 labeled with 2 mCi ^{125}I. In surgery, traditional exploration was followed by survey with a gamma-detecting probe. Sixty of 151 patients enrolled in the Neo2-14 Phase III study for recurrent colorectal cancer were diagnosed with liver metastases based on preoperative CT.

In 17/56 patients (30%), RIGS identified at least one tumor site confirmed by pathology (H&E). This resulted in 16 major changes in surgical plan. RIGS performance varied between lymphatic and non-lymphatic tissue, with positive predictive value (PPV) of 100% and negative predictive value (NPV) of 94% for non-lymphoid tissue, compared to PPV of 46.5% and NPV of 100% for the lymphoid tissue.

Thirty-five out of 60 patients were considered resectable after traditional evaluation. RIGS identified occult tumor in 10 of these patients (28.5%). 7/10 occult patients expired (70%), while only 7/25 of the non-occult patients expired (28%) ($P = 0.046$).

In localizing patients, no RIGS activity in lymph nodes signifies no tumor, while H&E confirmation is needed for decisions based on RIGS activity in the lymph nodes. RIGS provides important staging information, identifying patients for whom surgery may be done with curative intent.

Introduction

Surgery for recurrent colorectal cancer may be of a palliative nature or of curative intent. During curative surgery the surgeon is faced with two major questions. First, is the patient locally resectable, without underlying anatomical restrictions ruling out the possibility of resection. Second, is there a curative probability for surgery, where lymph node metastases play a most important prognostic role. The area where lymph node metastasis has gained general acceptance as a prognostic predictor in patients with liver metastasis, is where involvement of the periportal lymph nodes signifies no curative probability and is generally considered to be a contraindication for excision of liver metastasis [1]. Another subset of patients for whom this finding is of importance are those with pelvic recurrence and extrapelvic lymph node involvement, as pelvic surgery may result in morbidity or major changes in quality-of-life. Knowledge of lymph node status in these patients may be of major help.

Radioimmunoguided surgery (RIGS) is a surgical technique in which the patient is injected with a radiolabeled monoclonal antibody (MoAb) three weeks prior to surgery. The surgeon, using a gamma-detecting probe (GDP) in surgery, can better assess and stage the disease status of the patient. The technology was developed in order to compensate for the frustration of the surgeon doing CEA-directed second-look surgery and not being able to find the tumor causing the rise in CEA [2]. It has evolved into a technology capable of detecting occult metastasis, delineating tumor margins, and assessing completeness of resection [3–5] and has resulted in reports of better survival [6]. The use of anti-TAG (tumor-associated antigen) monoclonal antibodies, currently the 2nd generation CC49, has given the surgeon the advantage of locating lymph node metastases and identifying patterns of tumor spread [7, 8]. This technology identifies lymph node metastases that are occult to the surgeon, but may require more sophisticated pathology than the routine one-cut H&E for their confirmation. It also identifies tumor antigen [9] whose clinical significance is only beginning to be clarified. In this chapter, we report the results of using RIGS for recurrent colorectal cancer at our institute. We also review the results of a multicenter study for patients with liver metastasis and discuss the data supporting the value of the RIGS methodology in the identification of lymph node metastasis.

RIGS Methodology

Patients enrolled in the RIGS study were all diagnosed to have recurrent or metastatic colorectal cancer by clinical findings, abdominal CT or elevated CEA blood levels.

Prior to enrollment, all patients had CT of the chest to exclude extraabdominal disease, and CT of the abdomen and pelvis, as well as colonoscopy. All patients signed an informed consent approved by the local Institutional

Review Board. Starting two hours prior to injection, and then daily until surgery, all patients took a thyroid-blocking agent. This was either a saturated solution of potassium iodide (SSKI) or Thyro-block tablets (Wallace Laboratories, Cranbury, N.J.). Patients were injected with 1 mg CC49 (anti-TAG-72 tumor associated glycoprotein MoAb radiolabeled with ^{125}I). Patients were taken to surgery with precordial counts ≤20, usually 3–4 weeks after injection.

Surgery started with traditional exploration of inspection and palpation. In order to standardize exploration and abdominal assessment, the abdomen was divided into four zones: zone I – liver; zone II – upper abdomen, including stomach, spleen, periportal and celiac lymph nodes; zone III – mid-abdomen, including colon, small bowel, kidneys and lymph nodes along the aorta and vena cava as far as the bifurcation; zone IV – pelvis, including rectum, lymph nodes along both iliac artery and vein, female reproductive organs and urinary bladder. CT evaluation prior to surgery was also done according to the same zones. In all patients, the liver was examined with intraoperative ultrasound as part of the traditional evaluation. After exploration, the surgeon declared the resectability status, his findings and surgical plan. This was followed by survey with the GDP, Neoprobe 1000® (Neoprobe Corp. Dublin, Ohio, USA). The probe emits a sound whenever the measured radioactivity is significantly higher than a chosen reference point. The processor in the probe calculates the mean counts of the reference point, adding three standard deviations (square root) after which it starts to emit a sound. At the start of surgery, the surgeon "squelches" on the aortic bifurcation or any intra-abdominal major blood vessel with a count that correlates with the precordial count [10]. The blood vessel serves as a reference point "bloodpool background" for the lymph nodes. For parenchymatous organs, such as the liver, the surgeon may also squelch on an adjacent normal appearing area as a reference point. The surgeon then surveys the abdomen and whenever the probe emits a continuous sound, he stops and takes three two-second counts. Counts which are twice the reference point and greater than 20 are considered positive. At the end of the survey, the surgeon again declares the resectability status of the patient, surgical findings and surgical plan. Every suspicious tissue is biopsied or resected as some lymph node involvement may cause the surgeon to abandon resection. As shown in previous studies [7], some RIGS-positive lymph nodes are not always confirmed by hematoxylin and eosin (H&E). Resection was not abandoned based on RIGS-positive lymph nodes without frozen H&E confirmation. Data was analyzed according to abdominal zones and H&E confirmation.

The Tel-Aviv Sourasky Medical Center Experience [11]

Patients

As the RIGS methodology was introduced at the Tel-Aviv Sourasky Medical Center after the initiation of the phase III study, all surgery was done according to this protocol. Sixty-six patients with recurrent colorectal cancer were enrolled in phase III multicenter studies (Neo2-14, Neo2-12 and single center study Neo2-04 and compassionate use protocol Neo2-81).

Results

Eight of the 66 patients enrolled were inevaluable as they did not go to surgery. Three of them were injected but underwent emergency surgery for various reasons, without using the probe. Thus, 58 patients were evaluable and are the subjects of this study. Localization of CC49 on the tumor was observed in 54 of the 66 intent-to-treat patients (81.8%), or in 54 of the 58 evaluable patients (96.4%).

In Table 1, the tumor findings can be seen categorized according to the four zones, preoperative CT findings, surgeon findings first with traditional exploration and then RIGS methodology, as well as H&E pathology confirmation. The performance differed between the four zones. In zone I, using intraoperative ultrasound, the detection capability of the surgeon is quite high. In zones II and III, CT performance is poor, but there were also some false-positive findings by RIGS. In zone IV, RIGS identified many tumors, most of them H&E-positive. Altogether, CT identified 56 tumor sites, the surgeon using traditional exploration only 117, and with the RIGS methodology 177, while pathology confirmed 133.

A summary of RIGS findings can be seen in Table 2. In 17/58 patients (28.2%), RIGS exploration resulted in occult findings which changed the surgical plan in 16 patients: in 5 abandoning planned resection, 4 liver patients and one planned pelvic exenteration that had to be abandoned due to extra-

Table 1. CT, surgical (traditional), and RIGS-positive and H&E-positive findings of excised tumor sites (Adapted from Schneebaum et al. 1999, World J Surg, to be published)

	CT	Surgeon	RIGS	Pathology
I	19	34	35	35
II	2	5	23	5
III	13	42	68	48
IV	22	36	51	45
	56	117	177	133

CT, tumor sites identified before surgery; *Surgeon*, tumor sites identified by the surgeon using traditional methods; *RIGS*, tumor sites identified in surgery using the GDP; *Pathology*, excised tissue confirmed by pathology to be H&E-positive.

Table 2. Summary of biopsied RIGS-positive findings in 58 patients with metastatic colorectal cancer (adapted from Schneebaum et al. 1999, World J Surg, to be published)

Liver	34
Anastomotic recurrence	9
Pelvic tumor	19
Peritoneal metastasis	11
Uterus	6
Periaortic nodes	90
Ovary	6
Small bowel	2

Table 3. RIGS performance in 58 localizing and non-localizing patients (adapted from Schneebaum et al. 1999, World J Surg, to be published)

	Total	Localizing Patients
Sensitivity	95%	96.8%
Specificity	42.7%	44%
Positive predictive value	67.2%	67.9%
Negative predictive value	88%	91%

Table 4. RIGS performance in 58 patients (lymphatic and non-lymphatic nodes) (adapted from Schneebaum et al. 1999, World J Surg, to be published)

Performance	Non-lymphatic nodes	Lymphatic nodes
Sensitivity	95.6%	100%
Specificity	90%	7%
Positive predictive value	95.6%	40%
Negative predictive value	90%	100%

pelvic disease. In 11 patients, additional tissue was removed. In one patient found to be unresectable by traditional exploration, this additional finding did not cause any change in surgical plan.

Performance was also analyzed according to criteria of true-positive, false-positive, true-negative and false-negative. Calculations of sensitivity and specificity, positive predictive value (PPV) and negative predictive values (NPV) of all tumor sites are seen in Table 3 in the 54 localizing patients, and in all 58 patients. This was also calculated for the lymphatic and non-lymphatic tissue (Table 4). Non-lymphatic tissue had a sensitivity of 95.6% and a specificity of 90%, while lymphatic tissue had a sensitivity of 100% with a very low specificity of 7%, due to an high false-positive rate and no negative lymph node biopsied. On the other hand, the NPV of lymphatic tissue is 100%, due to no false-negative nodes, which means that in a localizing patient, a RIGS-negative lymph node implies no tumor. The only false-positive non-lymphatic tissue was in non-localizing patients (4 tumor sites) and in patients with peritoneal spread (2 tumor sites). There was no false-positive tissue in liver, pelvis nor parenchymatous organs. All true-negative tissue was tissue suspected by the surgeon, RIGS-negative and biopsied. The number of tumor sites was 2.7 per patient.

Subgroups According to Anatomic Location

Phase III Results: Liver Metastasis [12]

Patients

One hundred and fifty-five patients were enrolled in Neoprobe multicenter phase III study, Neo2–14, for recurrent and metastatic colorectal cancer, in the USA, Europe and Israel. Sixty patients were diagnosed with liver metastasis based on preoperative CT.

Results

Tumor was pathology-proven in 56 of the 60 patients (93.3%), while localization of antibody to tumor was observed in 52 patients (92.9%). After the traditional intraoperative assessment, 35 of the 60 patients were found to be resectable. Ten patients in this group of 35 resectable patients had RIGScan (surgeon using the RIGS methodology with CC49 MoAb) occult tumor (28.5%) versus 25 patients with no RIGScan occult tumor. Seven of the ten occult patients (70%) expired with a median survival time of 411.5 days, while 7 of the 25 non-occult patients expired (28.0%). The median for this group could not be computed due to the small proportion of observed deaths. The log rank test was significant at a p-value = 0.046 (Fig. 1).

Since prognosis of these patients is dependent on the occurrence of extra-hepatic tumor, and in particular tumor deposits in lymph nodes, an analysis of survival was performed only in patients with biopsied lymph nodes. Twenty-two patients were eligible for this analysis: ten patients in the occult group and 12 patients in the non-occult group. Seven of the 10 occult patients died (70%), while only two of the 12 non-occult patients expired (16.7%). The resultant p-value from the log rank statistic was 0.025 (Fig. 2). The efficacy of the RIGS methodology was also tested in patients whose liver resection margins were biopsied or excised during surgery, correctly identifying five positive and 33 negative resection margins.

Pelvic Recurrence [13]

Patients

At the Tel-Aviv Sourasky Medical Center, 21 patients diagnosed with recurrent pelvic cancer were operated using the RIGS methodology. In their pri-

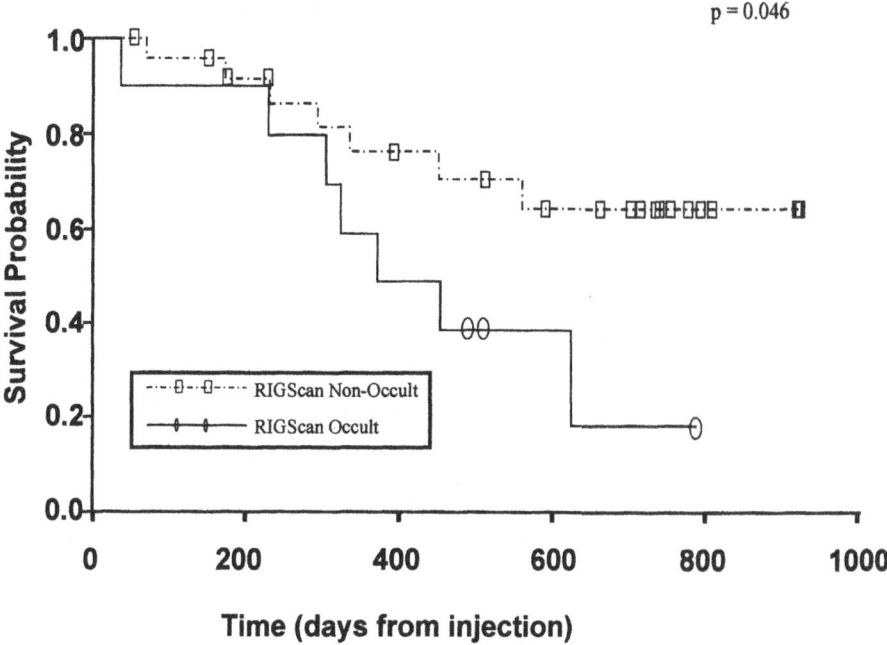

Fig. 1. Survival differences for surgically resectable patients with positive CT scan, hepatic lesions identified preoperatively, clinical study Neo2–14. Patient with RIGScan identified non-occult metastasis vs. patient with RIGScan identified occult metastasis. Log rank p-value = 0.046. (Adapted from [12])

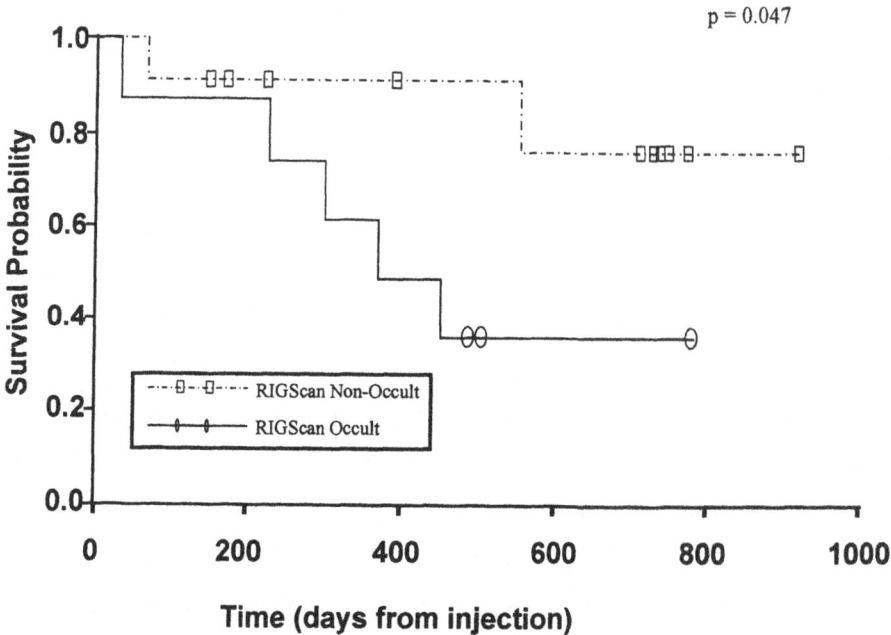

Fig. 2. Survival differences for surgically resectable patients with positive CT scan, hepatic lesions identified preoperatively, and biopsied lymph nodes, clinical study Neo2–14. Patients with RIGScan identified non-occult vs. RIGScan identified occult metastasis. Log rank p-value = 0.047. (Adapted from [12])

mary surgery, 14 of the patients had undergone anterior resection (AR) and seven patients abdomino-perineal resection (APR).

Results

Traditional exploration identified 8 intra-colorectal recurrences, 9 extra-colonic pelvic recurrences and 5 extra-pelvic lymph node metastases. RIGS exploration confirmed all intra-colorectal recurrences except for one (patient with no MoAb localization), identified 13 extra-colonic pelvic recurrences and 10 lymph node metastases. In all, seven patients had occult findings (33%). This resulted in changed surgical procedure in six by extending surgery and in one abandoning resection due to extra-pelvic disease. RIGS positivity at surgery end was also monitored. Out of the 20 patients who localized, 12 patients were RIGS-positive and eight patients RIGS-negative. At 36 months follow-up, actual survival of RIGS-negative patients was significantly better than that of RIGS-positive patients, p = 0.0337.

Comments

An important prognostic variable for colorectal cancer is the presence or absence of tumor in lymph nodes [14]. Yet, the assessment of lymph node involvement is not easy as size and consistency, the two parameters used by the surgeon in his/her traditional exploration, are not reliable indications for metastasis detection in lymph nodes [15].

RIGS has shown itself to be a technology capable of detecting lymph node metastasis in areas such as along the vena cava and hepato-duodenal ligament (portal) [4, 7, 8]. Biopsy of lymph nodes during surgery is part of colorectal cancer surgery, but random biopsies are of low yield. Even when concentrating on distinct areas, such as the periportal region, biopsy of only firm or >1 cm lymph nodes, results in only 11% positive findings [16]. In a recent study by Gibbs et al., periportal and celiac lymph node sampling resulted in 11% positive findings [17].

RIGS identifies lymph nodes with cancer, but using an anti-TAG MoAb may result in a high ratio of RIGScan-positive lymph nodes unconfirmed by H&E. The problem of RIGS-positive lymph nodes that are H&E-negative was first reported by Arnold [7] when using the MoAb CC49. He found that these lymph nodes have similar tumor-to-normal tissue ratio as the positive lymph node. It is accepted today that lymph nodes examined by routine analysis, i.e., one-cut H&E, can miss micrometastases and that when dealing with sentinel nodes, for example, more sophisticated pathology such as immune histochemistry (IHC) and PCR is advocated [18]. Arnold [8] has named these lymph nodes Type III lymph nodes. (Type I – RIGS-negative/H&E-negative, Type II – RIGS-negative/H&E-positive, and Type IV – obvious tumor RIGS-positive/H&E-positive). In a study done by Cote et al. [9], 57 lymph nodes were evaluated by routine analysis H&E staining, 17 were H&E-positive and 40 H&E-negative. Thirty-nine of the 57 were RIGS-positive, but only 14 of these were H&E-positive. Out of the 39 RIGS-positive nodes 25 were Type III lymph nodes (RIGS-positive/H&E-negative). These 25 Type III lymph nodes were subjected to multiple H&E sections and IMH with cytokeratin. Occult metastasis were found in 10/25 nodes (40%), showing that routine analysis signified tumor in 17/27 (63%) nodes while the probe signaled the presence of tumor in 24/27 (89%) of these lymph nodes. The clinical significance of these lymph nodes with metastasis identified by IMH with anti-cytokeratin was demonstrated in a study reported by Greenson et al. [19] where 448 lymph nodes of 41 Dukes' B patients were analyzed by IMH with anti-cytokeratin MoAb. After a five-year follow-up, 7/14 patients with cytokeratin-positive lymph nodes died of disease and only one died out of those 27 patients with no cytokeratin-lymph nodes.

In another study, that concentrated on periportal lymph nodes [20], Type III lymph nodes from 34 patients were subjected to multiple section and IMH analysis. Multiple section found tumor in 24%, IMH with cytokeratin in 48% and IMH with cytokeratin and IMH with CC49, found tumor and tumor antigen in 70%.

Further proof of the clinical significance of these findings can be seen in some of the data generated in the phase III study where prognostic variable data was analyzed including only patients with resectable disease after traditional survey (unpublished data).

Prognostic outcome of RIGS findings in lymph nodes was examined by contrasting survival data for three distinct groups: (a) patients with RIGS (+)/Pathology (+) lymph nodes, (b) patients with RIGS (+)/Pathology (-) lymph nodes, and (c) patients with RIGS (-)/Pathology (-) lymph nodes. Since patients may have presented with all three RIGS/Pathology combinations, assignment to the groups was made in the following manner: patients with ≥1 RIGS (+)/Pathology (+) node were classified as (+)/(+) patients; patients with no pathology (+) nodes, but one or more RIGS (+) nodes were classified (+)/(-); and lastly, patients in whom all nodes were RIGS (-)/Pathology (-) were assigned to the (-)/(-) group (Table 5, Fig. 3). The difference between RIGS (+)/Pathology (-) and RIGS (-)/Pathology (-) groups makes sense. RIGS is associated with high NPV especially in lymph nodes (94%). This outcome of the RIGS performance, coupled with the above analysis, tends to suggest that RIGS-negative findings reliably predict no tumor and may be of prognostic value. This high NPV is of major importance in surgery where decisions are taken whether to resect hepatic metastasis or do extensive pelvic surgery. This advantage is unique to the RIGS technology and its importance should not be underestimated, as the surgeon is often faced with this question and frozen section may be problematic, as sampling errors cannot be ruled out. This important attribute of RIGS enables the surgeon to continue with his surgical plan of curative probability. Our experience has taught us that extensive lymph node dissection in patients with widespread abdominal lymph node involvement cannot be translated into cure, most probably due to extra-abdominal spread not previously evaluated nor detected by RIGS as the patients develop thoracic metastasis within a short time.

Table 5. Overall survival (in days). Comparisons among RIGS findings in biopsied/resected lymph nodes traditionally resectable patients – Clinical study Neo2–14

	RIGS (+) Pathology (+)	RIGS (+) Pathology (–)	RIGS (–) Pathology (–)
No. of patients	12	29	7
No. of deaths	8	12	0
% deaths	66.7%	42.4%	0.0%
Median survival time (days)	460	699	–[a]
Log rank p-value	0.002		
Wilcoxon p-value	0.006		

[a] Median not computed due to small number of deaths.

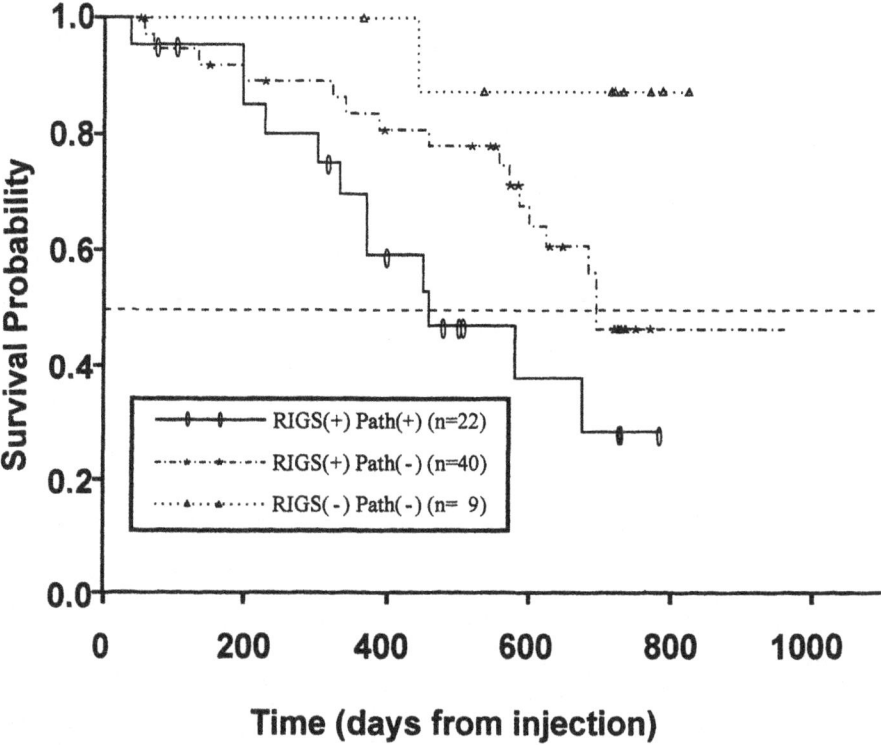

Fig. 3. Overall survival RIGS performance in lymph nodes (n = 71), clinical study Neo2–14. RIGS-positive / pathology-positive vs. RIGS-positive / pathology-negative vs. RIGS-negative / pathology-negative. Log rank p-value = 0.002. (Adapted from [12])

The data shown and reviewed suggest that RIGS-negative lymph nodes in a localizing patient signify no tumor. Major decisions based on RIGS-positive lymph nodes need H&E confirmation. RIGS-positive lymph nodes signify bad prognosis but not necessarily regional cancer. Using RIGS, the surgeon is better able to detect lymph node metastasis. RIGS provides the surgeon with additional information, resulting in better staging and prognostication and better intra- and post-operative decisions.

Additional molecular biology studies of RIGS (+)/H&E (-) are needed to further quantify the biological significance of these lymph nodes.

References

1. Hughes HS, Sugarbaker PH (1987) Resection of the liver for metastatic solid tumors. In: Rosenberg SA (ed) Surgical treatment of metastatic cancer, 1st edn. JB Lippincott, Philadelphia, pp 125–164
2. Thurston MO, Mojzisik CM (1995) History and development of radioimmunoguided surgery. Semin in Colon & Rectal Surg 6:185–191
3. Cohen AM, Martin EW Jr, Lavery I, Daly J, Sardi A, Aitken D, Bland K, Mojzisik C, Hinkle G (1991) Radioimmunoguided surgery using iodine 125 B72.3 in patients with colorectal cancer. 126:349–352
4. Schneebaum S, Papo J, Graif M, Baratz M, Baron J, Skornick Y (1997) Radioimmunoguided Surgery Benefits for Recurrent Colorectal Cancer. Ann Surg Oncol 4:371–376
5. Martin EW Jr, Carey LC (1991) Second-look surgery for colorectal cancer. The second time around. Ann Surg 214:321–325
6. Bertsch DJ, Burak WE, Young DC, Arnold MW, Martin EW Jr (1995) Radioimmunoguided surgery system improves survival for patients with recurrent colorectal cancer. Surgery 118:634–639
7. Arnold MW, Schneebaum S, Berens A, Petty L, Mojzisik C, Hinkle G, Martin EW Jr (1992) Intraoperative detection of colorectal cancer with radioimmunoguided surgery and CC49, a second-generation monoclonal antibody. Ann Surg 216:627–632
8. Arnold MW, Hitchcock CL, Young DC, Burak WE, Bertsch DJ, Martin EW (1996) Intra-abdominal patterns of disease dissemination in colorectal cancer identified using radioimmunoguided surgery. Dis Colon Rectum 39:509–515
9. Cote RJ, Houchens DP, Hitchcock CL, Saad AD, Nines RG, Greenson JK, Schneebaum S, Arnold MW, Martin EW (1996) Intraoperative detection of occult colon cancer micrometastases using ^{125}I-radiolabeled monoclonal antibody CC49. Cancer 77:613–620
10. Mojzisik CM, Cook CH, Schneebaum S (1994) Safety and performance factors in the development and clinical use of the RIGS system. In: Martin EW Jr (ed) Radioimmunoguided surgery (RIGS) in the detection and treatment of colorectal cancer, Landes RG Co, Austin, TX, pp 81–105
11. Schneebaum S, Troitsa A, Haddad R, Avital S, Kashtan H, Baratz M, Brazovsky E, Papo J, Skornick Y (1999) Immunoguided lymph node dissection in colorectal cancer: a new challenge? World J Surg (to be published)
12. Schneebaum S, Daly JM, Burak W, Lavery I, Chevinsky A, Martin EW, The RIGS Study Group (1998) RIGS efficacy in patients with colorectal cancer liver metastasis. Abstract, presented at the 9th Congress of European Society of Surgical Oncology, Lausanne, Switzerland, June 3–6
13. Haddad R, Avital S, Baratz M, Brazovsky E, Skornick Y, Schneebaum S (1998) Benefits of radioimmunoguided surgery for pelvic recurrence. Abstract presented at 3rd Meeting of the Israel Society of Colon and Rectal Surgery, November 11–14, Dead Sea, Israel.

14. Cohen AM, Minsky BD, Schilsky RL (1997) Cancer of the Colon. In: De Vita VT Jr, Hellman S, Rosenberg S (eds) Cancer principles and practice of oncology, 5th edn. Lippincott-Raven, Philadelphia, New York, pp 1144–1197
15. Herrera-Ornelas L, Justiniano J, Castillo N, Petrelli NJ, Stule JP, Mittelman A (1987) Metastases in small lymph nodes from colon cancer. Arch Surg 122:1253–1256
16. Fuhrman GM, Curley SA, Hohn DC, Roh MS (1995) Improved survival after resection of colorectal liver metastases. Ann Surg Oncol (2) 6:537–541
17. Gibbs JF, Weber TK, Rodriguez-Bigas MA, Driscoll DL, Petrelli NJ (1998) Intraoperative determinants of unresectability for patients with colorectal hepatic metastases. Cancer 82:1244–1249
18. Reintgen D, Albertini J, Berman C, Cruse CW, Fenske N, Glass F, Puleo C, Wang X, Wells K, Rapaport D, DeConti R, Messina J, Heller R (1995) Accurate nodal staging of malignant melanoma. Cancer Control 405–414
19. Greenson JK, Isenhart CE, Rice R, Mojzisik C, Houchens D, Martin EW Jr (1994) Identification of occult micrometastasis in pericolic lymph nodes of Dukes' B colorectal cancer patients using monoclonal antibodies against cytokeratin and CC49. Cancer 73:563–569
20. Schneebaum S, Arnold MW, Houchens DP, Greenson JK, Cote RJ, Hitchcock CL, Young DC, Mojzisik CM, Martin EW Jr (1995) The significance of intraoperative periportal lymph node metastasis identification in patients with colorectal carcinoma. Cancer 75:2809–2817

Fluorescence as a Concept
in Colorectal Lymph Node Diagnosis

K. T. Moesta[1], B. Ebert[2], T. Handke[1], H. Rinneberg[2], and P. M. Schlag[1]

[1] Robert-Roessle-Hospital, Charité, Humboldt Universität, Lindenberger Weg 80, 13125 Berlin, Germany
[2] Division of Medical Physics and Metrological Information Technology, Section of Biomedical Optics and NMR-Measuring Techniques, Physikalisch-Technische Bundesanstalt, Berlin, Germany

Abstract

Fluorescence detection may constitute an appropriate means in gastrointestinal cancers to diagnose lymphatic tumor spread as opposed to gamma-scintillation methods. Photodiagnostic tracers have been shown to localize rapidly in malignant cells and may enable sensitive detection of small cell aggregates in lymph nodes. To reach a detection depth of several millimeters, a broad banded unspecific tissue autofluorescence may be controlled by so-called background subtracting techniques, generally based either on fluorescence observation at several wavelengths or on dual-wavelength fluorescence excitation. Using such comparative fluorescence detection techniques, some tumor entities can be differentiated soley based upon autofluorescence characteristics. Introducing a further enhancement in sensitivity for longer life-time fluorophores by time delayed fluorescence detection we ran a pilot trial comprising 174 lymph nodes from colorectal cancer specimen from 9 patients. Metastatically involved lymph nodes could be differentiated from all other palpable nodes in the mesenteric fat at a specificity of 85% with a sensitivity of 65%. Specific fluorescence features may be useful to preselect tissue samples for further histological analysis.

Introduction

Lymphatic spread is a major prognostic factor in colorectal cancer [1, 2]. Adequate surgical clearing of the tumor draining lymphatics is accepted as improving survival [3, 4]. However, the extent of lymphatic dissection has been determined more or less empirically and may be questioned in view of the impressive results of the sentinel node technique in other human cancers. However, a sentinel node procedure is certainly more difficult to realize in colorectal cancer due to reduced access to the primary tumor, as well for the injection of the tracer substance as for the intra-operative identification

Recent Results in Cancer Research, Vol. 157
© Springer-Verlag Berlin · Heidelberg 2000

of the draining lymph node. It is also questionable whether a single tumor draining lymph node can be expected in a tumor entity that is regularly detected at a rather large primary tumor extension. On the other hand, there is already considerable experience with radioimmunolabeling of colorectal cancer metastases by monoclonal CEA-antibodies [5, 6]. However, this technique, called radioimmunoguided surgery, has not found general acceptance so far. The reason may be that the monoclonal preparation must be administered more than one week prior to surgery, and that the procedure generates a considerable number of false positive readings. Instead of working with radioactive tracers it may be promising to exploit the fluorescence properties of certain biological molecules in order to detect lymphatic metastases by optical means. Light is advantageous over radioactive radiation in terms of its biological compatibility and its detectability by our natural senses. On the other hand, light is readily scattered and absorbed by human tissues, requiring a specific technology for sensitive detection and precise reproducibility.

Fluorescence

Light backscattered from a biological surface contains only a very small proportion of photons originating from deeper tissue layers. It is, thus, technically very difficult to gain diagnostic information on deeper tissue levels from the bulk of backscattered light. However, if the incident light excites fluorescence, i.e., the emission of photons of longer wavelength, filters or dichroic mirrors may remove any reflected light and enable a deep 'view' into the tissue. Furthermore, fluorescing molecules (fluorophores) are rare in the biological milieu and may, thus, be rather precisely identified based upon their spectral fluorescence characteristics. Fluorescence, thus, is an ideal optical tool to determine the presence of specific fluorophores in biological tissues to a depth of several millimeters.

Fluorophores are characterized by absorption and emission spectra. These spectral characteristics allow us to sensitively detect endogenous as well as exogenous fluorophores in human tissues. The depth in tissue at which fluorophores can be detected is dependent on the tissue absorption at both the exciting and the emitted light wavelengths. Figure 1 illustrates the absorption characteristics of the major biological absorbers, hemoglobin and melanin. The main absorption occurs in the blue part of the visible spectrum, while above 600 nm in the red and near infrared, a so-called transparent window exists. Thus, for diagnosis of superficial lesions, fluorescence excitation techniques using blue or ultraviolet light excitation are well suited. However, if deeper structures are to be investigated such as for lymphatic metastases detection, longer excitation wavelengths are required.

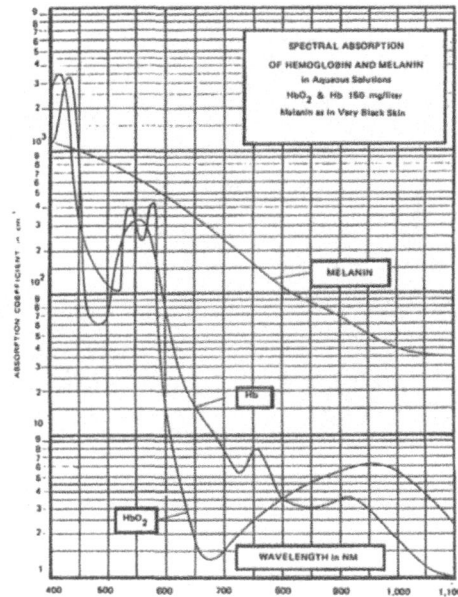

Fig. 1. Absorption characteristics of the major biological absorbers, hemoglobin and melanin. Maximum light absorption occurs in the blue part of the visible spectrum, while above 600 nm in the red and near infrared, a so-called transparent window exists

Photodiagnostic Tracers

A number of artificial fluorophores have been determined to accumulate in malignant disease [7–10]. The most prominent of these substances is hematoporphyrin derivative (HpD). A more purified version thereof, polyporphimer sodium, is well known under the trade name Photofrin and is commercialized for photodynamic therapy in most western countries now. The substance seems to accumulate even in very small tumor deposits to a level detectable by fluorimetry [9, 10]. The fluorescence micrograph (Fig. 2) of an experimental lymph node metastasis illustrates this accumulation (image courtesy of T.S. Mang, Buffalo, N.Y., USA). Figure 3 reveals the absorption spectra of the substance. Fluorescence may be excited at several wavelengths ranging from 405 to 630 nm (Soret- and Q-bands). The fluorescence emission spectra consist of a main band at about 630 nm and a minor peak at about 700 nm. Considering the wavelength dependence of light penetration in tissue, different diagnostic applications may require appropriate excitation wavelengths. If the Q-band at 630 nm is chosen for fluorescence excitation, of course, only the minor 700 nm peak can be monitored. A number of diagnostic studies have been published using hematoporphyrin derivative as a diagnostic tracer [9–13]. However, the procedure has not entered regular clinical practice. Another procedure leading to porphyrin fluorescence in malignant tissues actually finds more widespread acceptance [14–16], the exogenous supplementation of 5-aminolevulinic acid (ALA). ALA is not a fluorescent marker in the common sense of the term [17]. It functions as a sub-

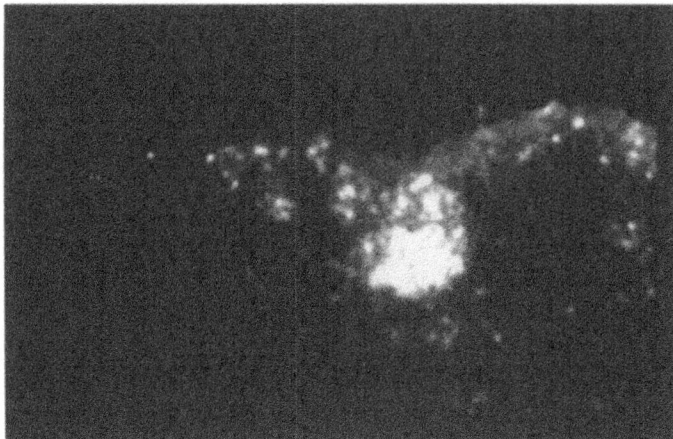

Fig. 2. Fluorescence micrograph of an experimental lymph node metastasis demonstrating the accumulation of polyporphimer sodium by the metastatic cells (image courtesy of T.S. Mang, Buffalo, N.Y.)

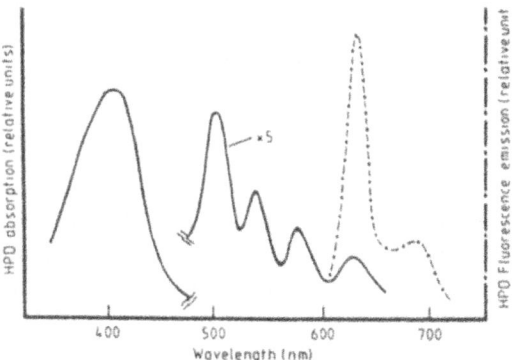

Fig. 3. Absorption spectra of the hematoporphyrin derivative (HpD). Fluorescence may be excited at several wavelengths ranging from 405 to 630 nm. The fluorescence emission spectra present a primary fluorescence at about 630 nm and a secondary peak at about 690 nm

strate in the heme synthetic pathway (Fig. 4). In the last step of heme synthesis, the enzyme ferrochelatase catalyzes the incorporation of an iron atom into a protoporphyrin IX molecule. Since this step is directly inhibited by the heme concentration, an excess of 5-ALA leads to an accumulation of protoporphyrin IX. It is not yet entirely understood why this occurs to a much higher degree in tumors than in normal tissue. Protoporphyrin IX is fluorescent and may even be used as a photosensitizer. Thus, the most common fluorescence diagnostic systems are both based on porphyrin fluorescing tracers for diagnostic purposes.

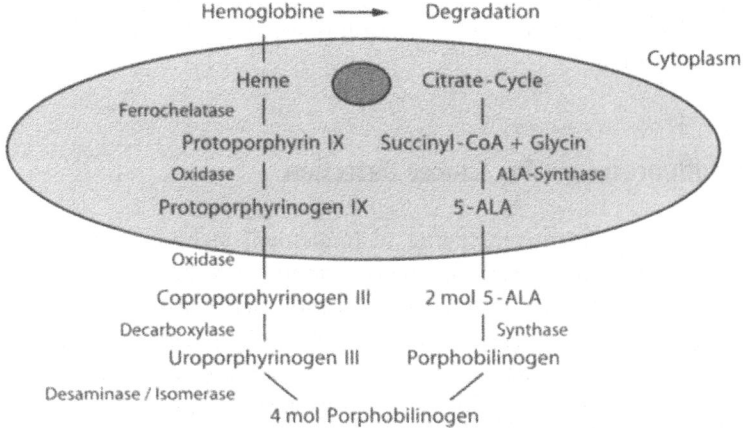

Fig. 4. The heme synthetic pathway. In the last step of heme synthesis, the enzyme ferrochelatase catalyzes the incorporation of an iron atom into a protoporphyrin IX molecule. Since this step is directly inhibited by the heme concentration, an excess of 5-ALA leads to an accumulation of protoporphyrin IX

Autofluorescence Reduction

Unspecific tissue autofluorescence represents a background that renders the detection of small concentrations of tumor localizing fluorophores difficult, especially if these are embedded at a considerable tissue depth [18]. Biological molecules like elastin, collagen, NADH, FADH do fluoresce and contribute to a broad tissue fluorescence background. In order to sensitively detect selected fluorophores, the instrumentation for fluorescence detection must account for this autofluorescence and, if possible, provide algorithms to reduce this autofluorescence background [18]. The most often used technique is based on the selection of specific emission bands of the fluorophore which are not pronounced in the rather homogenous autofluorescence background [19, 20]. Thus, as a relative measure, exciting fluorescence by a single wavelength, the amount of autofluorescence contributing to the specific band may be estimated from the fluorescence intensity outside the specific band. Otherwise, the autofluorescence background may be estimated using two alternating excitation wavelengths, one exciting the specific fluorescence and the other rather close to it but outside the absorption band of the photodiagnostic tracer, thus, exciting only autofluorescence [10, 21]. Subtracting the response to both excitations at a given specific emission wavelength resolves the photodiagnostic tracer fluorescence. Both methods exploit the spectral characteristics of the tumor localizing fluorophore. There is a third way to increase the sensitivity of fluorescence detection [22, 23]. It is based on fluorophore-specific fluorescence decay times. Fluorescence decay time of porphyrins are considerably longer than for the majority of the physiological fluorophores. Thus, a time-delayed detection of fluorescence after excitation with nanosecond laser pulses leads to a strong decrease of the background fluorescence in the derived spectra. This last method may be combined with any of the others resulting in the highest possible sensitivity within the biological milieu.

Autofluorescence for Cancer Detection

A group in Vancouver, trying to implement techniques for background subtraction for HpD-based diagnosis of lung cancer, observed that the autofluorescence background differed significantly between tumors and healthy mucosa. Tumors are characterized by a reduction in connective tissue mediated autofluorescence [24] because these tissues are covered by several layers of malignant cells. Instead of using an exogenous tracer, an imaging system was developed based on autofluorescence characteristics only [25]. This system has been commercialized in the meantime under the name 'light-induced fluorescence endoscopy' (LIFE) and is gaining widespread acceptance [26, 27]. In a recently published multicenter evaluation [28], the sensitivity of white light bronchoscopy (WLB) enhanced by LIFE versus WLB alone was 6.3 times higher for intraepithelial neoplastic lesions and 2.7 times higher still for invasive cancers. The positive predictive value was 0.33.

Autofluorescence of Colorectal Cancers and Lymph Node Metastases

To detect a cancer metastasis within a macroscopically unsuspicious lymph node requires sensitivity at a depth of several millimeters.

Furthermore, several groups have reported natural occurrence of porphyrins in colorectal primary tumors in considerable concentrations [29, 30]. With the aim to develop a porphyrin-based fluorescence technique for the detection of colorectal lymph nodes it was necessary to systematically characterize autofluorescence properties of these targets.

Methods

In a pilot trial we investigated 174 lymph nodes taken from the pericolic fat of 9 patients with colorectal cancers (rectal cancers, n = 2; colonic cancers, n = 7; pT3, n = 8; pT4, n = 1). All nodes were individually dissected, fluorimetrically characterized and histologically investigated.

The histological investigation of every single lymph node was based primarily on a single H&E stained equatorial section. Those lymph nodes that were fluorescence positive but negative in routine pathology were submitted to an extensive histological work-up comprising at least ten serial sections (n = 25). For comparison, a random sample of the same size of fluorescence apparently true negative lymph nodes were investigated by the same way.

Fluorescence Instrumentation

The experimental set-up used for detection of time-delayed fluorescence spectra is shown in Fig. 5. An optical parametric oscillator (OPO, Model A-1, GWU-Lasertechnik, Germany) with β-BaB$_2$O$_4$ as optical non-linear medium, pumped by the third harmonic ($\lambda = 355$ nm, $E_{pulse} \approx 100$–140 mJ) of a Q-switched Nd:YAG laser (GCR 230-50, Spectra-Physics, USA), provided pulsed laser radiation at a rate of 50 pulses per second, tunable between 410 nm and 2.2 μm. The energy and the duration of the OPO-output pulses amounted typically to 15 mJ and 3 ns, respectively. The remaining pump laser radiation ($\lambda = 355$ nm) was removed from the OPO output by means of two dichroic beam splitters (HR 355, Laseroptik GmbH, Germany), the idler wave (720 nm–2.2 μm) by a corresponding short-wave pass filter. The energy of the OPO output pulses was reduced to about 300 μJ using neutral density filters. The laser beam was coupled into a 600 μm hard-clad silica fiber. The laser induced fluorescence of the tissue was collected by the same fiber and guided to the entrance slit of an optical multichannel analyzer (see Fig. 5), consisting of an imaging polychromator (Spectra Pro-150, Acton Research Corp., USA) and a cooled, intensified CCD camera (Princeton Instruments Inc., USA). A dichroic beam splitter (550 DRLPO2, Omega Optical Inc., USA)

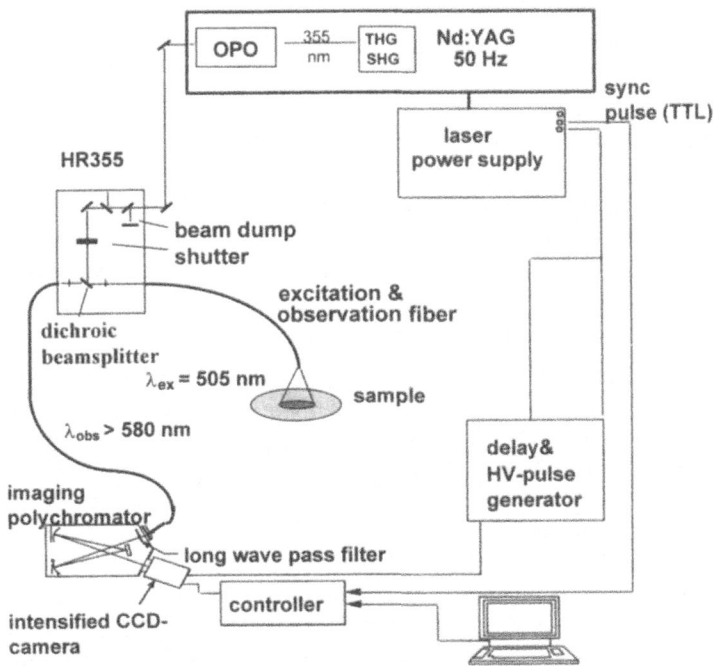

Fig. 5. The experimental set-up used for recording time-delayed fluorescence spectra from colorectal tissues (for details, see text)

served to separate excitation and observation optical paths, and to suppress backscattered laser light. In addition, a long wave pass filter ($\lambda_{50\%} = 550$ nm, LL 550 Corion Corp., USA) at the entrance slit of the polychromator was used to suppress the remaining backscattered excitation light. The intensifier of the diode array detector was gated by an electrical pulse (–180 V) of about 20 ns duration delivered by a high voltage (HV) pulse generator (Model 6040, Berkeley Nucleonics Corp., USA) synchronized and delayed to the laser pulse. For this purpose the HV pulse generator was triggered by an electrical (TTL) pulse provided by the power supply of the Nd:YAG laser.

The fluorescence spectra of tissue specimen were recorded at zero delay ($t_d = 0$ ns) and at a delay of $t_d = 20$ ns. Subsequently, the spectra were corrected for the spectral transmittance of the polychromator and for the spectral sensitivity of the photocathode of the intensified CCD camera, but not for the transmittance of the long wave pass filter ($\lambda_{50\%} = 550$ nm) used to block off backscattered laser light. In addition, electronic background of the detector was subtracted from the raw data. Subsequently, the prompt ($I(\lambda, 0$ ns)) and delayed ($I(\lambda, 20$ ns)) spectra were normalized to the maximum intensity I(633 nm, 0 ns) of the corresponding prompt fluorescence spectrum. Since geometrical factors were unchanged when recording prompt and delayed fluorescence spectra, and fluorescence spectra were corrected for the number of laser pulses applied and for their pulse energy, normalized prompt ($t_d = 0$ ns) and delayed ($t_d = 20$ ns) fluorescence spectra $I_n(\lambda, t_d) = I(\lambda, t_d)/I(633$ nm, 0 ns) can be compared quantitatively. As a parameter for the porphyrin-like fluorescence intensity, the ratio $R = I(633$ nm, 20 ns)/I(595 nm, 20 ns) was used for quantification of the spectra recorded [23].

First Clinical Results

Routine pathology revealed 31 lymph nodes as metastatically involved. Three further metastases were identified by step sections resulting in total of 34 of 174 lymph nodes being pathologically involved. A typical example of the measured fluorescence spectra is shown in Figs. 6 and 7. Without time delay, no significant peak appears in the spectral range between 600 and 700 nm. The spectra recorded with a 20 ns delay show a distinct peak at 630 and a very weak secondary peak at 700 nm indicative of the metastatic lymph nodes. These peaks are not distinguishable in the normal lymph node from the same patient shown for comparison. Figure 8 shows the cumulative frequencies of the R-values between the noninvolved and metastatically involved lymph nodes. Based on a discriminator of 1 for the parameter R a total of 43 lymph nodes were determined fluorescence positive, 22 of these were pathologically positive. 171 were fluorescence negative ($R > 1$), 119 of these were pathologically negative. In the initially 24 fluorescence false positive lymph nodes, there were three further metastases diagnosed by stepwise sectioning. In the random sample of the same size of fluorescence true negative lymph nodes no metastases were identified. The discriminator $R = 1$ thus results at a specificity of 85%

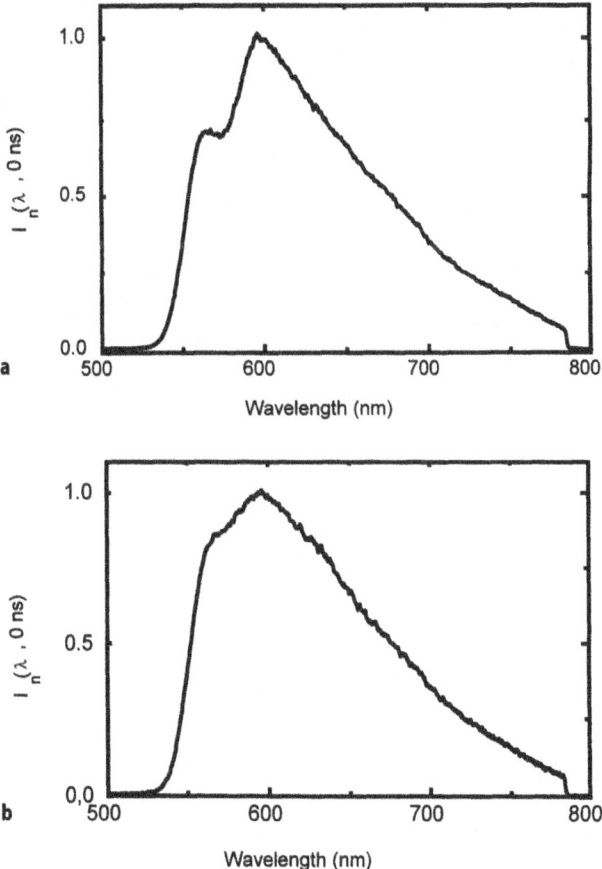

Fig. 6. Undelayed autofluorescence spectra of normal (**a**) and metastatically involved (**b**) colorectal lymph nodes. Fluorescence was excited at 505 nm

in a sensitivity of 65%, a positive predictive value of 52%, and a negative predictive value of 91%. The fluorescence emission and excitation spectra of the endogenous chromophore detected correspond well to spectra of porphyrins.

Conclusion

There is obviously an accumulation or induction of endogenous porphyrins in colorectal tumors and in their metastases. This might be the basis for an intraoperative detection of lymph node metastases without the use of exogenous markers. The relatively low sensitivity of 65% is not an obstacle for a surgical technique. Using this technique it is possible just to select lymph nodes of high fluorescence for frozen section analysis. Furthermore, these specific fluorescence features can be used to select a certain subset of lymph nodes for in-depth pathological investigation.

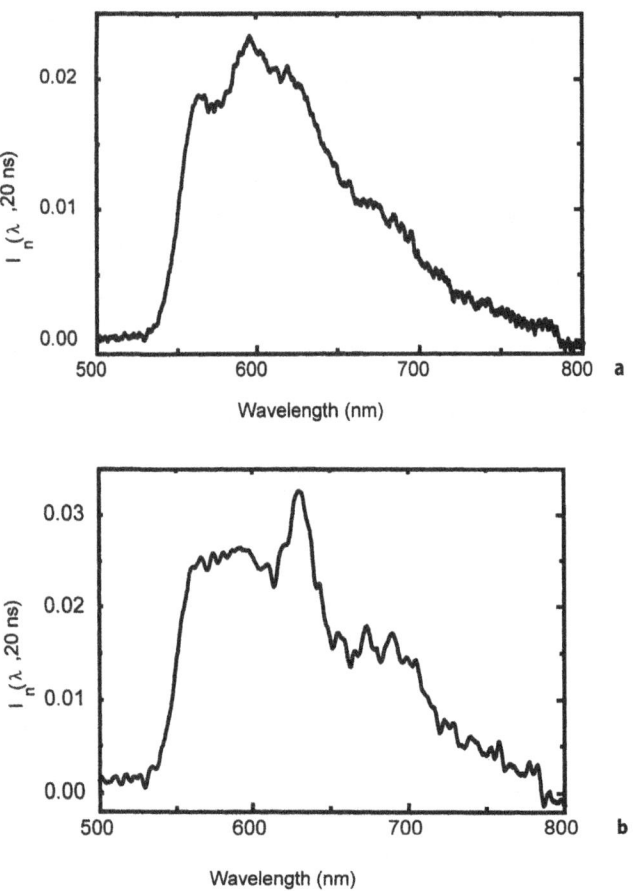

Fig. 7. Time-delayed autofluorescence spectra of normal (**a**) and metastatically involved (**b**) colorectal lymph nodes. Fluorescence was excited at 505 nm. The fluorescence spectra were recorded at a delay of $t_d = 20$ ns

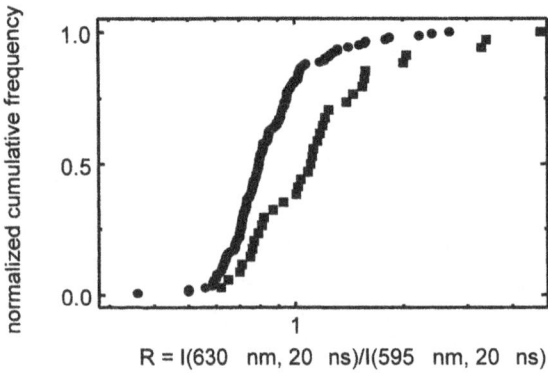

Fig. 8. Cumulative frequencies of the autofluorescence parameter R for normal (●) and pathologically involved lymph nodes (■)

References

1. Malassagne B, Valleur P, Serra J, Sarnacki S, Galian A, Hoang C, Hautefeuille P (1993): Relationship of apical lymph node involvement to survival in resected colon carcinoma. Dis Colon Rectum 36:645–653
2. Hermanek P, Wiebelt H, Staimmer D, Riedl S (1995): Prognostic factors of rectum carcinoma – experience of the German Multicentre Study SGCRC. German Study Group Colo-Rectal Carcinoma. Tumori 81:60–64
3. Wiggers T, Jeekel J, Arends JW, Brinkhorst AP, Kluck HM, Luyk CI, Munting JD, Povel JA, Rutten AP, Volovics A, et al (1988): No-touch isolation technique in colon cancer: a controlled prospective trial. Br J Surg 75:409–415
4. Herfarth C, Hohenberger P (1989): Lymphadenektomie bei der Primartherapie colorectaler Carcinome. Chirurg 60:139–147
5. Aftab F, Stoldt HS, Testori A, Imperatori A, Chinol M, Paganelli G, Geraghty J (1996): Radioimmunoguided surgery and colorectal cancer. Eur J Surg Oncol 22:381–388
6. Schneebaum S, Papo J, Graif M, Baratz M, Baron J, Skornik Y (1997): Radioimmuno-guided surgery benefits for recurrent colorectal cancer. Ann Surg Oncol 4:371–376
7. Svanberg K, Wang I, Colleen S, Idvall I, Ingvar C, Rydell R, Jocham D, Diddens H, Bown S, Gregory G, Montan S, Andersson Engels S, Svanberg S (1998): Clinical multi-colour fluorescence imaging of malignant tumours–initial experience. Acta Radiol 39:2–9
8. Mlkvy P, Messmann H, Regula J, Conio M, Pauer M, Millson CE, MacRobert AJ, Bown SG (1998): Photodynamic therapy for gastrointestinal tumors using three photosensitizers – ALA induced PPIX, Photofrin and MTHPC. A pilot study. Neoplasma 45:157–161
9. Lam S, Palcic B, McLean D, Hung J, Korbelik M, Profio AE (1990): Detection of early lung cancer using low dose Photofrin II. Clin Chest Med 97:333–337
10. Mang TS, McGinnis C, Liebow C, Nseyo UO, Crean DH, Dougherty TJ (1993): Fluorescence detection of tumors. Early diagnosis of microscopic lesions in preclinical studies. Cancer 71:269–276
11. Lipson RL, Baldes EJ, Gray MJ (1967): Hematoporphyrin derivative for detection and management of cancer. Cancer 20:2255–2257
12. Kato H, Cortese DA, Lam S, Palcic B, McLean D, Hung J, Korbelik M, Profio AE (1990): Early detection of lung cancer by means of hematoporphyrin derivative fluorescence and laser photoradiation Detection of early lung cancer using low dose Photofrin II. Clin Chest Med 97:333–337
13. Baert L, Berg R, Van Damme B, D'Hallewin MA, Johansson J, Svanberg K, Svanberg S (1993): Clinical fluorescence diagnosis of human bladder carcinoma following low-dose Photofrin injection. Urology 41:322–330
14. Kriegmair M, Stepp H, Steinbach P, Lumper W, Ehsan A, Stepp HG, Rick K, Knuchel R, Baumgartner R, Hofstetter A (1995): Fluorescence cystoscopy following intravesical instillation of 5-aminolevulinic acid: a new procedure with high sensitivity for detection of hardly visible urothelial neoplasias. Urol Int 55:190–196
15. Jichlinski P, Forrer M, Mizeret J, Glanzmann T, Braichotte D, Wagnieres G, Zimmer G, Guillou L, Schmidlin F, Graber P, van den Bergh H, Leisinger HJ (1997): Clinical evaluation of a method for detecting superficial surgical transitional cell carcinoma of the bladder by light-induced fluorescence of protoporphyrin IX following the topical application of 5-aminolevulinic acid: preliminary results. Lasers Surg Med 20:402–408
16. Baumgartner R, Huber RM, Schulz H, Stepp H, Rick K, Gamarra F, Leberig A, Roth C (1996): Inhalation of 5-aminolevulinic acid: a new technique for fluorescence detection of early stage lung cancer. J Photochem Photobiol B 36:169–174
17. Kennedy JC, Marcus SL, Pottier RH (1996): Photodynamic therapy (PDT) and photo-diagnosis (PD) using endogenous photosensitization induced by 5-aminolevulinic acid (ALA): mechanisms and clinical results. J Clin Laser Med Surg 14:289–304
18. Profio AE, Balchum OJ, Carstens F (1986): Digital background subtraction for fluorescence imaging. Med Phys 13:717–721

19. Andersson Engels S, Johansson J, Svanberg K, Svanberg S (1991): Fluorescence imaging and point measurements of tissue: applications to the demarcation of malignant tumors and atherosclerotic lesions from normal tissue. Photochem Photobiol 53:807–814
20. Monnier P, Savary M, Fontolliet C, Wagnieres G, Chatelain A, Cornaz P, Depeursigne C, Van den Berg H (1990): Photodetection and photodynamic therapy of 'early' squamous cell carcinomas of the pharynx, oesophagus and tracheo-bronchial tree. Lasers Med Sci 5:149–169
21. Baumgartner R, Unsold E (1987): High contrast fluorescence imaging using two-wavelength laser excitation and image processing. J Photochem Photobiol B 1:130–132
22. Kohl M, Neukammer J, Sukowski U, Rinneberg H, Sinn HJ, Friedrich EA (1993): Delayed observation of laser-induced fluorescence for imaging of tumours. Appl Phys 56:131–138
23. Ebert B, Nolte D, Rinneberg H, Moesta KT, Nowack C, Schlag PM (1995): Characteristic porphyrin-like autofluorescence in primary colon tumours and lymph nodes. SPIE 2627:57–67
24. Hung J, Lam S, Leriche JC, Palcic B (1991): Autofluorescence of normal and malignant bronchial tissue. Lasers Surg Med 11:99–105
25. Lam S, MacAulay C, Hung J, LeRiche J, Profio AE, Palcic B (1993): Detection of dysplasia and carcinoma in situ with a lung imaging fluorescence endoscope device. J Thorac Cardiovasc Surg 105:1035–1040
26. Kurie JM, Lee JS, Morice RC, Walsh GL, Khuri FR, Broxson A, Ro JY, Franklin WA, Yu R, Hong WK (1998): Autofluorescence bronchoscopy in the detection of squamous metaplasia and dysplasia in current and former smokers. J Natl Cancer Inst 90:991–995
27. Diaz Jimenez JP, Sans Torres J, Domingo C, Martinez Ballarin I, Castro MJ, Manresa F (1998): [The 1st case in Spain of detection of occult squamous carcinoma using LIFE system] Primer caso en Espana de deteccion de un carcinoma escamoso oculto mediante la utilizacion del sistema LIFE. Med Clin Barc 110:217–219
28. Lam S, Kennedy T, Unger M, Miller YE, Gelmont D, Rusch V, Gipe B, Howard D, Leriche JC, Coldman A, Gazdar AF (1998): Localization of bronchial intraepithelial neoplastic lesions by fluorescence bronchoscopy. Clin Chest Med 113:696–702
29. Policard A (1924): Etudes sur les aspects offerts par les tumeurs experimentales examinees a la lumiere de woods. CR Soc Biol 91:1423–1425
30. Harris DM, Werkhaven J (1987): Endogenous porphyrin fluorescence in tumors. Lasers Surg Med 7:467–472

Subject Index

The manufacturer's authorised representative in the EU is Springer
Nature Customer Service Centre GmbH, Europaplatz 3, 69115 Heidelberg,
Germany. If you have any concerns regarding our products, please
contact ProductSafety@springernature.com

Printed and bound by CPI Group (UK) Ltd, Croydon, CR0 4YY
28/04/2026
02098453-0003